Computational Models for Biomedical Reasoning and Problem Solving

Chung-Hao Chen
Old Dominion University, USA

Sen-Ching Samson Cheung
University of Kentucky, USA

A volume in the Advances in
Bioinformatics and Biomedical
Engineering (ABBE) Book Series

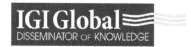

Published in the United States of America by
    IGI Global
    Medical Information Science Reference (an imprint of IGI Global)
    701 E. Chocolate Avenue
    Hershey PA, USA 17033
    Tel: 717-533-8845
    Fax: 717-533-8661
    E-mail: cust@igi-global.com
    Web site: http://www.igi-global.com

Library of Congress Cataloging-in-Publication Data

Names: Chen, Chung-Hao, 1974- editor. | Cheung, Sen-Ching Samson, 1969-
  editor.
Title: Computational models for biomedical reasoning and problem solving /
  Chung-Hao Chen and Sen-Ching Samson Cheung, editors.
Description: Hershey PA : Medical Information Science Reference, [2019] |
  Includes bibliographical references.
Identifiers: LCCN 2018028564| ISBN 9781522574675 (hardcover) | ISBN
  9781522574682 (ebook)
Subjects: | MESH: Patient-Specific Modeling | Computational Biology--methods
  | Decision Making, Computer-Assisted | Image Interpretation,
  Computer-Assisted--methods
Classification: LCC R855.3 | NLM W 26.5 | DDC 610.285--dc23 LC record available at https://
lccn.loc.gov/2018028564

This book is published in the IGI Global book series Advances in Bioinformatics and Biomedical Engineering (ABBE) (ISSN: 2327-7033; eISSN: 2327-7041)

British Cataloguing in Publication Data
A Cataloguing in Publication record for this book is available from the British Library.

All work contributed to this book is new, previously-unpublished material.
The views expressed in this book are those of the authors, but not necessarily of the publisher.

For electronic access to this publication, please contact: eresources@igi-global.com.

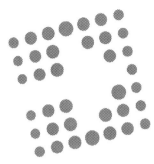

Advances in Bioinformatics and Biomedical Engineering (ABBE) Book Series

ISSN:2327-7033
EISSN:2327-7041

Editor-in-Chief: Ahmad Taher Azar, Benha University, Egypt

MISSION

The fields of biology and medicine are constantly changing as research evolves and novel engineering applications and methods of data analysis are developed. Continued research in the areas of bioinformatics and biomedical engineering is essential to continuing to advance the available knowledge and tools available to medical and healthcare professionals.

The **Advances in Bioinformatics and Biomedical Engineering (ABBE) Book Series** publishes research on all areas of bioinformatics and bioengineering including the development and testing of new computational methods, the management and analysis of biological data, and the implementation of novel engineering applications in all areas of medicine and biology. Through showcasing the latest in bioinformatics and biomedical engineering research, ABBE aims to be an essential resource for healthcare and medical professionals.

COVERAGE

- Drug Design
- DNA Sequencing
- Biostatistics
- Orthopedic Bioengineering
- Neural Engineering
- Databases
- Tissue Engineering
- Prosthetic Limbs
- Genomics
- Bayesian methods

IGI Global is currently accepting manuscripts for publication within this series. To submit a proposal for a volume in this series, please contact our Acquisition Editors at Acquisitions@igi-global.com or visit: http://www.igi-global.com/publish/.

The Advances in Bioinformatics and Biomedical Engineering (ABBE) Book Series (ISSN 2327-7033) is published by IGI Global, 701 E. Chocolate Avenue, Hershey, PA 17033-1240, USA, www.igi-global.com. This series is composed of titles available for purchase individually; each title is edited to be contextually exclusive from any other title within the series. For pricing and ordering information please visit http://www.igi-global.com/book-series/advances-bioinformatics-biomedical-engineering/73671. Postmaster: Send all address changes to above address. ©© 2019 IGI Global. All rights, including translation in other languages reserved by the publisher. No part of this series may be reproduced or used in any form or by any means – graphics, electronic, or mechanical, including photocopying, recording, taping, or information and retrieval systems – without written permission from the publisher, except for non commercial, educational use, including classroom teaching purposes. The views expressed in this series are those of the authors, but not necessarily of IGI Global.

Titles in this Series

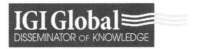

701 East Chocolate Avenue, Hershey, PA 17033, USA
Tel: 717-533-8845 x100 • Fax: 717-533-8661
E-Mail: cust@igi-global.com • www.igi-global.com

Table of Contents

Detailed Table of Contents

    Karla Conn Welch, University of Louisville, USA
    Uttama Lahiri, Indian Institute of Technology Gandhinagar, India
    Zachary E. Warren, Vanderbilt University, USA
    Nilanjan Sarkar, Vanderbilt University, USA

This chapter presents work aimed at investigating interactions between virtual reality (VR) and children with autism spectrum disorder (ASD) using physiological sensing of affective cues. The research objectives are two-fold: 1) develop VR-based social communication tasks and integrate them into the physiological signal acquisition module to enable the capture of one's physiological responses in a time-synchronized manner during participation in the task and 2) conduct a pilot usability study to evaluate a VR-based social interaction system that induces an affective response in ASD and typically developing (TD) individuals by using a physiology-based approach. Physiological results suggest there is a different physiological response in the body in relation to the reported level of the affective states. The preliminary results from a matched pair of participants could provide valuable information about specific affect-eliciting aspects of social communication, and this feedback could drive individualized interventions that scaffold skills and improve social wellbeing.

Chapter 2
Electroencephalogram (EEG) for Delineating Objective Measure of Autism
Spectrum Disorder 34

Sampath Jayarathna, Old Dominion University, USA
Yasith Jayawardana, Old Dominion University, USA
Mark Jaime, Indiana University-Purdue University Columbus, USA
Sashi Thapaliya, California State Polytechnic University – Pomona,
*   USA*

Autism spectrum disorder (ASD) is a developmental disorder that often impairs a child's normal development of the brain. According to CDC, it is estimated that 1 in 6 children in the US suffer from development disorders, and 1 in 68 children in the US suffer from ASD. This condition has a negative impact on a person's ability to hear, socialize, and communicate. Subjective measures often take more time, resources, and have false positives or false negatives. There is a need for efficient objective measures that can help in diagnosing this disease early as possible with less effort. EEG measures the electric signals of the brain via electrodes placed on various places on the scalp. These signals can be used to study complex neuropsychiatric issues. Studies have shown that EEG has the potential to be used as a biomarker for various neurological conditions including ASD. This chapter will outline the usage of EEG measurement for the classification of ASD using machine learning algorithms.

Chapter 3
Predicting ADHD Using Eye Gaze Metrics Indexing Working Memory
Capacity 66

Anne M. P. Michalek, Old Dominion University, USA
Gavindya Jayawardena, Old Dominion University, USA
Sampath Jayarathna, Old Dominion University, USA

ADHD is being recognized as a diagnosis that persists into adulthood impacting educational and economic outcomes. There is an increased need to accurately diagnose this population through the development of reliable and valid outcome measures reflecting core diagnostic criteria. For example, adults with ADHD have reduced working memory capacity (WMC) when compared to their peers. A reduction in WMC indicates attention control deficits which align with many symptoms outlined on behavioral checklists used to diagnose ADHD. Using computational methods, such as machine learning, to generate a relationship between ADHD and measures of WMC would be useful to advancing our understanding and treatment of ADHD in adults. This chapter will outline a feasibility study in which eye tracking was used to measure eye gaze metrics during a WMC task for adults with and without ADHD and machine learning algorithms were applied to generate a feature set unique to the ADHD diagnosis. The chapter will summarize the purpose, methods, results, and impact of this study.

Chapter 4

The quickly extending field of huge information examination has begun to assume a crucial part in the advancement of human services practices and research. In this chapter, challenges like gathering information from complex heterogeneous patient sources, utilizing the patient/information relationships in longitudinal records, understanding unstructured clinical notes in the correct setting and efficiently dealing with expansive volumes of medicinal imaging information, and removing conceivably valuable data is shown. Healthcare and IoT and machine learning along with data mining are also discussed. Image analysis and segmentation methods comparative study is given for the examination of computer vision, imaging handling, and example acknowledgment has gained considerable ground amid the previous quite a few years. Examiners have distributed an abundance of essential science and information reporting the advance and social insurance application on medicinal imaging.

Chapter 5

Biomedical image analysis has become critically important to the public health and welfare. However, analyzing biomedical images is time-consuming and labor-intensive, and has long been performed manually by highly trained human experts. As a result, there has been an increasing interest in applying machine learning to automate biomedical image analysis. Recent progress in deep learning research has catalyzed the development of machine learning in learning discriminative features from data with minimum human intervention. Many deep learning models have been designed and achieved superior performance in various data analysis applications. This chapter starts with the basic of deep learning models and some practical strategies for handling biomedical image applications with limited data. After that, case studies of deep feature extraction for gene expression pattern image annotations, imaging data completion for brain disease diagnosis, and segmentation of infant brain tissue images are discussed to demonstrate the effectiveness of deep learning in biomedical image analysis.

This chapter was developed with a view to present a predictive model for the classification of the level of CD4 count of HIV patients receiving ART/HAART treatment in Nigeria. Following the review of literature, the pre-determining factors for determining CD4 count were identified and validated by experts while historical data explaining the relationship between the factors and CD4 count level was collected. The predictive model for CD4 count level was formulated using C4.5 decision trees (DT), support vector machines (SVM), and the multi-layer perceptron (MLP) classifiers based on the identified factors which were formulated using WEKA software and validated. The results showed that decision trees algorithm revealed five (5) important variables, namely age group, white blood cell count, viral load, time of diagnosing HIV, and age of the patient. The MLP had the best performance with a value of 100% followed by the SVM with an accuracy of 91.1%, and both were observed to outperform the DT algorithm used.

In drug-delivery systems containing nano-drug structures, targeting the tumorous tissue by anthraquinone molecules with high biological activity, and reaching and destroying tumors by their tumor-killing effect reveals remarkable results for the treatment of tumors. The various biological activities of anthraquinones and their derivatives depend on molecular conformation; hence, their intra-cell interaction mechanisms including deoxyribonucleic acid (DNA), ribonucleic acid (RNA), enzymes, and hormones. Computer-based drug design plays an important role in the design of drugs and the determination of goals for them. Molecular docking has been widely used in structure-based drug design. The effects of anthraquinone analogues in tumor cells as a result of their interaction with DNA strand has increased the number of studies done on them, and they have been shown to have a wide range of applications in chemistry, medicine, pharmacy, materials, and especially in the field of biomolecules.

Ionic liquids are salts with melting points generally below 100 °C made of entirely ions by the combination of a large cation and a group of anions. Some ionic liquids are found to have therapeutic properties due to their toxic effects (e.g., anticancer, antibacterial, and antifungal properties). The determination of the most stable molecular structures, that is, the lowest energy conformer of these ionic liquids with versatile biological activities, is of particular importance. Density function theory (DFT) based on quantum mechanical calculation method, one of the molecular modeling methods, is widely used in physics and chemistry to determine the electronic structures of these stable geometries and molecules. With the theory, the energy of the molecule is determined by using the electron density instead of the wave function. It is observed that the theoretical models developed on the ionic liquids in the literature are in agreement with the experimental results because of electron correlations included in the calculation.

Chapter 9

Logistic regression is one of the most popular models to classify in data science, and in general, it is easy to use. However, in order to conduct a goodness-of-fit test, we cannot apply asymptotic methods if we have sparse datasets. In the case, we have to conduct an exact conditional inference via a sampler, such as Markov Chain Monte Carlo (MCMC) or Sequential Importance Sampling (SIS). In this chapter, the authors investigate the rejection rate of the SIS procedure on a multiple logistic regression models with categorical covariates. Using tools from algebra, they show that in general SIS can have a very high rejection rate even though we apply Linear Integer Programming (IP) to compute the support of the marginal distribution for each variable. More specifically, the semigroup generated by the columns of the design matrix for a multiple logistic regression has infinitely many "holes." They end with application of a hybrid scheme of MCMC and SIS to NUN study data on Alzheimer disease study.

Preface

A biomedical computational model contains numerous variables that characterize the biological system being studied. The results of model simulations help researchers and clinicians make predictions about what will happen in the biological system in response to the changing conditions, especially for a complex disease or disorder. With a well-developed computational model, researchers and clinicians can better understand the cause of a disease or a disorder and predict treatment outcomes. The purpose of this book is to bring multidisciplinary researchers together to discuss challenging issues and state-of-the-art approaches when developing a biomedical computational model. With the advent of big data health analytics and emerging personalized medicine paradigm, this book should be a valuable addition to anyone interested in building and applying computational models for different biomedical applications.

The target audience of this book are practitioners and researchers working in the field of biomedical or behavioral sciences in various disciplines, e.g. psychology, engineering, and clinicians. A particular focus of the book is on providing insight and support concerned with the customized treatments to individuals, and prediction of responses to newly developed treatments.

Chapter 1 presents work aimed at investigating interactions between virtual reality (VR) and children with autism spectrum disorder (ASD) using physiological sensing of affective cues. The research objectives are two-fold: 1) Develop VR-based social communication tasks and integrate them into the physiological signal acquisition module to enable the capture of one's physiological responses in a time-synchronized manner during participation in the task, and 2) conduct a pilot usability study to evaluate a VR-based social interaction system that induces an affective response among ASD and typically-developing (TD) individuals by using a physiology-based approach.

Chapter 2 presents new modeling techniques of electroencephalogram (EEG) signals. EEG measures electric signals of the brain via electrodes placed on various places on the scalp. These signals can be used to study complex neuropsychiatric issues. Studies have shown that EEG has the potential to be used as a biomarker for various neurological conditions including ASD. This chapter will outline the usage of EEG measurement for the classification of ASD using machine learning algorithms.

Chapter 3 presents new approaches in understanding and treating attention deficit hyperactivity disorder (ADHD) in adults by applying machine learning to study its relationship with measures of working memory components (WMC). The authors outlined a feasibility study in which eye tracking was used to measure eye gaze metrics during a WMC task for adults with and without ADHD. Machine learning algorithms were then applied to generate a feature set unique to the ADHD diagnosis.

Chapter 4 presents new directions in understanding unstructured clinical notes. The focus is on how to efficiently deal with expansive volumes of medicinal imaging information and mitigate the risks in removing conceivably valuable data. Healthcare and machine learning along with data mining are also discussed.

Chapter 5 presents recent progress in Deep Learning research that has catalyzed discriminative feature learning from data with minimum human intervention. This chapter starts with the basic of deep learning models and some practical strategies for handling biomedical image applications with limited data. After that, case studies of deep feature extraction for gene expression pattern annotations, imaging data completion for brain disease diagnosis, and segmentation of infant brain tissue images were discussed to demonstrate the effectiveness of deep learning in biomedical image analysis.

Chapter 6 presents a predictive model for the classification of the CD4 count level among HIV patients receiving antiretroviral therapy (ART) or highly active antiretroviral therapy (HAART) treatment in Nigeria. Following the review of literature, the pre-determining factors for determining CD4 counts were identified and validated by experts while historical data explaining the relationship between the factors and CD4 count level was collected. The predictive model for CD4 count level was formulated using C4.5 decision trees (DT), support vector machines (SVM) and the multi-layer perceptron (MLP) classifiers based on the identified factors which were formulated and validated using WEKA machine learning software library.

Chapter 7 presents latest progresses in drug-delivery systems containing nano-drug structures that have shown remarkable results for the treatment of tumors. These structures can target the tumorous tissue by anthraquinone molecules with high biological activity, and destroy tumors by their tumor-killing effect. The various biological activities of anthraquinones and their derivatives depend on molecular conformation. Hence, their intra-cell interaction mechanisms including deoxyribonucleic acid (DNA), ribonucleic acid (RNA), enzymes, and hormones have been increasing studied and widely applied. This chapter focuses on computer-based drug design, specifically molecular docking, which has played an important role in the design of drugs and the determination of goals for them.

Chapter 8 looks at mathematical models in determining stable molecular structures of ionic liquids. Ionic liquids are salts with melting points generally below 100 °C, made of entirely ions by the combination of a large cation and a group of anions. Some ionic liquids are found to have therapeutic properties such as anti-cancer, antibacterial and antifungal due to their toxic effects. The determination of the most stable molecular structures, that is, the lowest energy conformer of these ionic liquids with versatile biological activities, is of particular importance. Density function theory (DFT) based on quantum mechanical calculation method, one of the molecular modeling methods, is widely used in physics and chemistry to determine the electronic structures of these stable geometries and molecules. In this chapter, the authors explained the theory and their approaches in determining the energy of the molecule using the electron density instead of the wave function.

Chapter 9 presents new approach in using sequential importance sampling (SIS) in conducting goodness-of-fit tests for logical regression. Logistic regression is one of the most popular approaches for classification tasks in bioinformatics. However, datasets in biomedical domains are often sparse, making it difficult to use typical asymptotic methods to conduct goodness-of-fit tests. In this chapter, the authors investigated SIS to circumvent the problem by conducting an exact conditional inference via a sampler on multiple logistic regression models with categorical covariates. They found that SIS in general can have a very high rejection rate even after applying Linear Integer Programming (IP) to compute the support of the marginal distribution for each variable. More specifically, the semigroup generated by the columns of the design matrix for a multiple logistic regression has infinitely many "holes".

Acknowledgment

The editors would like to acknowledge the help of all the people involved in this project and, more specifically, to the authors and reviewers that took part in the review process. Without their support, this book would not have become a reality.

First, the editors would like to thank each of the authors for his/her contributions. Our sincere gratitude goes to the chapter's authors who contributed their time and expertise to this book.

Second, the editors wish to acknowledge the valuable contributions of the reviewers regarding the improvement of quality, coherence, and content presentation of chapters. Most of the authors also served as referees; we highly appreciate their double task.

Chung-Hao Chen
Old Dominion University, USA

Sen-Ching Samson Cheung
University of Kentucky, USA

Chapter 1

A System to Measure Physiological Response During Social Interaction in VR for Children With ASD

Karla Conn Welch
University of Louisville, USA

Zachary E. Warren
Vanderbilt University, USA

Uttama Lahiri
Indian Institute of Technology Gandhinagar, India

Nilanjan Sarkar
Vanderbilt University, USA

ABSTRACT

This chapter presents work aimed at investigating interactions between virtual reality (VR) and children with autism spectrum disorder (ASD) using physiological sensing of affective cues. The research objectives are two-fold: 1) develop VR-based social communication tasks and integrate them into the physiological signal acquisition module to enable the capture of one's physiological responses in a time-synchronized manner during participation in the task and 2) conduct a pilot usability study to evaluate a VR-based social interaction system that induces an affective response in ASD and typically developing (TD) individuals by using a physiology-based approach. Physiological results suggest there is a different physiological response in the body in relation to the reported level of the affective states. The preliminary results from a matched pair of participants could provide valuable information about specific affect-eliciting aspects of social communication, and this feedback could drive individualized interventions that scaffold skills and improve social wellbeing.

DOI: 10.4018/978-1-5225-7467-5.ch001

INTRODUCTION

Autism is a neurodevelopmental disorder characterized by core deficits in social interaction and communication accompanied by restricted patterns of interest and behavior (American Psychiatric Association, 2000). Currently, with Centers for Disease Control and Prevention (CDC) prevalence estimates for the broad autism spectrum as high as 1 in 59 children (Baio et al., 2018), identification and effective treatment of autism spectrum disorder (ASD) is often characterized as a public health emergency (Interagency Autism Coordinating Committee, 2009). While there is at present no single accepted intervention, treatment, or known cure for ASD, there is growing consensus that intensive behavioral and educational intervention programs can significantly improve short and long term outcomes for individuals with ASD and their families (Cohen, Amerine-Dickens, & Smith, 2006; National Research Council, 2001; Rogers, 1998). While such intervention paradigms have demonstrated significant effect in addressing basic early deficits in young children (i.e., preschool children), traditional interventions designed to address higher level social and adaptive impairments (i.e., communicating with others, processing and integrating information from the environment, establishing and sustaining social relationships, participating in new environments, learning skills related to functional independence) have been demonstrated to be minimally effective for school-aged children and adolescents with ASD. Specifically, low treatment effects and low generalization effects are typical for social and adaptive skill interventions and are thought to be a result of a failure of traditional methodologies to systematically match intervention strategies to specific skill deficits within and across naturalistic settings in appropriately intensive dosages (Bellini, Peters, Benner, & Hopf, 2007). With a lack of widely available efficacious treatment modes for addressing these complex skills at later points in childhood, adolescence, and early adulthood, it is not surprising that evidence suggests a majority of individuals with ASD (i.e., >70%) fail to achieve adaptive independence as adults (Billstedt, Gillberg, & Gillberg, 2005; Cederlund et al., 2007). Current intervention limitations are compounded by the lack of available resources in many areas and the fact that many children are not identified with ASD until later ages (Christensen et al., 2016; Croen, Grether, & Selvin, 2002; Mandell, Listerud, Levy, & Pinto-Martin, 2002; Yeargin-Allsopp et al., 2003). Thus, despite the urgent need and societal import of intensive treatment of social and adaptive impairment at later ages, effective and appropriate intervention resources for children, adolescents, and young adults with ASD are lacking (Rutter, 2006). Moreover, given the limitation on the availability of trained professional resources in ASD intervention, it is likely that emerging technology will play an important role in providing more accessible intensive individualized therapies in the future (Goodwin, 2008).

Therefore, researchers are recognizing that advancements in technology, particularly computer technology, can be effectively harnessed to provide important new directions in ASD intervention. Such technology is especially promising for making the treatment individualized and intensive, flexible and adaptive, and more easily accessible (Goodwin, 2008). In response to this need, a growing number of studies have been investigating the application of advanced interactive technologies to address core deficits related to ASD, namely computer technology (Bernard-Opitz, Sriram, & Nakhoda-Sapuan, 2001; Blocher & Picard, 2002; Swettenham, 1996), robotic systems (Dautenhahn & Werry, 2004; Duquette, Michaud, & Mercier, 2008; Kozima, Michalowski, & Nakagawa, 2009), and virtual reality (VR) environments (Parsons, Mitchell, & Leonard, 2004; Strickland, Marcus, Mesibov, & Hogan, 1996; Tartaro & Cassell, 2007). Increased amalgamation of technology in everyday life (1) increases the need for more intuitive systems that can interpret explicit as well as implicit means of communication and (2) provides increased opportunity for user/patient-centered computing to promote positive life skills. Research suggests that endowing technology with an ability to understand implicit interaction cues, such as the person's intention, attitude, and their likes and dislikes should permit a smooth, natural, and more productive interaction process (Gilleade, Dix, & Allanson, 2005; Kapoor, Mota, & Picard, 2001; Prendinger, Mori, & Ishizuka, 2005). Since emotions and affective expressions play a role in decision-making, learning, and other cognitive functions, human-computer interaction could be improved if affect recognition was part of that interaction. The design of affect-sensitive interactions between humans and computers, a research area known as affective computing, is an increasingly important discipline in the human-computer interaction community (Picard, 1997).

Specifically for users on the autism spectrum, there are several reasons why incorporating technology into intervention practices may be particularly relevant. VR-based systems, which are the focus of this work, have a number of advantages useful in ASD intervention. Over the last decade, studies have been exploring the capability of VR technologies to address social communication deficits of children with ASD. Initial results indicate that VR holds promise as a potential alternative intervention approach with broad accessibility (Parsons & Mitchell, 2002). VR-based systems have demonstrated the advantages of this technology to facilitate children with ASD to learn social skills in designed tasks (Strickland, Marcus, Mesibov, et al., 1996), thus allowing children to more-fully participate in our social world. VR paradigms may offer a way to combine the strengths from cognitive behavioral interventions as well as skills-based approaches (Parsons & Mitchell, 2002), while utilizing potential strengths for individuals with ASD (i.e., visual and auditory learning paradigms). A virtual world that allows for controllable complexity and minimized distractions may be less intimidating or confusing for children with ASD to interact with vs. direct human interactions for initial interventions. Hence, VR models simplified but embodied social interaction (Moore, McGrath, & Thorpe, 2000; Standen & Brown, 2005) but also retains the capability to increase complexity in an interaction in a controlled manner. Since VR mimics real environments in terms of imagery and contexts, it may allow for efficient generalization of skills from the VR environment to the real world (Cromby, Standen, & Brown, 1996). Furthermore, while changing and controlling environments is challenging during real-world interventions, VR possesses the advantage of being a robust but flexible system that can reliably repeat as well as adaptively modify environments across and within contexts (Sherman & Craig, 2003).

However, to date the capability of VR technology has not been fully explored to examine the factors that lead to difficulties in social communication, which could be critical in designing an efficient intervention plan that improves social well-being. The research presented in this paper begins the work of addressing this deficiency. Various computer software packages and VR environments have been developed and applied to address specific deficits associated with autism, e.g., understanding of false belief (Swettenham, 1996), attention (Trepagnier et al., 2006), expression recognition (Silver & Oakes, 2001), social problem-solving (Bernard-Opitz, Sriram, & Nakhoda-Sapuan, 2001), and social conventions (Parsons, Mitchell, & Leonard, 2005). These systems may be able to chain learning via aspects of performance; however they are not capable of a higher degree of affective analysis or individualized adaptation. Specifically, they cannot identify, predict, or respond to one's affective states such as, engagement, anxiety, or enjoyment and thus cannot automatically adapt reinforcement based on the affective needs of the children with ASD. However, given the importance of affective information in ASD intervention practice (Ernsperger, 2003; Seip, 1996; Wieder & Greenspan, 2005), a system using this information may be critical for developing intervention technology that can allow realistic adaptive interaction to challenge and expectantly promote scaffolded skill development in the particular areas of vulnerability, both social and adaptive, for individuals with ASD.

Although affective cues can be used to alter or optimize an intervention setting, children with ASD often have communicative impairments (both verbal and nonverbal), particularly regarding understanding and expression of explicit affective states (Schultz, 2005). Implicit cues of emotional responses can be measured as Autonomic Nervous System (ANS) activation even as explicit expressions are non-evident or mismatched, as is often the case for individuals with ASD (Picard, 2009). Physiological measurement provides a continuously-available channel to gather involuntary responses that have been shown to correlate with affective states (Groden et al., 2005; Herbelin et al., 2004; Mandryk, Inkpen, & Calvert, 2006; Rani, Liu, Sarkar, & Vanman, 2006). Such measurement can be useful with or without additional audio-visual measurements. Our research strategy utilizes a physiological approach to achieve the primary objective of developing technology-based assessment tools capable of identifying specific aspects of interaction that induce an affective response in individuals with ASD. The children could practice social situations within a realistic VR environment, interacting with a system that can also take into account the child's individual affective cues during skill training. Physiological signals can be mapped to one's affective states and thereby could indicate when to push the user (i.e., when to gradually introduce more complex interactions) to advance the user's skill training. The ultimate objective would then be to have those skills transfer to the real world. While initial results applying VR to the treatment of ASD have demonstrated improvements related to basic social skills (Parsons, Mitchell, & Leonard, 2004; Standen & Brown, 2005; Tartaro & Cassell, 2009), no existing VR-based system specifically addresses how to detect and flexibly respond to physiologically-derived affective cues of children with ASD within an intervention paradigm to address complex social impairment and related skills (Bernard-Opitz, Sriram, & Nakhoda-Sapuan, 2001; Dautenhahn & Werry, 2004; Duquette, Michaud, & Mercier, 2008; Kozima, Michalowski, & Nakagawa, 2009; Mitchell, Parsons, & Leonard, 2006; Parsons, Mitchell, & Leonard, 2005; Pioggia et al., 2005; Scassellati, 2005; Strickland, 1997; Swettenham, 1996; Tartaro & Cassell, 2007; Trepagnier et al., 2006).

The presented work is grounded in VR-based technology that applies a physiological approach for detecting subtle affective changes in individuals with ASD as well as typically-developing (TD) individuals during socially-based experimental paradigms. In the future, the system is planned to be developed into a closed-loop intervention tool (see Figure 1) for detecting and adaptively responding to the effects of components of social interaction that lead to struggles in social communication in children with ASD. The current research will be discussed within the broader context of ASD assessment and intervention as a potential technological mechanism to be implemented in the future for enhancing our ability to understand and tailor interventions to the specific vulnerabilities of individuals with ASD.

BACKGROUND

Previous work suggested that affective computing through use of physiological signals and support vector machine algorithms is a feasible approach for children with ASD and robot interactions (Liu, Conn, Sarkar, & Stone, 2008a). A body of research suggests physiological signals vary enough in individuals with ASD to carry out affective computing strategies (Groden et al., 2005; Lang, Greenwald, Bradley, & Hamm, 1993; Shalom et al., 2006; Toichi & Kamio, 2003). To our knowledge, (Liu, Conn, Sarkar, et al., 2008a) was the first work that experimentally demonstrated that real-time implementation of affective models during affect-sensitive human-robot interaction could have an impact with individuals with ASD. Interactions without a specified learning objective, such as the previously-used robot interactions similar to a performance-driven basketball game, do not address the core deficits of ASD. Therefore, they are not the most desirable to reflect the interactions during regular ASD intervention sessions. Consequently, in this work we examine a core deficit, *social interaction*. We continue to monitor physiological signals to test if significant reactions are statistically detectable during different social situations presented in VR. Our work presented in this paper suggests that VR can elicit significant changes in physiological signals similar to observations in real-world settings (i.e., increased eye contact is correlated to higher reports of anxiety). A detailed analysis examines which physiological signals are most significant between and within subjects (an exhaustive look). This detailed look highlights the usefulness of individualized modeling when possible and pinpoints defining features between the subject pair. Also, we offer what a future closed-loop system would look like, including an accompanying intervention protocol. Further study will include an expansion of the number of subjects for continued individual analysis as well as group analysis.

SYSTEM DESIGN TO CONSTRUCT COMPUTATIONAL MODELS

The future implementation of a completely closed-loop system could make significant strides in ASD intervention. The design of a VR-based environment that can be used to systematically explore different social interaction scenarios modulated by the affective states of the participants can be considered a success from the system design standpoint. The ability of the proposed system to sustain an increased engagement level from the participants, while maintaining their comfort level, may also mark the success of the proposed system.

The target age range would be 13-18 years. This range is a time not addressed by early-intervention strategies, which are imperative to a comprehensive ASD intervention strategy. Continued interventions are also important and can equip participants with additional social skills to build on previous treatments or address previously-unaddressed behaviors. Also, teenagers are less accepting of feedback from their parents and caregivers regarding social interactions. However, computer-based systems are highly-engaging for this age group, which will be to the advantage of the system being accepted by participants.

The schematic of our affect-based human-in-the-loop interaction between a participant and the VR environment is depicted in Figure 1. The physiological signals would be collected from the participant during the interaction, and processed in real time to extract features. These features constitute the input material for the developed affective model of the participant, which estimates the most-likely affective cues. The affective information would be used by a main controller, which is responsible for inferring an optimized, therapeutically relevant interaction trajectory and enforcing it during the interaction. The design allows for a person with ASD to participate in an interactive session with VR settings while his/her physiological data are measured using wearable biofeedback sensors (e.g. BIOPAC sensors, E4 sensor, in-house designed sensors). A therapist with experience in working with individuals with ASD and the participant's parent/caregiver/teacher would also observe, from the view of the video camera, how the task progresses on separate monitors. The system could potentially be programmed to teach a variety of discrete and chained tasks, thus reducing patient-to-therapist ratios and increasing learning opportunities during intervention sessions. Figure 1 shows the use of autonomic sensors to guide the selection of instructional targets during

Figure 1. Schematic of the affect-sensitive closed-loop interaction system

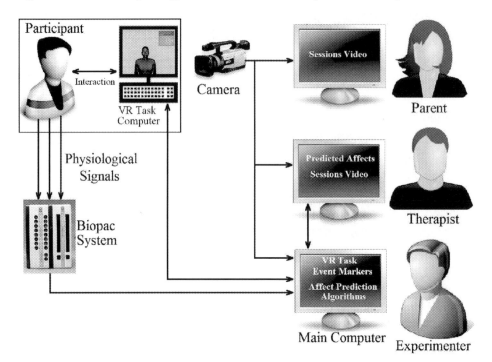

VR interactions, but robots are a possible platform as well. For example, in an affect-sensitive closed-loop system, a robot or character in VR would change the difficulty of instructional tasks in response to changes in users' physiological markers of anxiety, enjoyment, and engagement.

Method

Participants

Approval of the experimental protocol for this pilot study was sought and awarded through Vanderbilt University's Internal Review Board (IRB). IRB-approved language was used on flyers, websites, and e-mails to recruit participants. The flyers were posted around campus and Vanderbilt Treatment and Research Institute for Autism Spectrum Disorder (TRIAD). The information was listed on Vanderbilt Kennedy Center's "StudyFinder" website, which lists studies actively recruiting subjects. E-mails were sent to the Vanderbilt community at large. Participants had to be between 13-18 years old, have normal or corrected-to-normal hearing and vision in order to interact with the VR system, have at least average language understanding (i.e., score ≥80 on the Peabody Picture Vocabulary Test (PPVT) (Dunn & Dunn, 1997), and be able to interact with a computer for up to one hour. Participants with ASD meeting the inclusion/exclusion criteria would likely be described as high-functioning. The requirements were discussed with parents of all potential participants over the telephone prior to the sessions, to gauge general ability to complete the experiment. Participants were compensated with a $10 gift card for each completed session.

Two male children, one with ASD (A1) and one TD (T1), completed the experiment in this preliminary work. Their characteristics are shown in Table 1. The participants were matched by gender, age, and PPVT standard score (Dunn & Dunn, 1997). A1 had a confirmed diagnosis made by clinicians at the Vanderbilt Medical Center using DSM-IV criteria (American Psychiatric Association, 2000) as well as scores from ADOS-G (Autism Diagnostic Observation Schedule-Generic), ADI-R (Autism Diagnostic Interview-Revised), SRS (Social Responsiveness Scale) (Constantino, 2002), and SCQ (Social Communication Questionnaire) (Rutter et al., 2003) assessments. The SRS and SCQ represent widely-used standardized ASD assessment metrics for parental report of symptoms from a diagnostic capacity. Patients scoring above the cutoffs for ASD for SRS or SCQ would be recommended to complete the ADOS-G and ADI-R assessment for scores specific to social interaction, repetitive activities, etc. For the ADOS-G (Lord et al., 2000), the total score, combining Communication and Social Interaction scores, has a cutoff for autism spectrum of 7 and a cutoff for autism of 10. The total score, combining Social Interaction, Communication, Repetitive Activities, and Stereotyped Early Development scores, on the ADI-R (Rutter, Le Couteur, & Lord, 2003) has a cutoff for autism spectrum of 22. A1 had a total score

Table 1. Participant characteristics for initial analysis of system

Participant ID	Age (Years)	PPVT[a]	SRS[b]	SCQ[c]
A1 (male)	17.333	119	78	30
T1 (male)	17.667	118	37	3

[a]PPVT Standard score (Dunn & Dunn, 1997)
[b]SRS Total T-score (Constantino, 2002)
[c]SCQ Total score (Rutter et al., 2003)

on the ADOS-G and ADI-R of 9 and 63, respectively, and scored above ASD cutoffs on the SRS and SCQ. T1 did not complete an ADOS-G or ADI-R. T1's scores on the SRS and SCQ of 37 and 3, respectively, did not meet cutoffs for ASD. Both participants completed two sessions, each approximately one hour, with the VR system.

VR-Based Interactions and Procedure

For ASD intervention, VR is often effectively experienced on a desktop system using standard computer input devices (Parsons & Mitchell, 2002). Therefore, our participants also viewed the avatars in the VR environment on a computer monitor from the first-person perspective (see Figure 1). Vizard (worldviz.com), a commercially available VR design package, was employed to develop the environments. Dr. Jeremy Bailenson, director of the Virtual Human Interaction Lab at Stanford University, provided a set of distinct humanoid avatar heads for use in this work. Within the controllable VR environment, components of the interaction are systematically manipulated to allow users to explore different social compositions. The virtual social peers can make different eye contact and stand at varying distances from the participant in the virtual environment. They can converse by lip-synching with recorded sound files. The participant responds to the avatars using a keypad to select from transparent text boxes superimposed in the corner of the VR scene.

Physiological data were collected using a BIOPAC MP150 system (biopac. com) and wearable sensors placed on the participant, following a procedure close to (Liu, Conn, Sarkar, & Stone, 2008b). Data from cardiovascular, electrodermal, skin temperature, and electromyographic signals were collected. Features from these signals, such as the mean, standard deviation, and slope, were extracted. For example, the standard deviation of the third level coefficient of the Daubechies wavelet transform was extracted as a feature of the collected heart sound signal (Liu, Conn, Sarkar, et al., 2008b).

The experiments used an open-loop design, meaning physiological data and reports on affective states were collected, but the system was not automatically responding to the user in an affect-sensitive manner. Future work will implement a closed-loop design wherein the system reacts to users in an affect-sensitive way. For this current work and similar to previous work (Liu, Conn, Sarkar, et al., 2008b), the experiment was broken into multiple sessions, as not to overburden the subject with an excessive number of trials per session. The first session included obtaining assent and consent from the participants and their parents, explaining the sensors, completing two shorter example trials with the VR system, and completing eight trials of the experiment. The second session included the remaining 16 trials of the 24 trials in the experiment, discussed below. After each trial, the subject (i.e., child), the subject's parent, and the same therapist (i.e., clinical observer with ASD expertise but no previous contact with the subject) rated their perspective on the level of three affective states – anxiety, enjoyment, and engagement – experienced by the subject on a 9-point Likert scale, similar to (Liu, Conn, Sarkar, et al., 2008a) and (Liu, Conn, Sarkar, et al., 2008b). This paper focuses on social parameters studied in a VR-based system and its preliminary experiment, using techniques for measuring physiological signals and calculating physiological features developed in previous work (Liu, Conn, Sarkar, et al., 2008b). Additional details regarding the experimental setup and VR environment design can be found in our companion paper (Welch, Lahiri, Warren, & Sarkar, 2010).

The social parameters of interest for this preliminary work, namely eye gaze and social distance, are manipulated in a 4x2 experimental design, which makes possible eight distinct situations. These parameters are chosen because they play significant roles in social communication and interaction (Bancroft, 1995), and manipulation of these factors may elicit variations in affective reactions (Argyle & Dean, 1965) and physiological responses (Groden et al., 2005). Each situation is represented three times, which creates 24 trials in the experiment, following a Latin Square design to balance for sequencing and order effects (Keppel, 1991). Each trial of an experiment session includes one avatar for one-on-one interaction with the participant. Participants are asked to participate in a social communication task in VR. In each trial, participants are instructed to watch and listen as the virtual social peer tells a 2-min story. The stories are written in first-person. Thus, the task can be likened to having different people introduce themselves to the user, which is comparable to research on social anxiety and social conventions (Argyle & Dean, 1965; Schneiderman & Ewens, 1971; Sommer, 1962). Other social parameters, such as facial expression and vocal tone are kept as neutral as possible.

Detailed Specifications of the Social Parameters Studied

The two social parameters e.g., eye gaze and social distance of the virtual social peers of the participants are systematically manipulated in this study.

The eye gaze parameter dictates the percentage of time an avatar looks at the participant (i.e., staring straight out of the computer monitor). Four types of eye gaze are examined. These are defined as "direct," "averted," "speaking," and "listening." Direct gaze means looking straight ahead for the duration of the story (i.e., for the entire trial). Averted gaze means the avatar never attempts to make direct eye contact with the participant, but instead alternates between looking to the left, right, and up. Research represents averted gaze as looking more than 10° away from center in evenly-distributed, randomly-selected directions (Garau, Slater, Bee, & Sasse, 2001; Jenkins, Beaver, & Calder, 2006). Therefore, our averted gaze is an even distribution (33.3% each) of gazing left, right, and up more than 10° from the center. Based on social psychology literature from experimental observations of typical humans (Argyle & Cook, 1976) and algorithms adopted by the artificial intelligence community to create realistic virtual (Colburn, Drucker, & Cohen, 2000; Garau, Slater, Bee, & Sasse, 2001), normal eye gaze is defined as a mix of direct and averted gaze. A person displays varying mixes of direct and averted eye contact depending on if the person is speaking or listening during face-to-face conversations. Since the virtual social peer in the VR environment is speaking, we use the normal gaze definitions for a person speaking, which is approximately 30% direct gaze and 70% averted gaze (Argyle & Cook, 1976; Colburn, Drucker, & Cohen, 2000). Listening gaze is defined as the flip of a normal speaking gaze, which means looking direct approximately 70% of the time and averted 30% of the time, which is indicative of a person's normal gaze while listening.

The social distance parameter is characterized by the distance between the avatar and the participant. Two types of social distance, termed "invasive" and "decorum," are examined. In the VR environment, distance is simulated but can be appropriately represented to the view of the participant. For invasive distance, the avatar stands approximately 1.5 ft. from the main view of the scene. This social distance has been characterized as intimate space not used for meeting people for the first time or for having casual conversations with friends (Hall, 1955). A distance of 1.5 ft. apart has been investigated by several research groups in experiments with similar experimental setups to ours in which two people are specifically positioned while one introduces himself/herself to the other and discusses a personal topic for approximately 2 min (Argyle & Dean, 1965; Schneiderman & Ewens, 1971; Sommer, 1962) and this invasive distance is characterized by eliciting uncomfortable feelings and attempts to increase the distance to achieve a social equilibrium consistent with comfortable social interaction (Argyle & Dean, 1965). Decorum distance means the avatar stands approximately 4.5 ft. from the main view of the scene. This social distance is consistent with conversations when meeting a new person or a casual friend (Hall, 1966). Research indicates this distance results in a more comfortable conversation experience than the invasive distance (Argyle & Dean, 1965). Using Vizard software we project virtual social peers who display different eye gaze patterns at different distances. Two examples are shown in Figure 2.

Design of Menu-Driven Social Interactions

The interaction involves the virtual social peer telling a personal story while a participant listens. At the end of the story, the avatar asks the participant a question based on some basic facts narrated in the story. The questions are designed to facilitate interaction and to serve as a possible objective measure of engagement. The participant is not aware of the exact question before the story begins so that he/she engages in the task and is not focused on listening to one specific part of the discourse. The questions are intended to be easy to answer correctly if the participant listened to the story. Near the beginning of the first experiment session, the participant takes part in two demonstrations of the process of the VR task; therefore, any difficulty over correctly answering the questions that could be related to not understanding the process of the task is dealt with prior to starting the experiment and collecting data. Each question is accompanied by three possible answer choices (Figure 3). The correct choice is spoken at least five times during the story, which

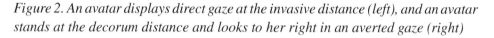

Figure 2. An avatar displays direct gaze at the invasive distance (left), and an avatar stands at the decorum distance and looks to her right in an averted gaze (right)

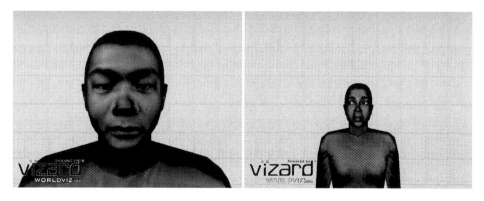

Figure 3. An example of a question asked at the end of a story is displayed as a semi-transparent dialog box overlaid on the VR scene

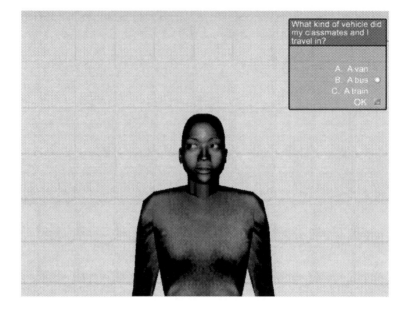

is sufficient for the information to be relayed (Jonides et al., 2008), and the incorrect choices are never spoken in the story. We expect that a participant who engages in the task would achieve near to or complete 100% accuracy on the questions; and consequently, a severely low percentage of correct answers would indicate a lack of engagement with the task.

SOLUTIONS AND RECOMMENDATIONS

Results from initial individual data analysis of A1 and T1 are presented in this section. Two participants are presented to go in depth on individual data results, similar to (Mandryk, Inkpen, & Calvert, 2006) and (Pioggia et al., 2005). Percent accuracy on correctly answering the story-related questions revealed that the participants attended to the task. A1 and T1 achieved 100% accuracy on the story-related questions.

Evidence of overt behaviors as well as more subtle reactions to the different experiment conditions was demonstrated. Participant A1 showed considerable reactions to the virtual social peers standing at the invasive distance or using increased amounts of eye contact by temporarily leaning far back from or looking away from the monitor when they appeared on screen. In post-interview, his mother was surprised to observe such a stark reaction to the change in stimuli. Although accustomed to withdrawing behavior in complex, overwhelming social situations, the mother agreed that the story content and avatars' facial expressions were neutral and was therefore perplexed to see such a reaction from her child to the change in distance or eye gaze alone. These reactions and reflections highlight an advantage that systems like the virtual environment system for social interaction described here can provide to autism intervention. Because such technology can focus on each element of an interaction, minimizing distractions, and can do so with realistic representations of real-world settings; the VR system can systematically manipulate each element of an interaction and observe the effect. Therefore, the VR system can go beyond identifying a broad scope of situations that are affect-inducing. This system can pinpoint what components of a situation bring about an affective reaction to identify which specific component could be a vulnerability during social interaction.

The results of the values of Kappa (K) statistics, averaged across the three affective states showed that among the three possible reporter pairs for A1 (Therapist-Parent (T/P), Therapist-Child (T/C), and Parent-Child (P/C)) the agreement between the therapist and A1's parent (T/P) had the largest value (mean K-statistic for A1, T/P = 0.34, T/C = 0.22, P/C = 0.27). T1's parent was unable to participate in the experiment sessions, but the T/C K-statistic for T1 was also small (mean K-statistic for T1, T/C = 0.18). The same therapist/ clinical observer was involved in all of the experiment sessions, which aided in establishing a consistent reporter. Based on (1) previous work from (Liu, Conn, Sarkar, et al., 2008a) and (Liu, Conn, Sarkar, et al., 2008b) on therapist reliability and consistency, (2) results from K analysis of current results, (3) previous observations of participants reporting constant ratings even as tasks varied, (4) the common use of an observer or parent for rating emotions of children (Eisenberg, 1995), and (5) the possible unreliability of self-reports on emotions from adolescents with and without ASD (Barkley, 1998; Hill, Berthoz, & Frith, 2004), as an experiment design methodology reports from the therapist were used whenever relating the objective physiological data to the children's affective states.

The overt reactions reflected numerical ratings on affective states, collected on a 9-point Likert scale from the clinical observer, and the subtle variations in physiological signals during the experiment trials. Reports on affective states across all 24 experiment trials were correlated with the 51 extracted physiological features from the raw signals. The correlation between the physiological features and subjective ratings for A1 and T1 as rated by the therapist are listed in Table 2. Note, only features with significant correlation ($p < 0.05$) are shown. The sign of the correlation defines a direct/positive or inverse/negative relationship. Bulleted features show a similar pattern of response across participants. Non-bulleted features show the unique differences. The physiological features are the same as listed in (Liu, Conn, Sarkar, & Stone, 2008b), and additional details on the features can be found in (Liu, Conn, Sarkar, & Stone, 2008b). Within Table 2, additional references, beyond the acknowledged (Liu, Conn, Sarkar, & Stone, 2008b), for each physiological feature's use in affective computing research are listed.

As suggested by previous work in (Groden et al., 2005; Herbelin et al., 2004; Mandryk, Inkpen, & Calvert, 2006; Rani, Liu, Sarkar, et al., 2006), A1 and T1 showed significant correlations in their variations of physiological reactions versus variations in affective states. For example, the standard deviation of the interbeat interval from the heart (i.e., IBI_ECGstd (Liu, Conn, Sarkar, & Stone, 2008b)) had a significant correlation to all three affective states for both participants. The relationship of the response was also in the same direction, positive correlation for anxiety but negative correlation for enjoyment and engagement. An increase in the mean of skin conductance (i.e., Tonicmean in Table 2) reflected a decrease in anxiety but increase in enjoyment and engagement for A1, and skin conductance responses have been shown to be very responsive to changes in emotion and variations to task difficulty (Liu, Conn, Sarkar, & Stone, 2008b; Pecchinenda & Smith, 1996; Rani, Sarkar, & Adams, 2007). Although skin temperature is a slow-moving signal, significant features can be extracted to relate to affect. For example, the mean of the skin temperature signal (Tempmean) had a strong negative correlation to T1's anxiety response, and the standard deviation of temperature (Tempstd) for T1 had strong responses (in opposite directions) to anxiety and enjoyment.

Therefore, the VR system shows it can elicit variations in both affective ratings and physiological signals to changes in social experimental stimuli. The findings are similar to observations in social anxiety research of TD adults in real-world settings (Argyle & Dean, 1965; Schneiderman & Ewens, 1971; Sommer, 1962) but have now been examined with observations and physiological signals for children in a virtual interaction. This is the first step towards examining how children react to and accept the virtual social peers as realistic to real-world settings. Establishing realistic interactions builds a basis for creating more complex settings for social communication intervention.

Table 2. Individual analysis of significant correlations between affective state ratings and physiological features for each participant (A1 and T1)

Participant	Affective State	Physiological Feature	Pearson Correlation, r	Significance, p-Value
A1	Anxiety	IBI_ECGstd (AlZoubi, D'Mello, & Calvo, 2012; Chanel, Rebetez, Bétrancourt, & Pun, 2011; Honig, Wagner, Batliner, & Noth, 2009; Rani, Sarkar, & Adams, 2007)	0.5893	0.0024
		PTTstd (Rani, Sarkar, & Adams, 2007)	0.4377	0.0325
		D3_HSstd	0.6273	0.0010
		D4_HSstd	0.5707	0.0036
		Tonicmean (Pecchinenda & Smith, 1996; Rani, Sarkar, & Adams, 2007)	-0.4387	0.0320
		Tonicslope (Pecchinenda & Smith, 1996; Rani, Sarkar, & Adams, 2007)	0.4289	0.0365
		Corstd (AlZoubi, D'Mello, & Calvo, 2012; Cacioppo et al., 2000; Rani, Sarkar, & Adams, 2007)	0.5835	0.0028
		Blink_Peakmean (Cacioppo et al., 2000)	0.6156	0.0014
		Blinkstd (Cacioppo et al., 2000)	0.4819	0.0171
		Trapstd (Cacioppo et al., 2000)	0.4659	0.0218
	Enjoyment	IBI_ECGstd (AlZoubi, D'Mello, & Calvo, 2012; Chanel, Rebetez, Bétrancourt, et al., 2011; Honig, Wagner, Batliner, et al., 2009; Rani, Sarkar, & Adams, 2007)	-0.6589	0.0005
		IBI_PPGstd	-0.5715	0.0035
		PTTstd (Honig, Wagner, Batliner, & Noth, 2009)	-0.5798	0.0030
		D3_HSstd	-0.6798	0.0003
		D4_HSstd	-0.7154	8.5223e-5
		Tonicmean (Pecchinenda & Smith, 1996; Rani, Sarkar, & Adams, 2007)	0.5741	0.0034
		Tonicslope (Pecchinenda & Smith, 1996; Rani, Sarkar, & Adams, 2007)	-0.4996	0.0129
		Corstd (AlZoubi, D'Mello, & Calvo, 2012; Cacioppo et al., 2000; Rani, Sarkar, & Adams, 2007)	-0.5692	0.0037

continued on following page

Table 2. Continued

Participant	Affective State	Physiological Feature	Pearson Correlation, r	Significance, *p*-Value
		Blink_Peakmean (Cacioppo et al., 2000)	-0.6938	0.0002
		Blinkstd (Cacioppo et al., 2000)	-0.4730	0.0196
		Trapstd (Cacioppo et al., 2000)	-0.4828	0.0169
		Tempmean (Chanel, Rebetez, Bétrancourt, et al., 2011; Kataoka et al., 1998; Rani, Sarkar, & Adams, 2007)	0.5204	0.0091
	Engagement	Para (Chanel, Rebetez, Bétrancourt, et al., 2011; Fagundes et al., 2011)	-0.4421	0.0306
		IBI_ECGstd (AlZoubi, D'Mello, & Calvo, 2012; Chanel, Rebetez, Bétrancourt, et al., 2011; Honig, Wagner, Batliner, et al., 2009; Rani, Sarkar, & Adams, 2007)	-0.6803	0.0003
		IBI_PPGstd	-0.4845	0.0164
		PTTstd (Honig, Wagner, Batliner, et al., 2009)	-0.4335	0.0343
		D3_HSstd	-0.5952	0.0022
		D4_HSstd	-0.5995	0.0020
		Tonicmean (Pecchinenda & Smith, 1996; Rani, Sarkar, & Adams, 2007)	0.5003	0.0128
		Tonicslope (Pecchinenda & Smith, 1996; Rani, Sarkar, & Adams, 2007)	-0.4256	0.0381
		Corstd (AlZoubi, D'Mello, & Calvo, 2012; Cacioppo et al., 2000; Rani, Sarkar, & Adams, 2007)	-0.6586	0.0005
		Blink_Peakmean (Cacioppo et al., 2000)	-0.6000	0.0019
		Blinkstd (Cacioppo et al., 2000)	-0.5044	0.0120
		Zygstd (Cacioppo et al., 2000)	-0.4111	0.0460
		Trapstd (Cacioppo et al., 2000)	-0.4589	0.0241
		Tempmean (Chanel, Rebetez, Bétrancourt, et al., 2011; Kataoka et al., 1998; Rani, Sarkar, & Adams, 2007)	0.4313	0.0354

continued on following page

Table 2. Continued

Participant	Affective State	Physiological Feature	Pearson Correlation, r	Significance, *p*-Value
T1	Anxiety	Para (Chanel, Rebetez, Bétrancourt, et al., 2011; Fagundes et al., 2011)	0.4938	0.0142
		IBI_ECGstd (AlZoubi, D'Mello, & Calvo, 2012; Chanel, Rebetez, Bétrancourt, et al., 2011; Honig, Wagner, Batliner, et al., 2009; Rani, Sarkar, & Adams, 2007)	0.6111	0.0015
		PPG_Peakmean (Rani, Sarkar, & Adams, 2007)	-0.4541	0.0258
		IBI_PPGmean	-0.5547	0.0049
		PTTstd (Honig, Wagner, Batliner, et al., 2009)	0.4136	0.0445
		PEPstd (Cacioppo et al., 1994)	0.4672	0.0213
		IBI_ICGstd (Cacioppo et al., 1994)	0.6072	0.0017
		Trapstd (Cacioppo et al., 2000)	0.4768	0.0185
		Tempmean (Chanel, Rebetez, Bétrancourt, et al., 2011; Kataoka et al., 1998; Rani, Sarkar, & Adams, 2007)	-0.4344	0.0339
		Tempstd (Kataoka et al., 1998)	0.4492	0.0277
	Enjoyment	IBI_ECGstd (AlZoubi, D'Mello, & Calvo, 2012; Chanel, Rebetez, Bétrancourt, et al., 2011; Honig, Wagner, Batliner, et al., 2009; Rani, Sarkar, & Adams, 2007)	-0.4889	0.0153
		IBI_ICGstd (Cacioppo et al., 1994)	-0.4917	0.0147
		Trapstd (Cacioppo et al., 2000)	-0.4900	0.0151
		Tempstd (Kataoka et al., 1998)	-0.4238	0.0390
	Engagement	IBI_ECGstd (AlZoubi, D'Mello, & Calvo, 2012; Chanel, Rebetez, Bétrancourt, et al., 2011; Honig, Wagner, Batliner, et al., 2009; Rani, Sarkar, & Adams, 2007)	-0.6419	0.0007
		PEPstd (Cacioppo et al., 1994)	-0.5314	0.0075
		IBI_ICGstd (Cacioppo et al., 1994)	-0.6055	0.0017

continued on following page

Table 2. Continued

Participant	Affective State	Physiological Feature	Pearson Correlation, r	Significance, *p*-Value
		Corstd (AlZoubi, D'Mello, & Calvo, 2012; Cacioppo et al., 2000; Rani, Sarkar, & Adams, 2007)	-0.4390	0.0319
		Zygstd (Cacioppo et al., 2000)	-0.4146	0.0440
		Trapstd (Cacioppo et al., 2000)	-0.6060	0.0017

Also, the system has shown a capacity to detect differences between users, as evidenced by unique physiological features associated with each participant for changes in affect and experiment parameters. Therefore, measuring physiological response during social interaction in VR can tailor interventions to subtle, individual differences for patient-specific needs. However, the results of this pilot work cannot be directly generalized due to the small number of participants, and thus requires further study in the future. For TD individuals, potential benefits could include individualized care that this system holds promise for; but the idiosyncrasy inherent with ASD makes an even more compelling case for such systems to be implemented in ASD clinical settings. A physiologically-sensitive system that can interpret the changing emotions of a child with ASD and help them manage those emotions properly during social interactions could be transformative.

Social communication and social information processing are thought to represent core domains of impairment in children with ASD. This research may enhance our ability to understand the specific vulnerabilities in social communication of children with ASD as well as provide comparisons to a TD population. Investigation using avatars is not only cost and time efficient, it is also necessary to understand the complexity of social tasks. Systematic manipulation of facial expressions, eye gaze, social distance, vocal tone, and gestures need to be studied with virtual social peers where such manipulation is easy to perform, repeatable, and highly controllable. Questions on social communication can be exhaustively explored using controlled studies in virtual environments. Studies like the one presented here will provide insight on how virtual peers display intentions, how they should interact, and how their interactions with children with ASD should be regulated. In that sense, this work is one of the first that presents a design platform for virtual social peers for specific applications that is analogous to well-adopted practices in the manufacturing industry where computer-aided design inevitably precedes any manufacturing. The design of integrating VR social interaction tasks and biofeedback sensor technology is novel yet relevant to the current priorities of technology-assisted ASD intervention. With further development to equip the system with real-time affect recognition capabilities, an autism intervention paradigm could use the system in the future for adaptively responding to the effects of elements of social interaction that lead to struggles in social communication for children with ASD.

Pinpointing features that (1) show high correlation to affective states, (2) can be calculated with less sophisticated microprocessors, and (3) can be sent wirelessly sets up future work for mobile affect detection and in-home interventions. Future installments will focus on heart rate, skin conductance, and temperature data. These raw signals can be collected from smaller devices, using noninvasive and nonintrusive methods (e.g., Empatica's E4 wristband, empatica.com). For example, D3_HSstd (i.e., the standard deviation of the third level coefficient of the Daubechies wavelet transform; see Table 2) had a strong correlation for participant A1's anxiety, enjoyment, and engagement responses. This feature is extracted from a raw heart sound signal collected from a microphone taped to the skin of a user's chest in a position near the heart. Although a telling physiological signal in its relation to affective responses, the collection site would not fit into most user's daily routines. For example, a limit to this work is that it tested the system with a high-functioning user with ASD who wore the taped microphone without an issue, but a wider pool of lower-functioning individuals with ASD or other developmental disabilities may not tolerate that type of data collection. Furthermore, the extraction of this feature from the raw signal requires sophisticated numerical computation software. Other physiological signals, although informative and desirable to collect in laboratory settings, suffer from similar difficulties related to collection (e.g., impedance cardiogram requires four pairs of sensors – two on the sides of a person's neck and two on the torso) and vulnerabilities to settings (e.g., participants are asked not to talk in order to minimize interference with the heart sound signal). Therefore, although these results showcase a wide range of physiological reactions to VR, future work must find the signals most suited for settings outside a laboratory to be the most advantageous for broadening affective computing.

Additionally, interventions with the option of home implementation could significantly increase the presentation rate of social skills training tasks. If data collection and social skills training could be conducted remotely, the workload of trained clinicians could also be reduced. Clinicians could be freed to focus on analyzing performance measures and intervening when the system alters them to significant events such as an increase in anxiety; thus possibly increasing the number of individuals receiving interventions. Cyber distribution of appropriate tasks would have to be developed, which is a considerable undertaking. However, if the work described here can show the feasibility of physiological markers responding to VR-based social situations as well as pinpointing telling signals that can be robustly collected remotely, a future with remote data collection and automated intervention dosages is possible.

FUTURE RESEARCH DIRECTIONS

For future interventions, an affect-sensitive closed-loop system could adjust to the affective needs of individuals and promote positive social interactions. As part of an intervention protocol, participants would be initially screened with the SRS (Constantino, 2002) and SCQ (Rutter et al., 2003) to gauge behaviors. Approximately one-hour sessions with the system, focusing on social interaction tasks (e.g., cooperative scavenger hunts, conversations to find specific information with divergent and appropriate prompts, activities with unstructured waiting times and sympathetic or unresponsive avatars, etc.), would be conducted twice a week for twelve weeks. After each session, analysis of affective responses to the system and abilities to complete tasks would be evaluated. The potential of the system lies with its ability to identify and respond to the specific skill deficits of individual users, present scenarios in realistic settings, and offer intensive presentation rates. Results are expected to show decreases in social anxiety behaviors, as reported on SRS and SCQ, and an increase in performance on the social interaction tasks set in VR.

CONCLUSION

The ability to detect the physiological processes that are a part of impairments in social communication may also prove important for understanding the physiological mechanisms that underlie the presumed core impairments associated with ASD themselves. A description of the system and therapeutic protocol for use in future interventions is given. The pilot study makes comparisons between subjective reports, collected from three perspectives, about levels of anxiety, enjoyment, and engagement experienced while interacting with the current system. In addition, physiological results suggest there is a different physiological response in the body in relation to the reported level of the affective states, supporting the system evokes similar reactions to real-world environments. Despite the potential advantages, current VR technology as applied to assistive intervention for ASD are often designed without closed-loop feedback or even the intention of eventually implementing a closed-loop architecture (Parsons, Mitchell, & Leonard, 2004; Strickland, Marcus, Mesibov, et al., 1996; Tartaro & Cassell, 2007). Therefore, we believe that the presented research is a key step for ushering in a new generation of smart intervention systems that are (1) adaptive and responsive to the individual vulnerabilities of children and adolescents with ASD and (2) capable of enhancing specific intervention goals crucial to long-term independence. Accordingly, we believe that the design of an adaptive response system presented here has the potential to significantly improve overall performance in social tasks for users on the autism spectrum by utilizing an intelligent, adaptive, physiologically-sensitive VR-based technology.

ACKNOWLEDGMENT

This research was supported in part by the National Science Foundation [grant BRIGE-1228027].

REFERENCES

American Psychiatric Association. (2000). *Diagnostic and Statistical Manual of Mental Disorders: DSM-IV-TR* (4th ed.). Washington, DC: American Psychiatric Association.

Argyle, M., & Cook, M. (1976). *Gaze and Mutual Gaze*. Cambridge, MA: Cambridge University Press.

Asha, K., Ajay, K., Naznin, V., George, T., & Peter, D. (2005). *Gesture-based affective computing on motion capture data*. Paper presented at the International Conference on Affective Computing and Intelligent Interaction.

Barkley, R. A. (1998). *Attention Deficit Hyperactivity Disorder: A Handbook for Diagnosis and Treatment* (2nd ed.). New York: Guilford Press.

Bartlett, M. S., Littlewort, G., Fasel, I., & Movellan, J. R. (2003). *Real Time Face Detection and Facial Expression Recognition: Development and Applications to Human Computer Interaction*. Paper presented at the Conference on Computer Vision and Pattern Recognition Workshop. 10.1109/CVPRW.2003.10057

Ben Shalom, D., Mostofsky, S. H., Hazlett, R. L., Goldberg, M. C., Landa, R. J., Faran, Y., ... Hoehn-Saric, R. (2006). Normal physiological emotions but differences in expression of conscious feelings in children with high-functioning autism. *Journal of Autism and Developmental Disorders*, *36*(3), 395–400. doi:10.100710803-006-0077-2 PMID:16565884

Bernard-Opitz, V., Sriram, N., & Nakhoda-Sapuan, S. (2001). Enhancing social problem solving in children with autism and normal children through computer-assisted instruction. *Journal of Autism and Developmental Disorders*, *31*(4), 377–384. doi:10.1023/A:1010660502130 PMID:11569584

Bethel, C., Salomon, K., Murphy, R., & Burke, J. (2007). *Survey of psychophysiology measurements applied to human-robot interaction*. Paper presented at the IEEE International Symposium on Robot and Human Interactive Communication, Jeju, South Korea. 10.1109/ROMAN.2007.4415182

Bradley, M. M. (2000). Emotion and motivation. In J. T. Cacioppo, L. G. Tassinary, & G. Berntson (Eds.), *Handbook of Psychophysiology* (pp. 602–642). New York: Cambridge University Press.

Brown, R. M., Hall, L. R., Holtzer, R., Brown, S. L., & Brown, N. L. (1997). Gender and video game performance. *Sex Roles*, *36*(11/12), 793–812. doi:10.1023/A:1025631307585

Cantwell, D. P., Lewinsohn, P. M., Rohde, P., & Seeley, J. R. (1997). Correspondence between adolescent report and parent report of psychiatric diagnostic data. *Journal of the American Academy of Child and Adolescent Psychiatry*, *36*(5), 610–619. doi:10.1097/00004583-199705000-00011 PMID:9136495

Centers for Disease Control and Prevention (CDC). (2018). Prevalence of Autism Spectrum Disorder Among Children Aged 8 Years-ADDM Network, United States, 2014. *Morbidity and Mortality Weekly Report (MMWR) Surveillance Summaries, 67*, 1-23.

Chen, S. H., & Bernard-Opitz, V. (1993). Comparison of personal and computer-assisted instruction for children with autism. *Mental Retardation, 31*(6), 368–376. PMID:8152382

Cohen, H., Amerine-Dickens, M., & Smith, T. (2006). Early intensive behavioral treatment: replication of the UCLA model in a community setting. *Journal of Developmental & Behavioral Pediatrics, 27*(2), S145-155.

Colburn, A., Drucker, S., & Cohen, M. (2000). The role of eye-gaze in avatar-mediated conversational interfaces. Paper presented at SIGGRAPH Sketches and Applications, New Orleans, LA.

Conati, C., Chabbal, R., & Maclaren, H. (2003). *A study on using biometric sensors for detecting user emotions in educational games.* Paper presented at the Workshop on Assessing and Adapting to User Attitude and Affects: Why, When and How, Pittsburgh, PA.

Cowie, R., Douglas-Cowie, E., Tsapatsoulis, N., Votsis, G., Kollias, S., Fellenz, W., & Taylor, J. G. (2001). Emotion recognition in human-computer interaction. *IEEE Signal Processing Magazine, 18*(1), 32–80. doi:10.1109/79.911197

Cromby, J. J., Standen, P. J., & Brown, D. J. (1996). The potentials of virtual environments in the education and training of people with learning disabilities. *Journal of Intellectual Disability Research, 40*(6), 489–501. doi:10.1111/j.1365-2788.1996.tb00659.x PMID:9004109

Dautenhahn, K., & Werry, I. (2004). Towards interactive robots in autism therapy: Background, motivation and challenges. *Pragmatics & Cognition, 12*(1), 1–35. doi:10.1075/pc.12.1.03dau

Dautenhahn, K., Werry, I., Salter, T., & te Boekhorst, R. (2003). *Towards adaptive autonomous robots in autism therapy: Varieties of interactions.* Paper presented at the IEEE International Symposium on Computational Intelligence in Robotics and Automation, Kobe, Japan. 10.1109/CIRA.2003.1222245

Ernsperger, L. (2003). *Keys to Success for Teaching Students with Autism.* Arlington, TX: Future Horizons.

Fong, T., Nourbakhsh, I., & Dautenhahn, K. (2003). A survey of socially interactive robots. *Robotics and Autonomous Systems, 42*(3/4), 143–166. doi:10.1016/S0921-8890(02)00372-X

Gilleade, K., Dix, A., & Allanson, J. (2005). *Affective videogames and modes of affective gaming: Assist me, challenge me, emote me.* Paper presented at the Digital Games Research Association Conference.

Gillott, A., Furniss, F., & Walter, A. (2001). Anxiety in high-functioning children with autism. *Autism, 5*(3), 277–286. doi:10.1177/1362361301005003005 PMID:11708587

Goodwin, M. S. (2008). Enhancing and accelerating the pace of Autism Research and Treatment: The promise of developing Innovative Technology. *Focus on Autism and Other Developmental Disabilities, 23*(2), 125–128. doi:10.1177/1088357608316678

Green, D., Baird, G., Barnett, A. L., Henderson, L., Huber, J., & Henderson, S. E. (2002). The severity and nature of motor impairment in Asperger's syndrome: A comparison with specific developmental disorder of motor function. *Journal of Child Psychology and Psychiatry, and Allied Disciplines, 43*(5), 655–668. doi:10.1111/1469-7610.00054 PMID:12120861

Groden, J., Goodwin, M. S., Baron, M. G., Groden, G., Velicer, W. F., Lipsitt, L. P., ... Plummer, B. (2005). Assessing cardiovascular responses to stressors in individuals with autism spectrum disorders. *Focus on Autism and Other Developmental Disabilities, 20*(4), 244–252. doi:10.1177/10883576050200040601

Hill, E., Berthoz, S., & Frith, U. (2004). Brief report: Cognitive processing of own emotions in individuals with autistic spectrum disorder and in their relatives. *Journal of Autism and Developmental Disabilities, 34*(2), 229–235. doi:10.1023/B:JADD.0000022613.41399.14 PMID:15162941

Jacobson, J. W., Mulick, J. A., & Green, G. (1998). Cost-benefit estimates for early intensive behavioral intervention for young children with autism – General model and single state case. *Behavioral Interventions, 13*(4), 201–226. doi:10.1002/(SICI)1099-078X(199811)13:4<201::AID-BIN17>3.0.CO;2-R

Kapoor, A., Mota, S., & Picard, R. W. (2001). *Towards a learning companion that recognizes affect.* Paper presented at Emotional and Intelligent II: The Tangled Knot of Social Cognition AAAI Fall Symposium.

Kerr, S., & Durkin, K. (2004). Understanding of thought bubbles as mental representations in children with autism: Implications for theory of mind. *Journal of Autism and Developmental Disorders, 34*(6), 637–648. doi:10.100710803-004-5285-z PMID:15679184

Kleinsmith, A., Ravindra De Silva, P., & Bianchi-Berthouze, N. (2005). *Recognizing emotion from postures: cross-cultural differences in user modeling.* Paper presented at User Modeling. 10.1007/11527886_8

Kozima, H., Michalowski, M. P., & Nakagawa, C. (2009). Keepon: A playful robot for research, therapy, and entertainment. *International Journal of Social Robotics, 1*(1), 3–18. doi:10.100712369-008-0009-8

Kramer, A., Sirevaag, E., & Braune, R. (1987). A Psychophysiological Assessment of Operator Workload during Simulated Flight Missions. *Human Factors, 29*(2), 145–160. doi:10.1177/001872088702900203 PMID:3610180

Kulic, D., & Croft, E. (2007). Physiological and subjective responses to articulated robot motion. *Robotica, 25*(01), 13–27. doi:10.1017/S0263574706002955

Lee, C. M., & Narayanan, S. S. (2005). Toward detecting emotions in spoken dialogs. *IEEE Transactions on Speech and Audio Processing, 13*(2), 293–303. doi:10.1109/TSA.2004.838534

Liu, C., Conn, K., Sarkar, N., & Stone, W. (2008a). Physiology-based affect recognition for computer-assisted intervention of children with autism spectrum disorder. *International Journal of Human-Computer Studies, 66*(9), 662–677. doi:10.1016/j.ijhsc.2008.04.003

Liu, C., Conn, K., Sarkar, N., & Stone, W. (2008b). Online Affect Detection and Robot Behavior Adaptation for Intervention of Children with Autism. *IEEE Transactions on Robotics, 24*(4), 883–896. doi:10.1109/TRO.2008.2001362

Mandryk, R. L., Inkpen, K. M., & Calvert, T. W. (2006). Using physiological techniques to measure user experience with entertainment technologies. *International Journal of Human-Computer Studies, 25*(2), 141–158.

Meehan, M., Razzaque, S., Insko, B., Whitton, M., & Brooks, F. P. Jr. (2005). Review of four studies on the use of physiological reaction as a measure of presence in stressful virtual environments. *Applied Psychophysiology and Biofeedback, 30*(3), 239–258. doi:10.100710484-005-6381-3 PMID:16167189

Michaud, F., & Theberge-Turmel, C. (2002). Mobile robotic toys and autism. In K. Dautenhahn, A. H. Bond, L. Canamero, & B. Edmonds (Eds.), *Socially Intelligent Agents: Creating Relationships With Computers and Robots* (pp. 125–132). Norwell, MA: Kluwer. doi:10.1007/0-306-47373-9_15

Mitchell, P., Parsons, S., & Leonard, A. (2007). Using virtual environments for teaching social understanding to adolescents with autistic spectrum disorders. *Journal of Autism and Developmental Disorders, 37*(3), 589–600. doi:10.100710803-006-0189-8 PMID:16900403

Moore, D. J., McGrath, P., & Thorpe, J. (2000). Computer aided learning for people with autism - A framework for research and development. *Innovations in Education & Training International, 37*(3), 218–228. doi:10.1080/13558000050138452

Myers, S. M., & Johnson, C. P. (2007). Management of children with autism spectrum disorders. *Pediatrics, 120*(5), 1162–1182. doi:10.1542/peds.2007-2362 PMID:17967921

Nasoz, F., Alvarez, K., Lisetti, C., & Finkelstein, N. (2004). Emotion recognition from physiological signals using wireless sensors for presence technologies. *International Journal of Cognition, Technology, and Work, 6*(1), 4-14.

NRC (National Research Council). (2001). *Educating Children with Autism.* Washington, DC: National Academy Press.

Pantic, M., & Rothkrantz, L. J. M. (2003). Toward an affect-sensitive multimodal human–computer interaction. *Proceedings of the IEEE, 91*(9), 1370–1390. doi:10.1109/JPROC.2003.817122

Papert, S. (1993). *Mindstorms: Children, Computers, and Powerful Ideas* (2nd ed.). New York: Basic Books.

Parsons, S., & Mitchell, P. (2002). The potential of virtual reality in social skills training for people with autistic spectrum disorders. *Journal of Intellectual Disability Research, 46*(5), 430–443. doi:10.1046/j.1365-2788.2002.00425.x PMID:12031025

Parsons, S., Mitchell, P., & Leonard, A. (2004). The use and understanding of virtual environments by adolescents with autistic spectrum disorders. *Journal of Autism and Developmental Disorders, 34*(4), 449–466. doi:10.1023/B:JADD.0000037421.98517.8d PMID:15449520

Parsons, S., Mitchell, P., & Leonard, A. (2005). Do adolescents with autistic spectrum disorders adhere to social conventions in virtual environments? *Autism, 9*(1), 95–117. doi:10.1177/1362361305049032 PMID:15618265

Pecchinenda, A., & Smith, C. A. (1996). The affective significance of skin conductance activity during a difficult problem-solving task. *Cognition and Emotion, 10*(5), 481–504. doi:10.1080/026999396380123

Picard, R. W. (1997). *Affective Computing*. Cambridge, MA: MIT Press.

Pioggia, G., Igliozzi, R., Ferro, M., Ahluwalia, A., Muratori, F., & De Rossi, D. (2005). An android for enhancing social skills and emotion recognition in people with autism. *IEEE Transactions on Neural Systems and Rehabilitation Engineering, 13*(4), 507–515. doi:10.1109/TNSRE.2005.856076 PMID:16425833

Prendinger, H., Mori, J., & Ishizuka, M. (2005). Using human physiology to evaluate subtle expressivity of a virtual quizmaster in a mathematical game. *International Journal of Human-Computer Studies, 62*(2), 231–245. doi:10.1016/j.ijhcs.2004.11.009

Rani, P., Sarkar, N., Smith, C. A., & Kirby, L. D. (2004). Anxiety detecting robotic system – towards implicit human-robot collaboration. *Robotica, 22*(1), 85–95. doi:10.1017/S0263574703005319

Robins, B., Dickerson, P., & Dautenhahn, K. (2005). *Robots as embodied beings – Interactionally sensitive body movements in interactions among autistic children and a robot*. Paper presented at the IEEE International Workshop on Robot and Human Interactive Communication, Nashville, TN. 10.1109/ROMAN.2005.1513756

Rogers, S. J. (2000). Interventions that facilitate socialization in children with autism. *Journal of Autism and Developmental Disorders, 30*(5), 399–409. doi:10.1023/A:1005543321840 PMID:11098875

Ruble, L. A., & Robson, D. M. (2006). Individual and environmental determinants of engagement in autism. *Journal of Autism and Developmental Disorders, 37*(8), 1457–1468. doi:10.100710803-006-0222-y PMID:17151800

Rutter, M. (2006). Autism: Its recognition, early diagnosis, and service implications. *Journal of Developmental and Behavioral Pediatrics, 27*(Supplement 2), S54–S58. doi:10.1097/00004703-200604002-00002 PMID:16685186

Scassellati, B. (2005). *Quantitative metrics of social response for autism diagnosis*. Paper presented at the IEEE International Workshop on Robot and Human Interactive Communication, Nashville, TN. 10.1109/ROMAN.2005.1513843

Schneiderman, M. H., & Ewens, W. L. (1971). The Cognitive Effects of Spatial Invasion. *Pacific Sociological Review, 14*(4), 469–486. doi:10.2307/1388543

Schultz, R. T. (2005). Developmental deficits in social perception in autism: The role of the amygdala and fusiform face area. *International Journal of Developmental Neuroscience, 23*(2-3), 125–141. doi:10.1016/j.ijdevneu.2004.12.012 PMID:15749240

Seip, J. (1996). *Teaching the Autistic and Developmentally Delayed: A Guide for Staff Training and Development*. Delta, BC: Author.

Sharpe, D. L., & Baker, D. L. (2007). Financial issues associated with having a child with autism. *Journal of Family and Economic Issues, 28*(2), 247–264. doi:10.100710834-007-9059-6

Sherer, M. R., & Schreibman, L. (2005). Individual behavioral profiles and predictors of treatment effectiveness for children with autism. *Journal of Consulting and Clinical Psychology, 73*(3), 525–538. doi:10.1037/0022-006X.73.3.525 PMID:15982150

Sherman, W. R., & Craig, A. B. (2003). *Understanding virtual reality: interface, application, and design*. Boston: Morgan Kaufmann Publishers.

Silva, P. R. D., Osano, M., Marasinghe, A., & Madurapperuma, A. P. (2006). A computational model for recognizing emotion with intensity for machine vision applications. *IEICE Transactions on Information and Systems, E89-D*(7), 2171–2179. doi:10.1093/ietisy/e89-d.7.2171

Smith, C. A. (1989). Dimensions of appraisal and physiological response in emotion. *Journal of Personality and Social Psychology, 56*(3), 339–353. doi:10.1037/0022-3514.56.3.339 PMID:2926633

Standen, P. J., & Brown, D. J. (2005). Virtual reality in the rehabilitation of people with intellectual disabilities [review]. *Cyberpsychology & Behavior, 8*(3), 272–282, discussion 283–288. doi:10.1089/cpb.2005.8.272 PMID:15971976

Stokes, S. (2000). *Assistive technology for children with autism*. Published under a CESA 7 contract funded by the Wisconsin Department of Public Instruction.

Strickland, D. (1997). Virtual reality for the treatment of autism. In G. Riva (Ed.), *Virtual reality in neuropsycho-physiology* (pp. 81–86). Amsterdam: IOS Press.

Strickland, D., Marcus, L. M., Mesibov, G. B., & Hogan, K. (1996). Brief report: Two case studies using virtual reality as a learning tool for autistic children. *Journal of Autism and Developmental Disorders, 26*(6), 651–659. doi:10.1007/BF02172354 PMID:8986851

Swettenham, J. (1996). Can children with autism be taught to understand false belief using computers? *Journal of Child Psychology and Psychiatry, and Allied Disciplines, 37*(2), 157–165. doi:10.1111/j.1469-7610.1996.tb01387.x PMID:8682895

Tarkan, L. (2002). Autism therapy is called effective, but rare. *New York Times*.

Tartaro, A., & Cassell, J. (2007). Using virtual peer technology as an intervention for children with autism. In J. Lazar (Ed.), *Towards Universal Usability: Designing Computer Interfaces for Diverse User Populations*. Chichester, UK: John Wiley and Sons.

Toichi, M., & Kamio, Y. (2003). Paradoxical autonomic response to mental tasks in autism. *Journal of Autism and Developmental Disorders, 33*(4), 417–426. doi:10.1023/A:1025062812374 PMID:12959420

Trepagnier, C. Y., Sebrechts, M. M., Finkelmeyer, A., Stewart, W., Woodford, J., & Coleman, M. (2006). Simulating social interaction to address deficits of autistic spectrum disorder in children. *Cyberpsychology & Behavior, 9*(2), 213–217. doi:10.1089/cpb.2006.9.213 PMID:16640482

Vicente, K., Thornton, D., & Moray, N. (1987). Spectral-Analysis of Sinus Arrhythmia - a Measure of Mental Effort. *Human Factors, 29*(2), 171–182. doi:10.1177/001872088702900205 PMID:3610182

Wieder, S., & Greenspan, S. (2005). Can children with autism master the core deficits and become empathetic, creative, and reflective? *The Journal of Developmental and Learning Disorders, 9*, 1–29.

Wijesiriwardana, R., Mitcham, K., & Dias, T. (2004). *Fibre-meshed transducers based real time wearable physiological information monitoring system.* Paper presented at the International Symposium on Wearable Computers, Washington, DC. 10.1109/ISWC.2004.20

Zhai, J., Barreto, A., Chin, C., & Li, C. (2005). User Stress Detection in Human-Computer Interactions. *Biomedical Sciences Instrumentation*, *41*, 277–286. PMID:15850118

ADDITIONAL READING

Bolte, S., Feineis-Matthews, S., & Poustka, F. (2008). Emotional processing in high-functioning autism – physiological reactivity and affective report. *Journal of Autism and Developmental Disorders*, *38*(4), 776–781. doi:10.100710803-007-0443-8 PMID:17882540

Bradley, M. M. (1994). Emotional memory: a dimensional analysis. In S. Van Goozen, N. E. Van de Poll, & I. A. Sergeant (Eds.), *Emotions: Essays on emotion theory* (pp. 97–134). Hillsdale, NJ: Erlbaum.

Conn, K., Liu, C., Sarkar, N., Stone, W., & Warren, Z. (2008). Towards Affect-sensitive Assistive Intervention Technologies for Children with Autism. In J. Or (Ed.), *Affective Computing: Focus on Emotion Expression, Synthesis and Recognition* (pp. 365–390). Vienna, Austria: ARS/I-Tech Education and Publishing. doi:10.5772/6171

Ekman, P. (1993). Facial expression and emotion. *The American Psychologist*, *48*(4), 384–392. doi:10.1037/0003-066X.48.4.384 PMID:8512154

Frischen, A., Bayliss, A. P., & Tipper, S. P. (2007). Gaze cuing of Attention: Visual Attention, Social Cognition and Individual Differences. *Psychological Bulletin*, *133*(4), 694–724. doi:10.1037/0033-2909.133.4.694 PMID:17592962

Klin, A., Jones, W., Schultz, R., Volkmar, F., & Cohen, D. (2002). Visual fixation patterns during viewing of naturalistic social situations as predictors of social competence in individuals with autism. *Archives of General Psychiatry*, *59*(9), 809–816. doi:10.1001/archpsyc.59.9.809 PMID:12215080

Mandryk, R. L., & Atkins, M. S. (2007). A fuzzy physiological approach for continuously modeling emotion during interaction with play technologies. *International Journal of Human-Computer Studies*, *65*(4), 329–347. doi:10.1016/j.ijhcs.2006.11.011

Neumann, S. A., & Waldstein, S. R. (2001). Similar patterns of cardiovascular response during emotion activation as a function of affective valence and arousal and gender. *Journal of Psychosomatic Research*, *50*(5), 245–253. doi:10.1016/S0022-3999(01)00198-2 PMID:11399281

Picard, R. W. (2009). Future Affective Technology for Autism and Emotion Communication. *Philosophical Transactions of the Royal Society of London. Series B, Biological Sciences*, *364*(1535), 3575–3584. doi:10.1098/rstb.2009.0143 PMID:19884152

Zhai, J., & Barreto, A. (2006). Stress Detection in Computer Users through Noninvasive Monitoring of Physiological Signals. *Biomedical Sciences Instrumentation*, *42*, 495–500. PMID:16817657

KEY TERMS AND DEFINITIONS

Affective Computing: The study and development of systems and devices that can recognize, interpret, process, and simulate human affects.

Assistive Technologies: Devices for people with disabilities.

Human Affects: A human's experience of feeling or emotion.

Human-Centered Computing: The study of the design, development, and deployment of human-computer systems.

Human-Computer Interaction: The study of how people interact with computers, including the design and implementation of systems to study how successful those interactions are.

Physiological Measures: Measurements to assess how the human body functions. They be very simple, such as body temperature with a thermometer; or they may be more complicated, for example measuring how the heart is functioning by taking an ECG (electrocardiograph).

Virtual Reality: A computer-generated environment that simulates reality.

Chapter 2
Electroencephalogram (EEG) for Delineating Objective Measure of Autism Spectrum Disorder

Sampath Jayarathna
Old Dominion University, USA

Yasith Jayawardana
Old Dominion University, USA

Mark Jaime
Indiana University-Purdue University Columbus, USA

Sashi Thapaliya
California State Polytechnic University – Pomona, USA

ABSTRACT

Autism spectrum disorder (ASD) is a developmental disorder that often impairs a child's normal development of the brain. According to CDC, it is estimated that 1 in 6 children in the US suffer from development disorders, and 1 in 68 children in the US suffer from ASD. This condition has a negative impact on a person's ability to hear, socialize, and communicate. Subjective measures often take more time, resources, and have false positives or false negatives. There is a need for efficient objective measures that can help in diagnosing this disease early as possible with less effort. EEG measures the electric signals of the brain via electrodes placed on various places on the scalp. These signals can be used to study complex neuropsychiatric issues. Studies have shown that EEG has the potential to be used as a biomarker for various neurological conditions including ASD. This chapter will outline the usage of EEG measurement for the classification of ASD using machine learning algorithms.

DOI: 10.4018/978-1-5225-7467-5.ch002

INTRODUCTION

Autism Spectrum Disorder (ASD) is characterized by significant impairments in social and communicative functioning as well as the presence of repetitive behaviors and/or restricted interests. According to CDC estimates, the prevalence of ASD (14.6 per 1,000 children) has nearly doubled over the last decade and has a costly impact on the lives of families affected by the disorder. It is estimated that 1 in 6 children in the US suffer from developmental disorders. And 1 in 68 children fall under Autism Spectrum Disorder. ASD is a neurological and developmental disorder that has negative impact in a person's learning, social interaction and communication. It is a debilitating condition that affects brain development from early childhood creating a lifelong challenge in normal functioning. Autism is measured in spectrum because of the wide range of symptoms and severity. The total lifetime cost of care for an individual with ASD can be as high as $2.4 million (Buescher et al. 2014). In the U.S., the long-term societal costs are projected to reach $461 billion by 2025 (Leigh and Du 2015).

One of the main contributing factors for ASD is known to be genetics. And so far, no suitable cure has been found. However, early intervention has been shown to reverse or correct most of its symptoms (Dawson 2008). And this can only be possible by early diagnosis. Therefore, early diagnosis is crucial for successful treatment of ASD. Although progress has been made to accurately diagnose ASD, it is far from ideal. It often requires various tests such as behavioral assessments, observations from caretakers over a period to correctly determine the existence of Autism. Even with this tedious testing often individuals are misdiagnosed. However, there remains promise in the development of accurate detection using various modalities of Biomedical Images, EEG, and Eye movements.

Efforts to identify feasible, low-cost, and etiologically meaningful biobehavioral markers of ASD are thus critical for mitigating these costs through improvement in the objective detection of ASD. However, the phenotypic and genotypic heterogeneity of ASD presents a unique challenge for identifying precursors aligned with currently recognized social processing dimensions of ASD. One approach to unraveling the heterogeneity of ASD is to develop neurocognitive measures with shared coherence that map onto valid diagnostic tasks, like the Autism Diagnostic Observation Schedule Second Edition (ADOS-2) (Gotham et al. 2007), that are the gold standard in ASD identification. These measures can then be used to stratify children into homogeneous subgroups, each representing varying degrees of impaired social neurocognitive functioning. Despite the need for objective, physiological measures of social functioning, machine learning has not yet been widely applied to biobehavioral metrics for diagnostic purposes in children with ASD.

This chapter focuses on a social processing domain which, according to the NIMH Research Domain Criteria (RDoC), is a central deficit of ASD and lends itself to quantifiable neurocognitive patterns: social interactions during ADOS-2. The ability to socially coordinate visual attention, share a point of view with another person, and process self- and other-related information (Barresi and Moore 1996; Butterworth and Jarrett 1991; Mundy et al. 2009) is a foundational social cognitive capacity (Mundy 2016). Its emergence in infancy predicts individual differences in language development in both children with ASD and in typically developing children (Mundy et al. 1990; Mundy and Newell 2007). Moreover, attention is recognized in the diagnostic criteria of the DSM-V as one of the central impairments of early, nonverbal social communication in ASD. While the empirical evidence on the physiological nature of attention deficits in ASD is emerging that can index attention: social brain functional connectivity (FC) during real-life social interaction.

At the same time, it is well-established in the literature that the neural systems that subserve social cognition are functionally compromised in children with ASD (Baron-Cohen et al. 1985; Lombardo et al. 2011; Hill and Frith 2003; Kana et al. 2009; Mason et al. 2008). The research suggests there is a functional (frontal-temporal-parietal) overlap in neural system activity during ADOS-2 and social cognitive processing (Mundy 2016; Kennedy and Adolphs 2012; Redcay et al. 2012; Schurz et al. 2014; Lombardo et al. 2010; Caruana et al. 2015). Taken together, there is ample evidence to support that aberrant frontal temporal-parietal FC is a potential nexus for latent social cognitive disturbance in early ASD.

Many studies reveal either under- or over-connected areas in the autistic brain, depending on whether the subject is at rest or engaged in cognitive processing (Coben et al. 2008; Just et al. 2004; Just et al. 2006; Kana et al. 2014; Koshino et al. 2005; Koshino et al. 2007; Lazarev et al. 2015; Lynch et al. 2013; Uddin et al. 2013; Shih et al. 2010; Noonan et al. 2009; Jones et al. 2010; Damarla et al. 2010; Mohammad-Rezazadeh et al. 2016). Reduced FC within frontal, superior temporal, and temporal— parietal regions—regions that comprise the social brain system—have been consistently reported in most fMRI studies examining FC during social information processing

(Koshino et al. 2007; Castelli et al. 2002; Kleinhans et al. 2008; Rudie et al. 2011; Welchew et al. 2005). The presence of altered social brain system FC in early neurodevelopment can potentially reveal the onset of social difficulties (Keehn et al. 2013), as altered FC disrupts efficient information flow between parallel and distributed neural systems involved in the processing of social and communicative information (Mundy et al. 2009). Thus, children with ASD may develop with limited neurocognitive resources to efficiently deal with the processing demands of dynamic social exchanges. This social deficit may emerge as idiosyncratic patterns of EEG during bouts of joint social attention

LITERATURE SURVEY

Social Interaction Tasks

To date, the few studies that have examined FC during attention have done so using non-clinical paradigms that involve the observation of attention-eliciting videos; however, data from such paradigms may not reflect the true person-to-person interactive nature. More importantly, video paradigms may only tap into one of two facets of attention: responding to joint attention (RJA), which serves an imperative function. What is not represented in JA-eliciting video paradigms is initiating joint attention (IJA), which serves a declarative function and taps into social reward systems that are integral to the social sharing of experiences (Caruana et al. 2015; Schilbach et al. 2010; Gordon et al. 2013). Moreover, RJA and IJA show a developmental dissociation during the first and second years of life (Yoder et al. 2009; Ibañez et al. 2013; Mundy et al. 2007). Although RJA and IJA both have predictive value in infancy, IJA is a more stable marker of ASD than RJA in later childhood (Mundy et al. 1986). Some neuroimaging researchers have dealt with the above issues by using a live face-to-avatar paradigm to simulate IJA bids (Redcay et al. 2012; Gordon et al. 2013). However, the movement constraints inside the MRI scanner create testing conditions that can be difficult for younger children, with and without ASD.

Eye movement behavior is a result of complex neurological processes; therefore, eye gaze metrics can reveal objective and quantifiable information about the predictability and consistency of covert social cognitive processes, including social attention (Chita-Tegmark 2016; Guillon et al. 2014), emotion recognition (Bal et al. 2010; Black et al. 2017; Sawyer et al. 2012; Sasson et al. 2016; Tsang 2018; Wagner et al. 2016; Wieckowski and White 2017), perspective taking, (Symeonidou et al. 2016) and joint attention (Bedford et al. 2012; Billeci et al. 2016; Falck-Ytter et al. 2012; Falck-Ytter et al. 2015; Swanson et al. 2013; Thorup et al. 2016; Thorup et al. 2018; Vivanti et al. 2017) for children with and without ASD. Eye gaze measurement includes several metrics relevant to oculomotor control (Komogortsev et al. 2013) such as saccadic trajectories, fixations, and other relevant measures such as velocity, duration, amplitude, and pupil dilation (Krejtz et al. 2018a). We believe that combined analysis of fixations and saccades during natural and dynamic joint attention tasks, currently used as a reliable measure of ASD diagnostic criteria, will represent valid biomarkers for objectifying and delineating the dimensionality of ASD diagnosis in the future. Previous work in this area have successfully demonstrated development of Қ, the coefficient of ambient/focal attention (Krejtz et al. 2016) and previous work has supported the relationship between eye tracking metrics and severity of ASD diagnosis (Frazier et al. 2018; Del Valle Rubido et al. 2018) and communicative competence (Norbury et al. 2009). If visual attention influences stability of fixations dependent upon the demands of dynamic joint attention tasks, a natural next step is to look into how relevance may be reflected in similar neurophysiologic features for atypical social brain systems, such as in the context of ASD (Hotier et al. 2017).

EEG Based Machine Learning for ASD

Studies have shown that EEG has the potential to be used as biomarker for various neurological conditions including ASD (Wang et al. 2013). EEG measures the electrical signals of the brain via electrodes that are placed on various places on the scalp. These electrical signals are postsynaptic activity in the neocortex and can be used to study complex neuropsychiatric issues. EEG has various frequency bands and its analysis are performed on these varying bandwidths. Waves between 0.5 and 4 HZ are delta, between 4 and 8 HZ are theta, between 8 and 13 HZ are alpha, 13 to 35 HZ are beta and over 35 are gamma. Saccadic eye movement plays a big role in the attention and behavior of an individual which directly affects both language and social skills (Fletcher-Watson et al. 2009). Autistic children seem to have different eye movement behaviors than non-autistic children. They tend to avoid eye contact and looking at human face while focusing more on geometric shapes

(Klin et al. 2009). While a typical child doesn't find any interest in geometric shapes and tend to make more eye contact, and human face perception.

In Grossi et al. (2017), authors use a complex EEG processing algorithm called MSROM/I-FAST along with multiple machine learning algorithms to classify Autistic patients. In this study 15 ASD individuals and 10 non ASD were selected. ASD group comprised of 13 males and 2 females between 7 and 14 years of age. Control group comprised of 4 males and 6 females between 7 and 12 years of age. Resting State EEG of both closed and open eyes were recorded using 19 electrodes. Patients sat in a quiet room without speaking or performing any mentally demanding activity while the EEG was being recorded. The proposed IFAST algorithm consists of exactly three different phases or parts. In the first stage also called Squashing phase, the raw EEG signals are converted into feature vectors. Authors present a workflow of the system from raw data to classification to make comparison between different algorithms such as Multi Scale Entropy (MSE) and the Multi Scale Ranked Organizing Maps (MS-ROM). MSROM is a novel algorithm based on Single Organizing Map Neural Network. In this study, the dataset is randomly divided into 17 training consisting of 11 ASD, 6 controls and eight test records consisting of 4 ASD, 4 control. The noise elimination is performed only on the training set. Also, it completely depends on the algorithm selected for extraction of feature vectors. For MS-ROM features they utilize an algorithm called TWIST. In the final classification stage, they use multiple machine learning algorithms along with multiple validation protocols. The validation protocols are training-testing and leave one out cross validation. For classification purposes they make use of Sine Net Neural Network, Logistic Regression, Sequential Minimal Optimization, kNN, K-Contractive Map, Naive Bayes, and Random forest. With MSE feature extraction the best results were given by Logistic and Naive Bayes with exactly 2 errors. Whereas, MS-ROM with training test protocol had 0 errors (100% accuracy) with all the classification models.

Bosl et al. (2011), conduct a study using mMSE as feature vectors along with multiclass Support Vector Machine to differentiate developing and high-risk infant groups. In this study they use 79 different infants of which 49 were considered high risk and 33 typically developing infants. The 49 infants were high risk based on one of their older siblings having a confirmed ASD diagnosis. The other 39 infants were not high risk since no one in their family ever was diagnosed with ASD. Data was collected from each infant during multiple sessions with some interval. Data extracted from an infant in five different sessions in various months between 6 to 24-month period were considered unique. Resting state EEG with 64 electrodes was extracted by placing the infant in a dimly lit room in their mother's lap where the research assistant blew bubbles to catch their attention. The raw signals were preprocessed using Modified Multiscale Entropy. Low, high, and mean for each curve from mMSE were calculated to create a feature set of 192 values. The best fit for the classification for High risk and normal infants was at age 9 months with over 90% accuracy.

Abdulhay et al. (2017), use EEG intrinsic function pulsation to identify patterns in Autism. They mathematically compute EEG features and compare ASD with typically developing. In this study they selected 10 children with ASD and 10 non-autistic children within the age group of 4 to 13. They collected resting state EEG using 64 electrodes with a 500 HZ sampling frequency. Initially the signals were band pass filtered and all the artifacts including eye movements were removed by using Independent Component Analysis. Empirical Mode decomposition was applied to extract Intrinsic Mode Function from each of the channels of the participants. Then point by point pulsations of analytic intrinsic modes are computed which is then plotted to make comparison with the counterpart intrinsic mode in another channel. Any existing stability loops are analyzed for abnormal neural connectivity. In addition, they perform 3D mapping to visualize and spot unusual brain activities. In the first IMF of channel 3 versus the first IMF in channel 2 for typically developing and autistic child, it was found that the stability of local pulsation pathways maintained a consistency while it was random in typically developing. Similar patterns were seen in channels 1 and 2 and 36 and 37 of non-autistic and autistic children. Overall this computational method was able to differentiate the abnormal EEG activities between ASD and typically developing children.

Alie et al. (2011) use Markov Models with eye tracking to classify Autism Spectrum Disorder. Unlike most other studies that collected data from children who were 3 years or older, in this study they collect data from 6-month-old infants. There were in total 32 subjects out of which 6 were later at 3 years of age diagnosed with ASD and the rest were not. During the data collection the subjects were placed in front of their mothers and four different cameras from different angles recorded the video for about 3 minutes. The eye tracking was simply based on either the subject looked at the mother's face or not. Through this they get a binary sequence of subjects' eye pattern which is then converted into alphabet sequence of a specific length. Then the sequence was filtered using a low pass filter and down sampled by factor of 18. This is done to enhance Markov Models to produce effective results.

Using this data, they compare Hidden Markov Models and Variable-order Markov Models for the classification of ASD. Hidden Markov Models was able to correctly identify 92.03% of the typically developing subject while identifying only 33.33% of Autistic subject. Whereas the VMM correctly identified 100% of the Autistic and 92.03% of typically developing subjects. It was clear from this result that Variable-order Markov models are superior in finding Autistic eye pattern while both Markov Models are the same in finding typically developing. The authors point out this difference because of various spectrums of Autism with different eye patterns. Nevertheless, the VMM algorithm used in this study looks effective in identifying Autism in an early age. Similarly, Liu et al. (2015) propose a machine learning framework for the diagnosis of Autism using eye movement. They utilize two different datasets from previous studies. One of the datasets had 20 ASD children, 21 typically developing, and 20 typical developing IQ-matched children. The other dataset comprised of 19 ASD, 22 Intellectually disabled, and 28 typical young adults and adolescents. They compute Bag of Words for Eye Coordinates and Eye movement, N-Grams and AOI from the datasets. And they train five different Support Vector machine model with RBF kernel. Each of the model used different form of features like BOW of eye coordinates, BOW of eye movement, combination, N-Grams, and AOI. The result was good for both groups with Combination or fusion data. However, the children dataset with fusion was the best with around 87% accuracy.

Jiang and Zhao (2017) use eye movement with deep neural networks to identify individuals with Autism Spectrum Disorder. They used dataset from a previous study with 20 ASD and 19 health controls. Here the subjects observed around 700 images from the OSIE database. OSIE database is a popular eye tracking dataset used for image saliency benchmarking. First, they use Cluster Fix algorithm on the raw data to compute fixations and saccades. Next, they work on finding the discriminative images as the OSIE dataset is not specifically built for autism studies. So, both groups might have the same visual pattern for some of the images. For this purpose, they use Fisher score method by which they score each of the images and select only the one with the higher scores to be processed further. After this process of image selection, they compute fixation maps to differentiate fixations between two groups. Fixation maps are simply a probability distribution of all the eye fixations. In addition, they use a Gaussian Kernel for smoothing and normalize by their sum. Normalization is usually done when we are comparing two different fixation maps as is the case here. Then they compute difference of fixation map between the Autistic and non-Autistic group. This is the original target which they used to train a SALICON network to predict these values. SALICON network is one of the state-of-the-art image saliency prediction algorithms. Image saliency prediction is about predicting the visual pattern of users given an image. SALICON network uses two VGG with 16 layers. One of the VGG uses the original image to detect the small salient regions whereas the other VGG uses the down sampled image to detect the center of large salient regions. At the end both the outputs are combined to get a better result. This only predicts the image saliency. So, to predict the difference of fixation map they add another convolution layer with Cross Entropy Loss function using the original Difference of fixation map. Next, they send the predicted difference of fixation maps to the final prediction layer. In this part they first apply tanh function to the features then concatenate the feature vectors of all fixation to consider dynamic change of attention. After which they reduce the dimension by using local average pooling. At last they train an SVM to make the final classification between ASD and control. They make use of the popular leave-one-out cross validation to measure the performance of their model. The accuracy of this model showed real promise in eye tracking for ASD with about 92% accuracy.

METHODOLOGY

Current techniques in practice for identifying ASD are mostly subjective and prone to error and usually takes a lot of time for final diagnosis. Most of the children with ASD are diagnosed after 3 years of age. Early diagnosis is the key for reversing or treating ASD through early intervention. As time is of an essence we need a method of diagnosis that is fast, and efficient unlike the current practice that could take months to years. Medical Imaging and blood testing (Sparks et al. 2002; Spence et al. 2004) are promising and a lot of work is being done with these modalities to diagnose ASD. However, EEG and Eye movement are cost effective and hence can be accessible in consumer level. The aim of this research is to study the identification of Autism Spectrum Disorder using EEG during ADOS-2. Comparison of the classification performance between EEG features can potentially result in finding the better feature set. We hypothesize as the top performing signal most likely has more of the unique data points and pattern of ASD and similarly, the least performing signals have less of the data points and patterns relating to

Figure 1. EEG Processing Pipeline for Study 1. EEG Data preprocessed using Makoto Pipeline follows this pipeline to train SVM, Logistic, DNN and Gaussian Naïve Bayes Models

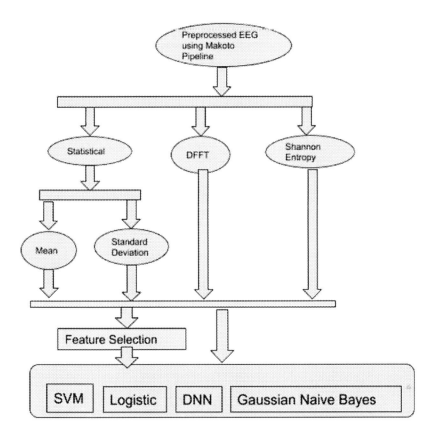

ASD. The secondary goal is to compare various machine learning algorithms for the classification purposes. Conditions like ADHD, and other learning disabilities can also share similar comparative patterns for different features.

Machine Learning With EEG Measures During Joint Attention

We have recently employed preliminary feature analysis on acquired raw EEG data from the work of Jaime et al. (2016), wherein the EEG was recorded from adolescents with ASD (N=24) and typically developing adolescents (N=28) while they watched a series of 30-second joint attention eliciting video clips.

Figure 2. EEG Feature Processing Pipeline for Deep Neural Network. Each layer of the deep neural network is shown in the figure, with its functionality

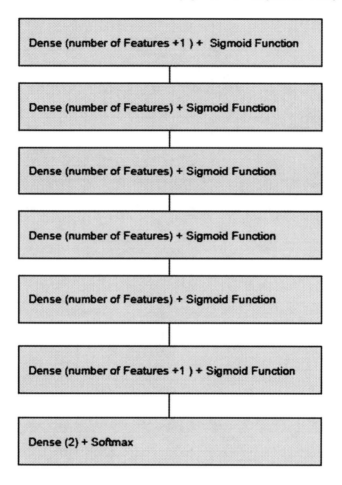

First, we applied the pre-processing pipeline (described in §3.3.1) on the raw EEG time series to remove noisy channels and data segments containing movement and ocular artifacts from the EEG data. The pre-processed data was then classified using *EEG Analytics Pipeline* (implemented in Python) (Thapaliya et al. 2018).

Joint attention is the ability to socially coordinate visual attention, share a point of view with another person, and process self and other-related information. Hence the data retrieval was performed while making the subjects watch video clips that would help in examining joint attention. There was a total of 12 videos each of which was 30 seconds. About one second gap was provided between each video. Both the EEG and Eye movement were collected while the participants watched the video. A total of 34 participants EEG data was used in this paper after the preprocessing step.

There are many ways to extract feature from EEG data. Entropies, wavelets, FFT and various other statistical methods are commonly computed features (Al-Fahoum and Al-Fraihat 2014). In this work we use Statistical and Entropy values. Statistical features comprise of Mean, Standard Deviation, and combined mean and standard deviation of the filtered data. For the feature analysis, we used statistical and entropy values including mean, standard deviation, and combined mean and standard deviation on the pre-processed data. Entropy is computed by using Shannon entropy function (Lin 1991), which is the average rate at which information is produced by a stochastic source of data given by, $H_e = -\sum p_i \log_2 p_i$. Mean function takes in a 2D matrix consisting of the EEG signal of a person and returns a feature vector with mean values for each channel over windows of signal. For the mean, each of the 128 channels were computed. For each subject a feature vector consisting of mean of single channel was created. So, the mean function takes in a 2D matrix consisting of the EEG signal of a person and returns a feature vector with mean values for each channel. For the standard deviation, each of the 128 channels were computed. For each subject a feature vector consisting of mean of single channel was created. So, the deviation function takes in a 2D matrix consisting of the EEG signal of a person and returns a feature vector with standard deviation values for each channel. This is shown in the Figure 1.

For classification SVM, Logistic, Deep Neural Network (DNN), and Gaussian Naive Bayes is used. For the deep neural network (see Figure 2) with five hidden layers with sigmoid activation function is used. For optimization categorical cross entropy for loss and Adamax optimizer (Freivalds and Liepins 2017) is used. We captured three different feature set; entropy features, FFT

Table 1. Classification Accuracy of EEG during Joint Attention Study. The Entropy, FFT, Mean and Standard Deviation values are given for each classifier used for this study

Classifier	Entropy	FFT	Mean	Std.
Gaussian Naive Bayes	0.26	0.53	0.55	0.55
Logistic Regression	0.11	0.78	0.58	0.50
SVM	0.11	0.56	0.55	0.55
DNN	0.20	0.52	0.58	0.45

and statistical features. We also calculate mean, and standard deviation. In total there are 4 different features from EEG and 4 different models for each type of classifier and, overall there are 16 different model variations based on the features (4 feature set x 4 classifiers). For each feature there are three models for each algorithm, two models using Feature Selection and the third one without using any feature selection. For Feature selection PCA and sequential feature selection is used.

Classification of EEG During Joint Attention: Results

The Table 1 presents an analysis and comparison of EEG data. Note that two models were created for each model with only EEG and combined data by using PCA and without using PCA. Like SVM with PCA and without PCA. For some models with PCA did better while for some without PCA did better. For example, DNN almost always without using PCA did worse because of the curse of dimensionality. The highest performing SVM with about 56% accuracy was using FFT with all the features without PCA. The highest performing Logistic regression with 78% accuracy was using FFT without PCA. SVM, Logistic Regression, and Gaussian Naive Bayes do better without PCA which means that with PCA it loses data points that these models find useful. This is interesting because PCA is supposed to find the most discriminant features and remove redundant or noisy features. And this is supposed to help machine learning models produce better results. For SVM most models with PCA did better except the highest performing model. This might mean that the Entropy data is more linear than the other datasets. For DNN the curse of dimensionality is obvious. Whereas for Gaussian Naive Bayes all the high performing models did not use PCA except the one with EEG mean. This is an exception and must be due to the nature of the EEG mean data. But in general case Naive Bayes does better without PCA. This might be since probabilistic models are able to make sense of higher dimensional dataset much easier than other models like DNN. Then with using Sequential Feature Selection algorithm almost all the models performed better than either PCA or no Feature Selection.

In this study we have used PCA, and Sequential Feature Selection algorithms. There are other Feature Selection algorithms like Genetic algorithm, Particle Swarm Optimization, and TWIST which can be compared to find features to optimize the performance of the models. Also, this will tell us which feature selection algorithm will work better for the combined data sets. Gaussian Naive Bayes with some of the features had perfect score. But we need to reproduce this result with large number of participants to be able to use this in a clinical setting. Current number of 34 participants is too low to confirm our results. However, this is a first step towards developing an optimal Autism Diagnosis system.

EEG Coherence During Live Social Interaction

The notion that social brain system FC may be a useful index of social impairment is suggested by both the literature (Mundy 2016; Jaime et al. 2016) and by our preliminary findings obtained from our pilot sample composed of individuals between the ages of 5 and 17 years who completed an ADOS-2 assessment while we simultaneously recorded their EEG. Despite a small sample size (ASD = 8; TD = 9), our preliminary results indicate a trending negative association between right hemisphere delta and theta band EEG coherence and level of social symptom severity (according to the ADOS-2 algorithm scoring) in children with ASD (see Table 2 below), but not in our pilot sample of typically developing (TD) children. Our preliminary results paint a conceptual picture that is in line with our prior work evaluating EEG coherence during joint social attention perception in ASD (Jaime et al. 2016), that there are diagnostic group differences in the association between right hemisphere frontal–temporal–parietal FC and standardized measures of social functioning. Such diagnostic group differences in FC association patterns reflect a tendency for children with impaired social capacity to have idiosyncratic patterns of social brain system functional organization relative to typical neurodevelopment. Thus, EEG measures of social brain system FC acquired during live social interaction shows promise as a candidate non-invasive biomarker of early emerging aberrant social neurocognitive dysfunction in ASD.

EEG Acquisition and Pre-Processing

Our preliminary FC measures were analyzed from each pilot subject's EEG recording, acquired throughout the entire duration of the ADOS-2. We used a 32-channel LiveAmp wireless EEG system with active electrodes and a digital sampling rate of 250 Hz (Brain Products GmbH) for EEG time series acquisition. Use of a wireless EEG system allowed for head movements

Figure 3. EEG Feature Processing and Classification. The raw signals acquired from an EEG are stored and is subjected to preprocessing to obtain clean time-series data. Once this completes, the clean data is passed through band pass filters and feature extraction is performed. Then the extracted features are fed into a classifier, which uses cross validation to evaluate its performance depending on how it predicts ASD and TD class labels.

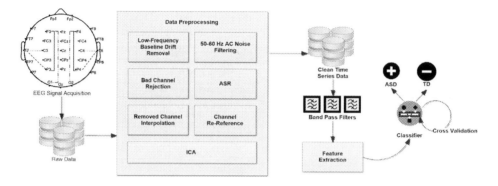

and the active electrodes increased speed of application thereby increasing probability of successful EEG data acquisition with special populations.

All 32 channels were continuously recorded using the FCz electrode as reference. To maximize the consistency of the recording quality across conditions, a single epoch was recorded per experimental condition. In between epoch recordings an impedance check will be performed. This was resulted in 6 different epochs per subject. Prior to the recording of each experimental epoch, a 90 second epoch of eyes closed while resting will be recorded. This served as a necessary baseline metric for the EEG analysis. After acquisition, the raw EEG data output was imported into the open-source MATLAB toolbox: EEGLAB (Delorme and Makeig 2004). Next, following preprocessing pipeline is applied:

1. Remove low frequency baseline drift with a 1 Hz high-pass filter.
2. Remove 50-60 Hz AC line noise by applying the CleanLine plugin.
3. Clean continuous raw data using the clean_rawdata plugin (Mullen et al. 2015). The clean_rawdata plugin first performs bad channel rejection based on two criteria: (1) channels that have flat signals longer than 5 seconds and (2) channels poorly correlated with adjacent channels. It

then applies artifact subspace reconstruction (ASR) — an algorithm that removes nonstationary, high variance signals from the EEG then uses calibration data (1 min sections of clean EEG) to reconstruct the missing data using a spatial mixing matrix.

4. Interpolate removed channels.
5. Re-reference channels to average reference.
6. Separate non-brain artifacts from the EEG recording via EEGLAB's Independent Component Analysis (ICA)[1]. Briefly, ICA involves the linear decomposition of the aggregate channel activity into a series of independent components that are spatially filtered from the recorded EEG time series. Components representing eye, cardiac, and muscle artifact are removed and components representing genuine brain activity are retained.

Table 2. ADOS-2 Score of the ASD vs TD subjects. Here, 8 subjects were diagnosed with ASD (above horizontal line) and the others were typically developing (TD)

Participant	Sex	Age	ADOS-2	ASD Diagnosis
2	M	10	19	ASD
4	M	17	12	ASD
11	M	6	11	ASD
12	M	16	16	ASD
13	F	11	16	ASD
15	F	10	7	ASD
18	M	5	20	ASD
20	M	15	9	ASD
5	M	11	5	TD
7	F	9	0	TD
8	F	6	5	TD
14	F	16	0	TD
16	M	8	4	TD
17	F	6	0	TD
19	M	15	2	TD
21	M	6	4	TD
22	F	8	0	TD

EEG Measures of Functional Connectivity

We first extracted 180-second epochs beginning from the middle one-third portion of each subject's pre-processed EEG time series to calculate a functional connectivity (FC) measure of the engaged social brain system. With each subject's epoched EEG time series treated as a discrete-time signal $u = x_i(t)$ for EEG channel i, we used EEG coherence as a variable of FC. EEG coherence, or normalized magnitude-squared coherence (MSC), $C^2_{uv}(\omega)$, is a statistical estimate of the amount of phase synchrony between two EEG time series, u and v: $C^2_{uv}(\omega) = \left|\phi_{uv}(\omega)\right|^2 / \left(\phi_{uu}(\omega)\phi_{vv}(\omega)\right)$ where the squared magnitude of the cross spectrum density $\left|\varphi_{uv}(\omega)\right|^2$ (a measure of co-variance) between the two signals u and v at a given frequency ω, is normalized by the Power Spectral Densities (PSDs) (variance) of each channel φ_{uu} and φ_{vv} so that $0 \leq C^2_{uv}(\omega) \leq 1$. Higher values represent greater synchronous activity between distinct channels whereas lower values represent reduced or non-synchronous activity (Nunez and Srinivasan 2006). Coherence is a function of frequency; to compute a single similarity metric between a pair of signals, we integrate over frequency to obtain total power (or variance in a statistical sense) $P_{ij} = \dfrac{1}{T}\int_0^T C^2_{uv}(\omega)$ where T is the extent of frequency components sampled. The MSC of a signal which itself produces no variance (in the statistical sense) and hence $P_{ii} = 1$, gives a convenient, normalized metric of similarity.

Accordingly, intra-hemispheric MSC between electrode positions that are spatially collocated over areas comprising the social brain system (Saxe 2006; Adolphs 2009) were examined. Electrode pairs were selected based on Homan et al.'s [1987] electrode placement correlates of cortical location. Using the international 10/20 placement system (Klem et al. 1999), the following electrodes were selected: F7, F8, T7, T8, TP9, TP10, P7, P8, C3, and C4.

Classification of EEG During ADOS-2: Results

We generated five feature sets categorized according to the frequency bands: 1) delta, 2) theta, 3) alpha, 4) beta and 5) gamma with each set representing the amplitude and power of the signal from each electrode. These feature sets were entered to 43 different classifiers yielding precision rates, recall rates, F1 scores, and percent accuracy. We identified six the top performing classifiers: Random Forest, Logistic, Bagging, JRIP, LMT and AdaBoostM1.

The six top performing classifiers for the 5-band feature set are listed in Table 3. The JRIP classifier yielded the highest percent accuracy with 98.06% indicating that a 5-band feature set collected during an ADOS-2 test classifies a diagnosis of ASD with greater than 90% accuracy. From these six classifiers, the AdaBoostM1 classifier yielded the lowest percent accuracy at 92.14%.

The evaluation results in Table 3 were calculated based on features from all electrodes. We also conducted an evaluation by selecting only F7, F8, T7, T8, TP9, TP10, P7, P8, C3 and C4 electrodes based on Homan et al.'s [1987] electrode placement correlates of cortical location. The results of this evaluation are listed in Table 4. When comparing the results, it was observed that the Random Forest classifier yielded the highest percent accuracy with 97.04%. The AdaBoostM1 classifier yielded the lowest percent accuracy at 79.75%.

Table 3. Precision, Recall, F1 and Accuracy of six classifiers used for classification of EEG during ADOS-2

Classifier	Precision	Recall	F1	Accuracy
Random Forest	0.98	0.98	0.98	**98.00%**
Logistic	0.96	0.96	0.96	96.63%
Bagging	0.95	0.95	0.95	95.66%
JRIP	0.98	0.98	0.98	**98.06%**
LMT	0.95	0.95	0.95	95.79%
AdaBoostM1	0.92	0.92	0.92	92.14%

Table 4. Precision, Recall, F1 and Accuracy of six classifiers used for classification of EEG during ADOS-2 using only a selected set of features

Classifier	Precision	Recall	F1	Accuracy
Random Forest	0.97	0.97	0.97	**97.04%**
Logistic	0.84	0.84	0.84	84.72%
Bagging	0.95	0.95	0.95	**95.50%**
JRIP	0.94	0.94	0.94	94.57%
LMT	0.83	0.82	0.82	82.94%
AdaBoostM1	0.80	0.79	0.79	79.75%

DISCUSSION AND FUTURE OUTLOOK

Due to its low cost and feasibility, electroencephalography (EEG) shows potential as an effective neurophysiological instrument in the classification of ASD (Lenartowicz and Loo 2014; Snyder et al. 2015; Gloss et al. 2016), and there is emerging evidence that——combined with machine learning approaches——quantitative measures of EEG can predict ASD with high levels of sensitivity and specificity (Bosl et al. 2018; Grossi et al. 2017; Djemal et al. 2017). An advantage of EEG is its ability to be applied to ecologically valid contexts (i.e., person-to-person social interaction) via wireless solutions thus allowing for the simultaneous acquisition of data from multiple participants in real-world settings.

To establish proof of concept—that our classifiers show utility to predict features in line with diagnostic criteria of ASD—we collect biobehavioral metrics within the context of standardized tasks used in a gold standard assessment of ASD symptomatology: The Autism Diagnostic Observation Schedule Second Edition (ADOS-2) (Gotham et al. 2007). The ADOS-2 has been carefully developed to create snapshots of naturalistic social scenarios that can reveal observable features central to ASD (i.e., joint attention, social overtures), thereby allowing us to measure brain activity that are temporally concurrent with these observable ASD features within relatively brief periods. It is also important to note that we did not use these ADOS-2 tasks as a clinical tool to diagnose participants; rather, we capitalized on the semi-structured and standardized nature of these social tasks in the ADOS-2 to create a context that engages the social brain system and elicits joint visual attention behavior for acquisition of biobehavioral metrics. Thus, participants recruited for this study have already received a diagnosis of ASD by a clinical professional prior to enrolling in this study.

Due to its high temporal resolution and feasibility, electroencephalography (EEG) shows potential as an effective neurophysiological instrument in the classification of ASD (Lenartowicz and Loo 2014; Snyder et al. 2015; Gloss et al. 2016). An advantage of EEG is its ability to be applied to ecologically valid contexts via wireless solutions that allow for the simultaneous acquisition of data from multiple participants. This makes EEG an appropriate choice for examining relevant neurophysiological features of ASD in real-world settings (Lee and Tan 2006). Despite these advantages, most EEG research occurs in highly controlled experimental environments, requiring data collected over many trials with minimal head movement. We will address this deficiency by combining EEG and eye tracker usage in the future studies.

Early diagnosis is crucial for successful treatment of ASD. Although progress has been made to accurately diagnose ASD, it is far from ideal (Dawson 2008). It often requires various subjective measures, behavioral assessments, observations from caretakers over a period to correctly diagnose ASD. Even with this tedious testing often individuals are misdiagnosed. However, there remains promise in the development of accurate detection using subjective modalities of EEG, and Eye movements. In the future we will obtain two sets of biobehavioral measures representing joint attention: functional integration of neurocognitive networks associated with the social brain (i.e., EEG metrics) and visual behavior (i.e. eye tracking metrics). Regarding visual behavior, we will collect, analyze, and produce a battery of traditional positional eye movement metrics thought to be potential indicators of joint attention, including number of fixations (Jacob and Karn 2003), fixation durations (Fitts et al. 1950; Just and Carpenter 1976), and number of regressions (Azuma et al. 2014), during naturalistic, dynamic communication tasks.

REFERENCES

Abdulhay, E., Alafeef, M., Hadoush, H., & Alomari, N. (2017). Frequency 3d mapping and inter-channel stability of EEG intrinsic function pulsation: Indicators towards autism spectrum diagnosis. In *Electrical and Electronics Engineering Conference (JIEEEC), 2017 10th Jordanian International.* IEEE. 10.1109/JIEEEC.2017.8051416

Adolphs, R. (2009). The social brain: Neural basis of social knowledge. *Annual Review of Psychology, 60*(1), 693–716. doi:10.1146/annurev. psych.60.110707.163514 PMID:18771388

Al-Fahoum, A. S., & Al-Fraihat, A. A. (2014). Methods of EEG signal features extraction using linear analysis in frequency and time-frequency domains. *ISRN Neuroscience, 2014,* 1–7. doi:10.1155/2014/730218

Alie, D., Mahoor, M. H., Mattson, W. I., Anderson, D. R., & Messinger, D. S. (2011). Analysis of eye gaze pattern of infants at risk of autism spectrum disorder using Markov models. In *Applications of Computer Vision (WACV), 2011 IEEE Workshop on.* IEEE. 10.1109/WACV.2011.5711515

Azuma, M., Minamoto, T., Yaoi, K., Osaka, M., & Osaka, N. (2014). Effect of memory load in eye movement control: A study using the reading span test. *Journal of Eye Movement Research, 7*(5), 1–9.

Bal, E., Harden, E., Lamb, D., Van Hecke, A. V., Denver, J. W., And Porges, S. W. 2010. Emotion Recognition in Children with Autism Spectrum Disorders: Relations to Eye Gaze and Autonomic State. *Journal of Autism and Developmental Disorders, 40*(3), 358–370.

Baron-Cohen, S., Leslie, A. M., & And Frith, U. (1985). Does the autistic child have a "theory of mind"? *Cognition, 21*(1), 37–46. doi:10.1016/0010-0277(85)90022-8 PMID:2934210

Barresi, J., & And Moore, C. (1996). Intentional relations and social understanding. *Behavioral and Brain Sciences, 19*(1), 107–122. doi:10.1017/S0140525X00041790

Bedford, R., Elsabbagh, M., Gliga, T., Pickles, A., Senju, A., Charman, T., & Johnson, M. H. (2012). Precursors to Social and Communication Difficulties in Infants At-Risk for Autism: Gaze Following and Attentional Engagement. *Journal of Autism and Developmental Disorders, 42*(10), 2208–2218.

Billeci, L., Narzisi, A., Campatelli, G., Crifaci, G., Calderoni, S., Gagliano, A., ... Muratori, F. (2016). Disentangling the initiation from the response in joint attention: An eye-tracking study in toddlers with autism spectrum disorders. *Translational Psychiatry, 6*(5), e808. doi:10.1038/tp.2016.75 PMID:27187230

Black, M. H., Chen, N. T. M., Iyer, K. K., Lipp, O. V., Bölte, S., Falkmer, M., ... Girdler, S. (2017). Mechanisms of facial emotion recognition in autism spectrum disorders: Insights from eye tracking and electroencephalography. *Neuroscience and Biobehavioral Reviews, 80*, 488–515. doi:10.1016/j.neubiorev.2017.06.016 PMID:28698082

Bosl, W., Tierney, A., Tager-Flusberg, H., & Nelson, C. (2011). EEG complexity as a biomarker for autism spectrum disorder risk. *BMC Medicine, 9*, 1, 18.

Bosl, W. J., Tager-Flusberg, H., & Nelson, C. A. (2018). EEG analytics for early detection of autism spectrum disorder: a data-driven approach. *Scientific Reports, 8*(1), 6828.

Buescher, A. V., Cidav, Z., Knapp, M., & Mandell, D. S. (2014). Costs of autism spectrum disorders in the United Kingdom and the united states. *JAMA Pediatrics*, *168*(8), 721–728. doi:10.1001/jamapediatrics.2014.210 PMID:24911948

Butterworth, G., & Jarrett, N. (1991). What minds have in common is space: Spatial mechanisms serving joint visual attention in infancy. *British Journal of Developmental Psychology*, *9*(1), 55–72. doi:10.1111/j.2044-835X.1991. tb00862.x

Caruana, N., Brock, J., & Woolgar, A. (2015). A front temporoparietal network common to initiating and responding to joint attention bids. *NeuroImage*, *108*, 34–46. doi:10.1016/j.neuroimage.2014.12.041 PMID:25534111

Castelli, F., Frith, C., Happé, F., & Frith, U. (2002). Autism, Asperger syndrome and brain mechanisms for the attribution of mental states to animated shapes. *Brain*, *125*(8), 1839–1849. doi:10.1093/brain/awf189 PMID:12135974

Chita-Tegmark, M. (2016). Social attention in ASD: A review and meta-analysis of eye-tracking studies. *Research in Developmental Disabilities*, *48*, 79–93. doi:10.1016/j.ridd.2015.10.011 PMID:26547134

Coben, R., Clarke, A. R., Hudspeth, W., & Barry, R. J. (2008). EEG power and coherence in autistic spectrum disorder. *Clinical Neurophysiology*, *119*(5), 1002–1009. doi:10.1016/j.clinph.2008.01.013 PMID:18331812

Damarla, S. R., Keller, T. A., Kana, R. K., Cherkassky, V. L., Williams, D. L., Minshew, N. J., & Just, M. A. (2010). Cortical underconnectivity coupled with preserved visuospatial cognition in autism: Evidence from an FMRI study of an embedded figures task. *Autism Research*, *3*(5), 273–279. doi:10.1002/aur.153 PMID:20740492

Dawson, G. (2008). Early behavioral intervention, brain plasticity, and the prevention of autism spectrum disorder. *Development and Psychopathology*, *20*(3), 775–803. doi:10.1017/S0954579408000370 PMID:18606031

Del Valle Rubido, M., Mccracken, J. T., Hollander, E., Shic, F., Noeldeke, J., Boak, L., ... Umbricht, D. (2018). In Search of Biomarkers for Autism Spectrum Disorder. *Autism Research*, *11*(11), 1567–1579. doi:10.1002/aur.2026 PMID:30324656

Delorme, A., & Makeig, S. (2004). EEGLab: An open source toolbox for analysis of single-trial EEG dynamics including independent component analysis. *Journal of Neuroscience Methods, 134*(1), 1, 9–21. doi:10.1016/j.jneumeth.2003.10.009 PMID:15102499

Djemal, R., Alsharabi, K., Ibrahim, S., & Alsuwailem, A. (2017). EEG-based computer aided diagnosis of autism spectrum disorder using wavelet, entropy, and ann. *BioMed Research International*. PMID:28484720

Duchowski, A. T., Krejtz, K., Krejtz, I., Biele, C., Niedzielska, A., Kiefer, P., ... Giannopoulos, I. (2018). The Index of Pupillary Activity: Measuring Cognitive Load Vis-à-vis Task Difficulty with Pupil Oscillation. In *Proceedings of the 2018 CHI Conference on Human Factors in Computing Systems*. ACM. 10.1145/3173574.3173856

Falck-Ytter, T., Fernell, E., Hedvall, L., Von Hofsten, C., & Gillberg, C. (2012). Gaze Performance in Children with Autism Spectrum Disorder when Observing Communicative Actions. *Journal of Autism and Developmental Disorders, 42*(10), 2236–2245.

Falck-Ytter, T., Thorup, E., & Bölte, S. (2015). Brief Report: Lack of Processing Bias for the Objects Other People Attend to in 3-Year-Olds with Autism. *Journal of Autism and Developmental Disorders, 45*(6), 1897–1904.

Fitts, P. M., Jones, R. E., & Milton, J. L. (1950). Eye Movements of Aircraft Pilots During Instrument-Landing Approaches. *Aeronautical Engineering Review, 9*(2), 24–29.

Fletcher-Watson, S., Leekam, S. R., Benson, V., Frank, M., & Findlay, J. (2009). Eye-movements reveal attention to social information in autism spectrum disorder. *Neuropsychologia, 47*(1), 248–257. doi:10.1016/j.neuropsychologia.2008.07.016 PMID:18706434

Frazier, T. W., Klingemier, E. W., Parikh, S., Speer, L., Strauss, M. S., Eng, C., ... Youngstrom, E. A. (2018). Development and Validation of Objective and Quantitative Eye Tracking-Based Measures of Autism Risk and Symptom Levels. *Journal of the American Academy of Child and Adolescent Psychiatry, 57*(11), 858–866. doi:10.1016/j.jaac.2018.06.023 PMID:30392627

Freivalds, K., & Liepins, R. (2017). *Improving the neural GPU architecture for algorithm learning*. arXiv preprint arXiv:1702.08727

Gloss, D., Varma, J. K., Pringsheim, T., & Nuwer, M. R. (2016). Practice advisory: The utility of EEG theta/beta power ratio in ADHD diagnosis report of the guideline development, dissemination, and implementation subcommittee of the American academy of neurology. *Neurology*, 10–1212. PMID:27760867

Gordon, I., Eilbott, J. A., Feldman, R., Pelphrey, K. A., & Vander Wyk, B. C. (2013). Social, reward, and attention brain networks are involved when online bids for joint attention are met with congruent versus incongruent responses. *Social Neuroscience*, 8(6), 544–554. doi:10.1080/17470919.201 3.832374 PMID:24044427

Gotham, K., Risi, S., Pickles, A., & Lord, C. (2007). The autism diagnostic observation schedule: revised algorithms for improved diagnostic validity. *Journal of Autism and Developmental Disorders, 37*(4), 613.

Grossi, E., Olivieri, C., & Buscema, M. (2017). Diagnosis of autism through EEG processed by advanced computational algorithms: A pilot study. *Computer Methods and Programs in Biomedicine, 142*, 73–79. doi:10.1016/j. cmpb.2017.02.002 PMID:28325448

Guillon, Q., Hadjikhani, N., Baduel, S., & Rogé, B. (2014). Visual social attention in autism spectrum disorder: Insights from eye tracking studies. *Neuroscience and Biobehavioral Reviews, 42*, 279–297. doi:10.1016/j. neubiorev.2014.03.013 PMID:24694721

Hill, E. L., & Frith, U. (2003). Understanding autism: insights from mind and brain. *Philosophical Transactions of the Royal Society B: Biological Sciences, 358*(1430), 281.

Homan, R. W., Herman, J., & Purdy, P. (1987). Cerebral location of international 10–20 system electrode placement. *Electroencephalography and Clinical Neurophysiology*, 66(4), 376–382. doi:10.1016/0013-4694(87)90206-9 PMID:2435517

Hotier, S., Leroy, F., Boisgontier, J., Laidi, C., Mangin, J.-F., Delorme, R., ... Houenou, J. (2017). Social cognition in autism is associated with the neurodevelopment of the posterior superior temporal sulcus. *Acta Psychiatrica Scandinavica, 136*(5), 517–525. doi:10.1111/acps.12814 PMID:28940401

Ibañez, L. V., Grantz, C. J., & Messinger, D. S. (2013). The development of referential communication and autism symptomatology in high-risk infants. *Infancy*, *18*(5), 687–707. doi:10.1111/j.1532-7078.2012.00142.x PMID:24403864

Jacob, R. J. K., & Karn, K. S. (2003). Eye Tracking in Human-Computer Interaction and Usability Research: Ready to Deliver the Promises. In The Mind's Eye: Cognitive and Applied Aspects of Eye Movement Research. Elsevier Science.

Jaime, M., Mcmahon, C. M., Davidson, B. C., Newell, L. C., Mundy, P. C., & And Henderson, H. A. (2016). Brief report: Reduced temporal-central EEG alpha coherence during joint attention perception in adolescents with autism spectrum disorder. *Journal of Autism and Developmental Disorders*, *46*(4), 1477–1489. doi:10.100710803-015-2667-3 PMID:26659813

Jiang, M., & Zhao, Q. (2017). Learning visual attention to identify people with autism spectrum disorder. *Proceedings of the IEEE International Conference on Computer Vision*, 3267–3276. 10.1109/ICCV.2017.354

Jones, T. B., Bandettini, P. A., Kenworthy, L., Case, L. K., Milleville, S. C., Martin, A., & And Birn, R. M. (2010). Sources of group differences in functional connectivity: An investigation applied to autism spectrum disorder. *NeuroImage*, *49*(1), 401–414. doi:10.1016/j.neuroimage.2009.07.051 PMID:19646533

Just, M. A., & Carpenter, P. A. (1976). Eye Fixations and Cognitive Processes. *Cognitive Psychology, 8*(4), 441–480.

Just, M. A., Cherkassky, V. L., Keller, T. A., Kana, R. K., & Minshew, N. J. (2006). Functional and anatomical cortical underconnectivity in autism: Evidence from an FMRI study of an executive function task and corpus callosum morphometry. *Cerebral Cortex*, *17*(4), 951–961. doi:10.1093/cercor/bhl006 PMID:16772313

Just, M. A., Cherkassky, V. L., Keller, T. A., & Minshew, N. J. (2004). Cortical activation and synchronization during sentence comprehension in high-functioning autism: Evidence of underconnectivity. *Brain*, *127*(8), 1811–1821. doi:10.1093/brain/awh199 PMID:15215213

Kana, R. K., Keller, T. A., Cherkassky, V. L., Minshew, N. J., & Just, M. A. (2009). Atypical frontal-posterior synchronization of theory of mind regions in autism during mental state attribution. *Social Neuroscience*, *4*(2), 135–152. doi:10.1080/17470910802198510 PMID:18633829

Kana, R. K., Uddin, L. Q., Kenet, T., Chugani, D., & Müller, R.-A. (2014). Brain connectivity in autism. *Frontiers in Human Neuroscience*, *8*, 349. doi:10.3389/fnhum.2014.00349 PMID:24917800

Keehn, B., Müller, R.-A., & Townsend, J. (2013). Atypical attentional networks and the emergence of autism. *Neuroscience and Biobehavioral Reviews*, *37*(2), 164–183. doi:10.1016/j.neubiorev.2012.11.014 PMID:23206665

Kennedy, D. P., & Adolphs, R. (2012). The social brain in psychiatric and neurological disorders. *Trends in Cognitive Sciences*, *16*(11), 559–572. doi:10.1016/j.tics.2012.09.006 PMID:23047070

Kleinhans, N. M., Richards, T., Sterling, L., Stegbauer, K. C., Mahurin, R., Johnson, L. C., ... Aylward, E. (2008). Abnormal functional connectivity in autism spectrum disorders during face processing. *Brain*, *131*(4), 1000–1012. doi:10.1093/brain/awm334 PMID:18234695

Klem, G. H., Lüders, H. O., Jasper, H., & Elger, C. (1999). The ten-twenty electrode system of the international federation. *Electroencephalography and Clinical Neurophysiology*, *52*(3), 3–6. PMID:10590970

Klin, A., Lin, D. J., Gorrindo, P., Ramsay, G., & Jones, W. (2009). Two-year-olds with autism orient to non-social contingencies rather than biological motion. *Nature*, *459*(7244), 257.

Komogortsev, O., Holland, C., Jayarathna, S., & Karpov, A. (2013). 2d linear oculomotor plant mathematical model: Verification and biometric applications. *ACM Transactions on Applied Perception (TAP)*, *10*(4), 27.

Koshino, H., Carpenter, P. A., Minshew, N. J., Cherkassky, V. L., Keller, T. A., & Just, M. A. (2005). Functional connectivity in an FMRI working memory task in high-functioning autism. *NeuroImage*, *24*(3), 810–821. doi:10.1016/j.neuroimage.2004.09.028 PMID:15652316

Koshino, H., Kana, R. K., Keller, T. A., Cherkassky, V. L., Minshew, N. J., & Just, M. A. (2007). FMRI investigation of working memory for faces in autism: Visual coding and underconnectivity with frontal areas. *Cerebral Cortex*, *18*(2), 289–300. doi:10.1093/cercor/bhm054 PMID:17517680

Krejtz, K., Duchowski, A., Szmidt, T., Krejtz, I., Perilli, F. G., Pires, A., Vilaro, A., & Villalobos, N. (2015). Gaze transition entropy. *Transactions on Applied Perception, 13*(1), 4:1–4:20.

Krejtz, K., Duchowski, A. T., Krejtz, I., Szarkowska, A., & Kopacz, A. (2016). Discerning Ambient/Focal Attention with Coefficient K. *Transactions on Applied Perception, 13*, 3.

Krejtz, K., Duchowski, A. T., Niedzielska, A., Biele, C., & Krejtz, I. (2018a). Eye tracking cognitive load using pupil diameter and micro saccades with fixed gaze. *PloS One, 13*(9).

Krejtz, K., Duchowski, A. T., Niedzielska, A., Biele, C., & Krejtz, I. (2018b). Eye tracking cognitive load using pupil diameter and micro saccades with fixed gaze. *PloS One, 13*(9), 1–23.

Lazarev, V. V., Pontes, A., Mitrofanov, A. A., & deAzevedo, L. C. (2015). Reduced interhemispheric connectivity in childhood autism detected by electroencephalographic photic driving coherence. *Journal of Autism and Developmental Disorders, 45*(2), 537–547. doi:10.100710803-013-1959-8 PMID:24097142

Lee, J. C., & Tan, D. S. (2006). Using a low-cost electroencephalograph for task classification in HCI research. In *Proceedings of the 19th annual ACM symposium on User interface software and technology*. ACM. 10.1145/1166253.1166268

Leigh, J. P., & Du, J. (2015). Brief report: Forecasting the economic burden of autism in 2015 and 2025 in the united states. *Journal of Autism and Developmental Disorders, 45*(12), 4135–4139. doi:10.100710803-015-2521-7 PMID:26183723

Lenartowicz, A., & Loo, S. K. (2014). Use of EEG to diagnose ADHD. *Current Psychiatry Reports, 16*(11), 498.

Lin, J. (1991). Divergence measures based on the Shannon entropy. *IEEE Transactions on Information Theory, 37*(1), 145–151. doi:10.1109/18.61115

Liu, W., Yu, X., Raj, B., Yi, L., Zou, X., & And Li, M. (2015). Efficient autism spectrum disorder prediction with eye movement: A machine learning framework. In *Affective Computing and Intelligent Interaction (ACII), 2015 International Conference on*. IEEE. 10.1109/ACII.2015.7344638

Lombardo, M. V., Chakrabarti, B., Bullmore, E. T., Baron-Cohen, S., & Consortium, M. A. (2011). Specialization of right temporo-parietal junction for mentalizing and its relation to social impairments in autism. *NeuroImage*, *56*(3), 1832–1838. doi:10.1016/j.neuroimage.2011.02.067 PMID:21356316

Lombardo, M. V., Chakrabarti, B., Bullmore, E. T., Wheelwright, S. J., Sadek, S. A., Suckling, J., ... Baron-Cohen, S. (2010). Shared neural circuits for mentalizing about the self and others. *Journal of Cognitive Neuroscience*, *22*(7), 1623–1635. doi:10.1162/jocn.2009.21287 PMID:19580380

Lynch, C. J., Uddin, L. Q., Supekar, K., Khouzam, A., Phillips, J., & Menon, V. (2013). Default mode network in childhood autism: Posteromedial cortex heterogeneity and relationship with social deficits. *Biological Psychiatry*, *74*(3), 212–219. doi:10.1016/j.biopsych.2012.12.013 PMID:23375976

Mason, R. A., Williams, D. L., Kana, R. K., Minshew, N., & Just, M. A. (2008). Theory of mind disruption and recruitment of the right hemisphere during narrative comprehension in autism. *Neuropsychologia*, *46*(1), 269–280. doi:10.1016/j.neuropsychologia.2007.07.018 PMID:17869314

Mohammad-Rezazadeh, I., Frohlich, J., Loo, S. K., & Jeste, S. S. (2016). Brain connectivity in autism spectrum disorder. *Current Opinion in Neurology*, *29*(2), 137.

Mullen, T. R., Kothe, C. A., Chi, Y. M., Ojeda, A., Kerth, T., Makeig, S., ... Cauwenberghs, G. (2015). Real-time neuroimaging and cognitive monitoring using wearable dry EEG. *IEEE Transactions on Biomedical Engineering*, *62*(11), 2553–2567. doi:10.1109/TBME.2015.2481482 PMID:26415149

Mundy, P., Block, J., Delgado, C., Pomares, Y., Van Hecke, A. V., & Parlade, M. V. (2007). Individual differences and the development of joint attention in infancy. *Child Development*, *78*(3), 938–954. doi:10.1111/j.1467-8624.2007.01042.x PMID:17517014

Mundy, P., & Newell, L. (2007). Attention, joint attention, and social cognition. *Current Directions in Psychological Science*, *16*(5), 269–274. doi:10.1111/j.1467-8721.2007.00518.x PMID:19343102

Mundy, P., Sigman, M., & Kasari, C. (1990). A longitudinal study of joint attention and language development in autistic children. *Journal of Autism and Developmental Disorders*, *20*(1), 115–128. doi:10.1007/BF02206861 PMID:2324051

Mundy, P., Sigman, M., Ungerer, J., & Sherman, T. (1986). Defining the social deficits of autism: The contribution of non-verbal communication measures. *Journal of Child Psychology and Psychiatry, and Allied Disciplines, 27*(5), 657–669. doi:10.1111/j.1469-7610.1986.tb00190.x PMID:3771682

Mundy, P., Sullivan, L., & Mastergeorge, A. M. (2009). A parallel and distributed-processing model of joint attention, social cognition and autism. *Autism Research, 2*(1), 1, 2–21. doi:10.1002/aur.61 PMID:19358304

Mundy, P. C. (2016). *Autism and joint attention: Development, neuroscience, and clinical fundamentals.* Guilford Publications.

Noonan, S. K., Haist, F., & Müller, R.-A. (2009). Aberrant functional connectivity in autism: Evidence from low frequency bold signal fluctuations. *Brain Research, 1262*, 48–63. doi:10.1016/j.brainres.2008.12.076 PMID:19401185

Norbury, C. F., Brock, J., Cragg, L., Einav, S., Griffiths, H., & Nation, K. (2009). Eye-movement patterns are associated with communicative competence in autistic spectrum disorders. *Journal of Child Psychology and Psychiatry, and Allied Disciplines, 50*(7), 834–842. doi:10.1111/j.1469-7610.2009.02073.x PMID:19298477

Nunez, P. L., & Srinivasan, R. (2006). A theoretical basis for standing and traveling brain waves measured with human EEG with implications for an integrated consciousness. *Clinical Neurophysiology, 117*(11), 2424–2435. doi:10.1016/j.clinph.2006.06.754 PMID:16996303

Redcay, E., Kleiner, M., & Saxe, R. (2012). Look at this: The neural correlates of initiating and responding to bids for joint attention. *Frontiers in Human Neuroscience, 6*, 169. doi:10.3389/fnhum.2012.00169 PMID:22737112

Rudie, J. D., Shehzad, Z., Hernandez, L. M., Colich, N. L., Bookheimer, S. Y., Iacoboni, M., & Dapretto, M. (2011). Reduced functional integration and segregation of distributed neural systems underlying social and emotional information processing in autism spectrum disorders. *Cerebral Cortex, 22*(5), 1025–1037. doi:10.1093/cercor/bhr171 PMID:21784971

Sasson, N. J., Pinkham, A. E., Weittenhiller, L. P., Faso, D. J., & Simpson, C. (2016). Context Effects on Facial Affect Recognition in Schizophrenia and Autism: Behavioral and Eye-Tracking Evidence. *Schizophrenia Bulletin, 42*(3), 675–683. doi:10.1093chbulbv176 PMID:26645375

Sawyer, A. C. P., Williamson, P., & Young, R. L. (2012). Can Gaze Avoidance Explain Why Individuals with Asperger's Syndrome Can't Recognize Emotions from Facial Expressions? *Journal of Autism and Developmental Disorders, 42*(4), 606–618.

Saxe, R. (2006). Uniquely human social cognition. *Current Opinion in Neurobiology, 16*(2), 235–239. doi:10.1016/j.conb.2006.03.001 PMID:16546372

Schilbach, L., Wilms, M., Eickhoff, S. B., Romanzetti, S., Tepest, R., Bente, G., ... Vogeley, K. (2010). Minds made for sharing: Initiating joint attention recruits reward-related neurocircuitry. *Journal of Cognitive Neuroscience, 22*(12), 2702–2715. doi:10.1162/jocn.2009.21401 PMID:19929761

Schurz, M., Radua, J., Aichhorn, M., Richlan, F., & Perner, J. (2014). Fractionating theory of mind: A meta-analysis of functional brain imaging studies. *Neuroscience and Biobehavioral Reviews, 42*, 9–34. doi:10.1016/j.neubiorev.2014.01.009 PMID:24486722

Shih, P., Shen, M., Öttl, B., Keehn, B., Gaffrey, M. S., & Müller, R.-A. (2010). Atypical network connectivity for imitation in autism spectrum disorder. *Neuropsychologia, 48*(10), 2931–2939. doi:10.1016/j.neuropsychologia.2010.05.035 PMID:20558187

Snyder, S. M., Rugino, T. A., Hornig, M., & Stein, M. A. (2015). Integration of an EEG biomarker with a clinician's ADHD evaluation. *Brain and Behavior, 5*(4), 3–30. doi:10.1002/brb3.330 PMID:25798338

Sparks, B., Friedman, S., Shaw, D., Aylward, E., Echelard, D., Artru, A., ... Dager, S. R. (2002). Brain structural abnormalities in young children with autism spectrum disorder. *Neurology, 59*(2), 184–192. doi:10.1212/WNL.59.2.184 PMID:12136055

Spence, S. J., Sharifi, P., & Wiznitzer, M. (2004). Autism spectrum disorder: screening, diagnosis, and medical evaluation. In *Seminars in Pediatric Neurology* (Vol. 11, pp. 186–195). Elsevier. doi:10.1016/j.spen.2004.07.002

Swanson, M. R., Serlin, G. C., & Siller, M. (2013). Broad Autism Phenotype in Typically Developing Children Predicts Performance on an Eye-Tracking Measure of Joint Attention. *Journal of Autism and Developmental Disorders, 43*(3), 707–718.

Symeonidou, I., Dumontheil, I., Chow, W.-Y., & Breheny, R. (2016). Development of online use of theory of mind during adolescence: An eye-tracking study. *Journal of Experimental Child Psychology, 149*, 81–97. doi:10.1016/j.jecp.2015.11.007 PMID:26723471

Thapaliya, S., Jayarathna, S., & Jaime, M. (2018). *Evaluating the EEG and eye movements for autism spectrum disorder.* Academic Press.

Thorup, E., Nyström, P., Gredebäck, G., Bölte, S., & Falck-Ytter, T. (2016). Altered gaze following during live interaction in infants at risk for autism: an eye tracking study. *Molecular Autism, 7*(1), 12.

Thorup, E., Nyström, P., Gredebäck, G., Bölte, S., & Falck-Ytter, T. (2018). Reduced Alternating Gaze During Social Interaction in Infancy is Associated with Elevated Symptoms of Autism in Toddlerhood. *Journal of Abnormal Child Psychology, 46*(7), 1547–1561.

Tsang, V. (2018). Eye-tracking study on facial emotion recognition tasks in individuals with high-functioning autism spectrum disorders. *Autism, 22*(2), 161–170. doi:10.1177/1362361316667830 PMID:29490486

Uddin, L. Q., Supekar, K., Lynch, C. J., Khouzam, A., Phillips, J., Feinstein, C., ... Menon, V. (2013). Salience network–based classification and prediction of symptom severity in children with autism. *JAMA Psychiatry, 70*(8), 869–879. doi:10.1001/jamapsychiatry.2013.104 PMID:23803651

Vivanti, G., Fanning, P. A. J., Hocking, D. R., Sievers, S., & Dissanayake, C. (2017). Social Attention, Joint Attention and Sustained Attention in Autism Spectrum Disorder and Williams Syndrome: Convergences and Divergences. *Journal of Autism and Developmental Disorders, 47*(6), 1866–1877.

Wagner, J. B., Luyster, R. J., Tager-Flusberg, H., & Nelson, C. A. (2016). Greater Pupil Size in Response to Emotional Faces as an Early Marker of Social-Communicative Difficulties in Infants at High Risk for Autism. *Infancy, 21*(5), 560–581. doi:10.1111/infa.12128 PMID:27616938

Wang, J., Barstein, J., Ethridge, L. E., Mosconi, M. W., Takarae, Y., & Sweeney, J. A. (2013). Resting state EEG abnormalities in autism spectrum disorders. *Journal of Neurodevelopmental Disorders, 5*(1), 24.

Welchew, D. E., Ashwin, C., Berkouk, K., Salvador, R., Suckling, J., Baron-Cohen, S., & Bullmore, E. (2005). Functional Disconnectivity of the medial temporal lobe in Asperger's syndrome. *Biological Psychiatry, 57*(9), 991–998. doi:10.1016/j.biopsych.2005.01.028 PMID:15860339

Wieckowski, A. T., & White, S. W. (2017). Eye-Gaze Analysis of Facial Emotion Recognition and Expression in Adolescents with ASD. *Journal of Clinical Child and Adolescent Psychology, 46*(1), 110–124. doi:10.1080/15 374416.2016.1204924 PMID:27654330

Yoder, P., Stone, W. L., Walden, T., & Malesa, E. (2009). Predicting social impairment and ASD diagnosis in younger siblings of children with autism spectrum disorder. *Journal of Autism and Developmental Disorders, 39*(10), 1381–1391. doi:10.100710803-009-0753-0 PMID:19449096

ENDNOTE

[1]   Details regarding performing ICA in EEGLAB can be found here: Swartz Center for Computational Neuroscience (2018, September 19). Chapter 09: Decomposing Data Using ICA. EEGLAB Wiki. https://sccn.ucsd. edu/wiki/Chapter_09:_Decomposing_Data_Using_ICA

Chapter 3
Predicting ADHD Using Eye Gaze Metrics Indexing Working Memory Capacity

Anne M. P. Michalek

https://orcid.org/0000-0001-6850-3948
Old Dominion University, USA

Gavindya Jayawardena
Old Dominion University, USA

Sampath Jayarathna
Old Dominion University, USA

ABSTRACT

ADHD is being recognized as a diagnosis that persists into adulthood impacting educational and economic outcomes. There is an increased need to accurately diagnose this population through the development of reliable and valid outcome measures reflecting core diagnostic criteria. For example, adults with ADHD have reduced working memory capacity (WMC) when compared to their peers. A reduction in WMC indicates attention control deficits which align with many symptoms outlined on behavioral checklists used to diagnose ADHD. Using computational methods, such as machine learning, to generate a relationship between ADHD and measures of WMC would be useful to advancing our understanding and treatment of ADHD in adults. This chapter will outline a feasibility study in which eye tracking was used to measure eye gaze metrics during a WMC task for adults with and without ADHD and machine learning algorithms were applied to generate a feature set unique to the ADHD diagnosis. The chapter will summarize the purpose, methods, results, and impact of this study.

DOI: 10.4018/978-1-5225-7467-5.ch003

INTRODUCTION

Attention-Deficit/Hyperactivity Disorder is being recognized as a diagnosis which persists into adulthood impacting economic, occupational, and educational outcomes. Estimates indicate that 3-5% of adults have a diagnosis of ADHD (Willcutt 2012) with prevalence estimated to have increased from 6.1% of the United States population in 1997 to 10.2% of the population in 2016 (Xu et al. 2018). The disorder is behaviorally marked by difficulty with attention to important details, difficulty initiating and completing tasks, and difficulty modulating behaviors appropriately in relation to the situation (Fields et al. 2017; Fostick 2017). According to Barkley (1997), adult ADHD symptoms result from impairments of inhibition or the inability to regulate and modulate prepotent responses. While a diagnosis of adult ADHD presumes disinhibition, little is known about the physiological underpinnings of that cognitive skill in relation to an adult ADHD diagnosis. There is an increased need to accurately diagnose ADHD through the development and implementation of objective and reliable outcome measures which reflect core diagnostic criteria, like inhibition.

Researchers in cognitive psychology evidence attention control as the measurable psychological construct which facilitates inhibitory responses by allocating attention according to task demands, especially in the presence of distracting stimuli (Conway et al. 2005; Engle 2002; Kane et al. 2001). Attention control differentiates success during tasks requiring intentional and sustained constraints for effective inhibition, like dichotic listening (Colflesh and Conway 2007) or processing speech in noise (Rönnberg et al. 2013). Measurements of attention control are demonstrated through differences in working memory capacity (WMC) accounting for approximately 60% of the variance seen across people on measures of WMC, like complex span tasks (Engle et al. 1999). Adults with ADHD have reduced WMC when compared to their peers (Michalek et al. 2014) and, despite the understanding that disinhibition is central to an ADHD diagnosis and differences in WMC mathematically represent the resource which makes inhibition possible, there is a paucity of research investigating physiological responses during measures of WMC which could differentiate adults with and without ADHD.

The primary goal of this work is to determine the feasibility of identifying and integrating eye gaze metrics from a WMC task using machine learning to generate a valid and reliable feature set which indexes and predicts an ADHD diagnosis. This chapter investigates gaze measures that map onto these valid neurocognitive deficits that are central to ADHD within the context of a WMC task. The development of these objective measures of ADHD will facilitate its diagnosis and reveal strategies that can enhance the future design effective intervention strategies and accessible classroom environments.

BACKGROUND

Working Memory Capacity (WMC) Tasks

Working memory is the cognitive system which makes it possible to mentally hold and manipulate information simultaneously. Over a decade of work by Engle and colleagues Conway et al. (2008) supports the use of complex span tasks as not only measures of working memory but as a reflection of individual differences in WMC. Performance on complex span tasks generates a composite working memory score numerically indicating how well someone can manipulate and hold information. However, differences in WMC or that composite score represent a person's ability to moderate and control attention. Adults with ADHD have reduced working memory when compared to their peers demonstrating significant differences in WMC (Alderson et al. 2013). This finding suggests that adults with ADHD have a reduced ability to monitor and control attention, especially during situations with competing stimuli (Michalek et al. 2014) or that require response inhibition (Lee et al. 2015; Roberts et al. 2011). Little is known about the underlying covert processes engaged during inhibitory tasks which rely on attention allocation. Using physiological measures during a task which validly reflects attention control, like a complex span task, provides objective diagnostic information for adults with ADHD.

The reading span task (R-Span) is one complex span task widely used as a valid measure of working memory yielding a WMC score (Conway et al. 2005). The R-span was originally developed by Daneman and Carpenter (1983) as a predictor of reading comprehension and was subsequently modified by Engle and colleagues Engle et al. (1999). During the R-Span people see one sentence on a computer screen, read the sentence out loud, determine if the sentence is meaningful with a yes or no response, and then verbally identify a letter typed at the end of each sentence. After a set of sentences, the person is asked to verbally recall as many letters as possible in order of presentation.

This task represents the person's ability to hold and manipulate information simultaneously. To date, there have been no empirical studies investigating eye gaze metrics collected during this task which might differentiate performance and further explain diagnostic differences for adults with and without ADHD.

Machine Learning and ADHD

Typically, experts diagnose ADHD using subjective checklists and related academic and cognitive performance measures (Greenhill 1998). These comprehensive assessments can be time consuming, inconsistent, and can inaccurately represent deficits making differential diagnosis challenging. Ideally, it would be more efficient and reliable to develop predictive algorithms based on physiological metrics reflecting core diagnostic criteria. However, designing this type of computer program can be difficult because there is no existing set of confirmed mathematical features which accurately differentiate between adults with and without ADHD. Machine learning principles offer a solution to this barrier. While it is not practical to develop algorithms by providing a specific set of instructions, machine learning uses numeric features representing a cognitive skill to teach the computer data patterns and inferences which can be applied to groups of data for predicting accurate classifications.

In machine learning there are several varieties of sub categorical learning algorithms. Supervised learning is an example of such a subcategory. The core objective of supervised learning is to build a mathematical model which can be used to predict the outputs of new samples using the training data. Usually, the training data set is stored in a matrix. Each row of the training data matrix corresponds to one training instance which also contains the desired output. For example, in the ADHD/Non-ADHD literature, supervised learning algorithms are iterated through the training dataset to learn a mathematical model to predict or classify the output associated with unseen inputs. When determining whether a person does or does not have ADHD using eye gaze as the outcome metric, the training data would consist of eye tracking data of each person and each person would have a class specifying whether that person is identified as having ADHD or not having ADHD. Supervised learning algorithm will build a general mathematical model which covers the training data space. When a previously unseen person's eye gaze data is entered, the model will use its past experience to accurately predict whether or not that person has ADHD.

Some experts may question the reliability and validity of using machine learning for predicted outputs because those outputs do not consider experts knowledge from psychology or medicine in the decision process. Even with the involvement of expert physicians, it is reported that "diagnostic errors contribute to approximately 10% of patient deaths", by Institute of Medicine at the National Academies of Science, Engineering and Medicine (National Academies of Sciences et al. 2016). Causes for such diagnostic errors could be communication errors between patients and physicians and other failures of the healthcare system. These challenges could be addressed by identifying patterns of the symptoms patients confirm and use them to predict potential diagnostic codes. Even if there is a lack of communication between the patient and the physician or there is a failure in a healthcare system, the symptom patterns of the patient would be highlighted so that accurate diagnosis prediction could be facilitated.

Currently, machine learning is being used for diagnostic prediction not only based on reported symptoms, but also based on patient history and data extracted from wearable devices. Classification algorithms compare the symptoms pattern of the patient and other related data with the other patients in the training dataset in order to predict an accurate diagnosis. In literature using machine learning for ADHD diagnosis and classification, Mueller et al. (2010) attempt to classify adult ADHD patients and healthy controls using a machine learning algorithms. They conducted research to classify ADHD patients and healthy controls using support vector machine (SVM) learning based on event related potential (ERP) components. They examined data from 148 adult participants. Among them, 50% were diagnosed as ADHD while the rest did not have a diagnosis of ADHD. Both groups of adults were selected in a manner that age and gender did not vary between the two group. Each participant performed a visual two stimulus GO/NOGO task and ERP responses of participants were decomposed into independent components and created the feature set. Classification accuracy of assigning ADHD participants and healthy controls to the corresponding groups using a non-linear SVM with 10-fold cross-validation was 92%, whereas it was 90% for linear SVM. This research suggests that classification by means of non-linear methods is more accurate for experiments conducted in a clinical context. Even-though this study uses machine learning approaches to predict ADHD, it does not use eye gaze metrics nor working memory capacity.

Peng et al. (2013) shows that extreme learning machine (ELM), a machine learning algorithm, achieves 90.18% accuracy when predicting ADHD using structural MRI data. This study confirmed that linear support vector machine and support vector machine-RBF achieves an accuracy of 84.73% and 86.55% respectively when the same structural MRI dataset is used. Both extreme learning machine and support vector machine have been evaluated to find the classification accuracy using cross-validation. The goal of their study was proposing an ADHD classification model using the extreme learning machine (ELM) algorithm for ADHD diagnosis. They assessed the computational efficiency and the effect of sample size on both extreme learning machine and support vector machine. They acquired MRI images from 110 participants with 50% of them having a diagnosis of ADHD. This study gives us insight about how applying a machine learning model can accurately predict ADHD.

Marcano et al. (2016) aimed to classify people with ADHD and without ADHD using autoregressive models. They used EEG data collected using 26 electrodes from a group of children between the ages of 6 and 8 to discriminate between ADHD and Non-ADHD. Children participated in multiple experimental conditions, such as eyes open, eyes closed, and quiet video baseline tasks while collecting EEG data. This study verified that KNN classifier is able to provide high classification accuracy when classifying children as either ADHD or typically developing ADHD. The accuracy achieved in this study was high and varying between 85% and 95%. Abibullaev and An (2012) used EEG data with semi-supervised learning in order to predict a ADHD and Non-ADHD diagnosis. They had 10 children participants with 7 of them having a diagnosis of ADHD and 3 were typically. They trained and tested support vector machine with EEG data of each participant achieving an accuracy of 97% for ADHD prediction using support vector machine learning.

Taken together, the literature affirms the successful use of machine learning to accurately predicate a diagnosis of ADHD. However, an empirical gap exists with regard to the training dataset used to train the machine learning model. The majority of studies conducted have primarily used MRI, fMRI, or EEG data to train the machine learning model used to discriminate between ADHD and Non-ADHD. Our goal of this work is to predict diagnosis of ADHD using eye gaze metrics and measures of working memory as the training data for the machine learning algorithms. In this work we employ machine learning algorithms for a diagnosis of ADHD using eye gaze metrics collected during a WMC task. The output of our task is based on binary classes, ADHD and Non-ADHD. We employed supervised learning classification algorithms and evaluated the predicted output in terms of how close it is to the actual output. Our evaluation matrices include standard information retrieval domain evaluation measurements such as accuracy, precision, recall, and f1.

Eye Movements and ADHD

Eye movement behavior is a result of complex cognitive processes; therefore, eye gaze metrics can reveal objective and quantifiable information about the quality, predictability, and consistency of these covert processes (Van der Stigchel et al. 2007). Eye gaze measurement includes a number of metrics relevant to oculomotor control (Komogortsev et al. 2013) including saccadic trajectories, fixations, and other relevant measures - such as velocity, duration, amplitude, pupil dilation (Krejtz et al. 2018). A saccade (rapid eye movement from one fixation point to another) itself may not be an informative indicator of cognition since visual perception is suppressed during a saccade. However, fixations require preceding saccades to help place the gaze on target stimuli to gather salient and relevant information. We believe that analysis of these eye movements can provide important cumulative clues about the underlying physiological functions of attention control during a WMC task which can differentiate a diagnosis of ADHD for adults.

There is substantial overlap in brain systems that are involved in oculomotor control and cognitive dysfunction in ADHD. The precise measurements of eye movements during cognitively demanding tasks provide a window into underlying brain systems affected by ADHD. The neural substrates of oculomotor control are well established (Leigh and Kennard 2004) and show proximity to and overlap with the cortical and subcortical structures involved in cognitive dysfunction in ADHD. For example, the cortical structures that mediate saccadic programming as well as a number of saccadic behaviors include frontal-parietal areas such the frontal eye field (FEF), supplementary eye field (SEF), parietal eye field (PEF), and DLPC. These areas are also affected during cognitive control and WM in ADHD (Rubia 2018). With respect to subcortical structures, the accuracy of saccades is maintained via cerebellum. For example, saccadic hypometria is an undershooting of a saccade to a target that is typically seen in normal subjects, whereas saccadic hypermetria, overshooting the target, is a hallmark feature of cerebellar dysfunction (Leigh and Zee 2015). A study of saccades during visuo-spatial WM has reported significant diagnostic group differences in under- versus over-shooting to the target between boys with ADHD and non-affected controls, such that the ADHD group tended to overshoot the target and the control group tended undershoot the target (Rommelse et al. 2008). Studies have shown that individuals with ADHD also have deficits in the suppression of saccades relative to controls (Mostofsky et al. 2001; Munoz et al. 2003;

Rommelse et al. 2008). Similarly, people with ADHD demonstrate difficulties with intentionally inhibiting ocular responses when compared to their peers during tasks which require purposeful anti-saccade behaviors (Lee et al. 2015; Roberts et al. 2011). Eye gaze metrics, especially saccade features, reliably reveal important differences between adults with and without ADHD.

Based on the diagnostic utility of eye movements, Blazey et al. (2003) invented a method which determines whether an individual has ADHD by sampling the eye movements of participants when they are in an inactive state. This procedure includes a sampling device which has infrared radiation for brightening the eye of a participant and detecting reflections from the eye. The eye movement data collected using their device determines the value of a pre-selected parameter which has a threshold value indicating whether the participant has ADHD or not. According to their study, the most significant feature of the eye movement data is the angular acceleration of the eyeball (Blazey et al. 2003). They have measured ocular angular acceleration for the participants by asking them to stare at a blank screen (Blazey et al. 2003). The measurement data of the angular acceleration of the eye below the threshold value indicates diagnosis of ADHD and the data above the threshold value constitutes a classification of healthy/normal.

Eye Gaze and Machine Learning and ADHD

There is a paucity of empirical studies which implement machine learning to predict ADHD classification using a measures of attention control or WMC. However, there are a few investigations which use machine learning in combination with measures of inhibition. Hart et al. (2014) measured activation patterns using functional magnetic resonance imaging while adolescents with ADHD performed a Stop Task. During this task, participants had to suppress or inhibit the motoric response of pushing a button. The researchers used Gaussian process classifiers and whole activation pattern analysis and were able to predict the ADHD diagnosis with 77% accuracy. Likewise, in a study with adults with and without a diagnosis of ADHD, machine learning predicted the diagnosis with a specificity of .91 and sensitivity of .76 based on EEG metrics during a NoGo task measuring inhibition (Biederman et al. 2017). These results support collecting physiological metrics during tasks required attention control to generate pattern recognition analysis for the accurate classification of ADHD.

Similarly (Tseng et al. 2013) used eye movements in conjunction with machine learning to predict ADHD. This study included participants diagnosed with ADHD, fetal alcohol spectrum disorder (FASD), and Parkinson's disease (PD). Researchers presented short video clips to each participant and analyzed the resulting data sets for three specific types of eye movement features: 1) oculomotor-based features such as fixation durations and distributions of saccade amplitudes; 2) saliency-based features; and 3) group-based features. Results confirmed that saliency based features best differentiated children with ADHD and FASD from typically developing children. Machine learning algorithms predicted ADHD in the sample of children with 77.3% accuracy. Taken together, these empirical findings suggest that diagnostic biomarkers of ADHD could be generated from eye gaze metrics during a WMC task using machine learning.

As such, in this feasibility study, we examined patterns of saccades and stability of fixations generated when completing a measure of WMC to create a feature set which could be used to differentiate a diagnosis of ADHD for adults. Based on the evidence that WMC is reduced in adults with ADHD (Michalek et al. 2014), measurement of eye movements during a measure of WMC will address the following research question: 1) do eye gaze feature values indexing a WMC task predict the classification of ADHD in adults?

METHODOLOGY

Participants

A total of 14 adult participants without (n = 7) and with a diagnosis (n = 7) between the ages of 18-35 were recruited for this study from Old Dominion University. The seven adult participants were (6 F, 1 M, M_age=22.85, SD_age=3.01) diagnosed with ADHD by medical practitioners and that diagnosis was confirmed through formal and verified documentation. Each ADHD participant also completed an informational interview verbally confirming their diagnosis. Moreover, adults with ADHD remained medication free for the 12 hours prior to study participation. Prior to beginning study tasks, all adults were informed of their risks regarding remaining medication free and participating in the study. Participants provided their consent by signing forms outlining costs and benefits of participation approved the University's Institutional Review Board (IRB) in accordance with the Helsinki Declaration.

Participants who completed the protocol were given a ten-dollar Amazon or Chick-Fil-A gift card.

Working Memory Capacity Task

WMC is reflected through complex span tasks, including the Reading Span (R-Span). The R-Span is a validated task designed to reflect the cognitive system's ability to maintain activated representations (Engle et al. 1999; Engle 2002). In the R-Span task, participants are asked to read a sentence and letter they see on a computer screen. Sentences are presented in varying sets of 2-5 sentences. Participants are asked to judge sentence coherency by saying 'yes' or 'no' at the end of each sentence. Then, participants are asked to remember the letter printed at the end of the sentence. After a 2-5 sentence set, participants are asked to recall all the letters they can remember from that set. WMC scores are generated based on the number of letters accurately recalled divided by the total number of possible letters recalled in order. However, this work focused on measures of visual attention which could differentiate adults with and without ADHD.

Apparatus

Eye gaze metrics were recorded and analyzed using the Tobii Pro X2-60 computer screen-based eye tracker with Tobii Studio analysis software. The Tobii Pro X2-60 records eye movements using infrared corneal reflective technology at a sampling rate of 60 Hz (i.e. approximately once every 16.23 milliseconds). Gaze data accuracy was within 0.4 degrees of visual angle and precision was within 0.34 degrees of visual angle. Tobii's eye tracking technology is effective for generating reliable and valid brain/behavior outcomes for children and adolescents (Richmond and Nelson 2009).

All of the participants fulfilled the following inclusion criteria:

1. Between 18 and 65 years of age.
2. Spoke English as their first language.
3. Self-reported normal vision with or without corrective lenses.
4. No history of psychotic symptoms.
5. No comorbid cognitive impairments (e.g. documented learning disabilities, reading disabilities).

Eye Movement Features

The human oculomotor plant (OP) (Komogortsev et al. 2010) consists of the eye globe and six extraocular muscles and its surrounding tissues, ligaments each containing thick and thin filaments, tendon-like components and liquids. In general, there are six major eye movement types: fixations, saccades, smooth pursuits, optokinetic reflex, vestibule-ocular reflex and vergence (Leigh and Zee 2015). An eye-tracker provides eye gaze position information as well as other gaze related parameters (pupil dilation etc.) so that algorithmic derivation in terms of two primary eye movements, fixations (relative gaze position at one point on the screen) and saccades (rapid eye movements of gaze from one fixation point to another) can be analyzed to derive the users attention patterns.

We are interested in investigating number of eye fixation based features in the current framework. We developed a detailed saccade and fixation feature set using the following qualifiers: gender, number of fixations, fixation duration measured in milliseconds, average fixation duration in milliseconds, fixation standard deviation in milliseconds, pupil diameter left, pupil diameter right, and diagnosis label or class. Due to the sampling rate of the tracking system, we were not able to calculate microsaccades and overshoot/undershoot saccades as components of the feature set.

Measuring Attention During WMC

The data for this study was collected during a larger project involving adults with and without ADHD and an audiovisual listening in noise task where WMC scores were measured and used as a cognitive covariate without eye tracking metrics. The entire testing session for the study took approximately 45 minutes. The session began with the participant interview, explanation of the purpose of the study, and review of the consent form. During the interview, the participants provided demographic information and were screened to confirm that all inclusion criteria were satisfied. Once participants indicated they understood their rights and gave consent, they entered the testing area to begin the study. Participants sat at a desk in front of a Dell Computer with a 21-inch monitor. The distance and position of each participant was modified in order to maintain a 45 degree viewing angel of the monitor. For each participant, the experimental tasks began with eye gaze calibration. Once calibration was confirmed, participants viewed a welcome screen followed by the random presentation of several experimental tasks, including the R-SPAN task. The location of the R-SPAN in the order of experimental tasks was randomized and counterbalanced across participants in order to maintain validity. Participants were randomly assigned to a group determining the order of experimental task presentation prior to beginning the study. For all of the experimental tasks, participants were given practice trials.

MACHINE LEARNING ON DATA

We chose precision, recall, f-measure, and accuracy as the evaluation measures for our work. Prior studies (Manevitz and Yousef 2007) have already proven that these measures are independent of category distributions provided that precision and recall are measured at the same time. Intuitively, precision measures exactness of the system (i.e., out of all predicted data instances for a specific category label how many are predicted correctly) while recall indicates the completeness of the system (i.e., out of all labeled data for a specific a category label how many are predicted correctly). F value measures the balance between precision and recall in a single value. In our tables with results assessing classifiers, precision, and recall refers to their weighted average values. Accuracy specifies the fraction of the predictions that the classifier predicated correctly. We employed a grid search mechanism to identify the best parameter combination for optimal result. The optimal parameters are selected based on performance for each classifier after a 10-fold cross validation.

RESULTS

Table 1 shows the RSPAN score for the participants in the current study. An independent t-test statistical analysis (p=0.07) confirms that for this feasibility study there are no significant group differences on WMC scores and are predicted to be a result of the small sample size. The RSPAN is an individual differences measure and significance in variance is detected with large sample sizes. Additionally, WMC scores are typically generated through a composite score of two or more span tasks (Conway et al. 2005), for example, a previous investigation by one of the authors confirmed group differences in WMC using the RSPAN and operation span (OSPAN) to generate a WMC composite score for adults with ADHD (Michalek et al. 2014).

Table 1. RSPAN Score of the ADHD Vs Non-ADHD.

Participant	Age	Gender	RSPAN	Classification
3	18	Female	0.86	Non-ADHD
7	35	Male	0.88	Non-ADHD
9	19	Female	0.60	Non-ADHD
17	23	Male	0.55	Non-ADHD
20	21	Female	0.57	Non-ADHD
25	32	Male	0.88	Non-ADHD
26	20	Female	0.74	Non-ADHD
30	21	Female	0.51	ADHD
34	19	Male	0.67	ADHD
35	26	Female	0.76	ADHD
36	29	Female	0.71	ADHD
37	21	Female	0.60	ADHD
38	21	Female	0.40	ADHD
47	23	Female	0.62	ADHD

Visual Analysis

Figure 1 presents images of eye gaze patterns from two adult participants, one with and one without ADHD. Informal visual analysis indicates that the adult with ADHD is fixating primarily below the stimulus items with little direct fixation to sentence components including: the words, the decision point, or the item to be remembered. Unlike the adults with ADHD, the adult without ADHD has a majority of fixations which are in-line with all sentence components. Although this is a conclusion generated from informal visual inspection, it reveals that adults with ADHD are not visually scanning stimulus

Figure 1. Comparison of Eye Fixations for ADHD (Left) and Non-ADHD (Right) participant during WMC Task.

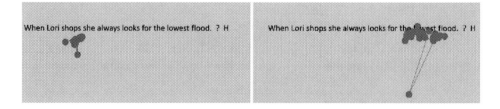

items in a path similar to adults without ADHD. The fixation cluster pattern is just below the stimulus sentence components. This is consistent with the findings of Krejtz et al. (2015) who suggest that while adults with ADHD had similar fixations to salient visual cues when compared to adults without ADHD, they demonstrated less structured and more chaotic scan patterns.

Machine Learning for Classification Prediction

We generated three feature sets categorized according to metric type:

1. Fixation feature set.
2. Saccade feature set.
3. Saccade and Fixation combination feature set.

Each of the three feature sets were individually entered into 43 different classifiers yielding precision rates, recall rates, F1 scores, and percent accuracy. We identified six of the top performing classifiers for each of the three feature sets: J48, LMT, RandomForest, REPTree, K Star, and Bagging. Results for each feature set are discussed individually.

Six of the top performing classifiers for the fixation feature set are listed in the Table 2. The Bagging classifier (ensemble meta-estimator) yielded the highest percent accuracy with 78.48% indicating that a fixation feature set collected during a RSPAN task classifies a diagnosis of ADHD with greater than 70% accuracy. The REPTree classifier yielded the lowest percent accuracy at 76.77%.

To further investigate the performance metrics for the 6 most effective classifiers for the fixation feature set we generated a Receiver Operating Characteristics (ROC) graph (see Figure 2). The ROC graph displays the

Table 2. Classification of Eye Fixation Features during WMC.

Classifier	Precision	Recall	F1	Accuracy
J48	0.77	0.76	0.77	77.79
LMT	0.77	0.77	0.77	77.92
RandomForest	0.76	0.76	0.76	76.79
REPTree	0.75	0.76	0.75	76.77
K*	0.76	0.76	0.76	76.92
Bagging	0.77	0.78	0.77	78.48

Figure 2. ROC Graph of the Top Performing Classifiers for Fixation Feature Set

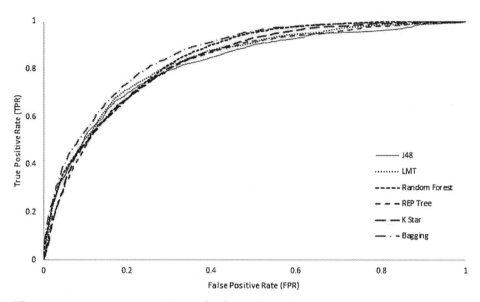

For a more accurate representation see the electronic version.

relative trade-off between benefits (true positive) rates on the Y axis and the costs (false positive) rate on the X axis. The graph shows the Bagging as our top performing classifier offering the best trade-off in terms of the cost and the benefits.

Table 3 outlines six of the top performing classifiers for the saccade feature set. The Random Forest classifier yielded the highest percent accuracy at 91.14% indicating that the saccade feature set collected during a RSPAN task classifies a diagnosis of ADHD with greater than 90% accuracy. The J48 classifier yielded the lowest percent accuracy at 88.95%.

Table 3. Classification of Saccade Features during WMC.

Classifier	Precision	Recall	F1	Accuracy
J48	0.89	0.89	0.89	88.95
LMT	0.89	0.89	0.89	89.51
RandomForest	0.91	0.91	0.91	91.14
REPTree	0.89	0.89	0.89	89.16
K*	0.86	0.86	0.86	85.98
Bagging	0.91	0.91	0.91	90.82

We generated a ROC graph (see Figure 3) for the classifiers we selected for the saccade feature set to investigate the performance metrics. The ROC curve shows that Random Forest classifier has the largest Area Under the Curve (AUC) meaning that it has the lowest error. The AUC of Random Forest classifier is 0.9114. Therefore, it has 91.14% chance of correctly distinguishing between ADHD and Non-ADHD. Random Forest is our top performing classifier offering the best trade-off in terms of the cost and the benefits for the saccade feature set.

Finally, table 4 provides results of the six top performing classifiers for the combination of saccade and fixations feature set. The Random Forest classifier yielded the highest percent accuracy at 91.11% indicating that the combination of fixation and saccade features collected during a RSPAN task classified a diagnosis of ADHD with greater than 90%accuracy. The K Star classifier yielded the lowest percent accuracy at 77.21%.

We generated a ROC graph (see Figure 4) to investigate the performance metrics for the classifiers we selected for the combination of saccade and

Figure 3. ROC Graph of the Top Performing Classifiers for Saccade Feature Set.

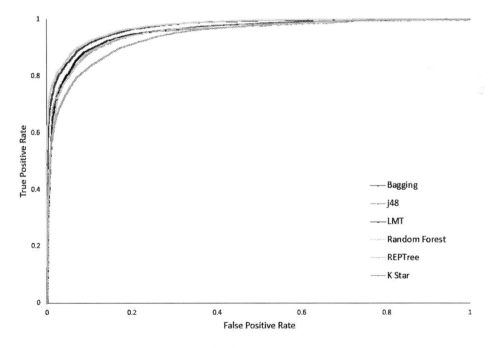

For a more accurate representation see the electronic version.

Table 4. Classification of Eye Fixation and Saccade Features during WMC.

Classifier	Precision	Recall	F1	Accuracy
J48	0.89	0.89	0.89	89.19
LMT	0.89	0.89	0.89	89.91
RandomForest	0.91	0.91	0.91	91.11
REPTree	0.89	0.89	0.89	89.16
K*	0.77	0.77	0.77	77.21
Bagging	0.91	0.91	0.91	90.83

fixations feature set as well. The graph shows that even for the combination of saccade and fixations feature set, Random Forest is the top most performing classifier offering the best trade-off in terms of the cost and the benefits. The AUC of Random Forest classifier is 0.9111 meaning that it has 91.11% chance of correctly distinguishing between ADHD and Non-ADHD.

Figure 4. ROC Graph of the Top Performing Classifiers for the Combination of Fixation and Saccade Features Set.

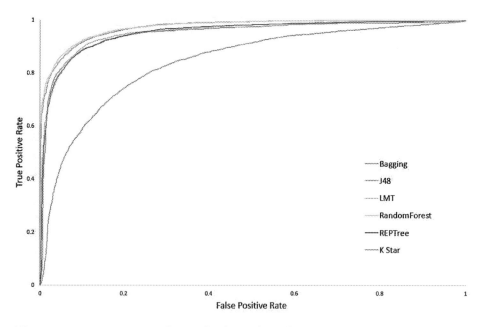

For a more accurate representation see the electronic version.

CONCLUSION

The purpose of this feasibility study was to determine if patterns of saccades and stability of fixations generated when completing a measure of WMC, the R-SPAN task, would create a feature set which could be used to differentiate a diagnosis of ADHD for adults. We used accuracy, precision, recall, and f-measure as the evaluation metrics. While fixation features, saccade features, and a combination of saccade and fixation features accurately predicted the classification of ADHD with an accuracy of greater than 78%, saccade features were the best predictors with an accuracy of 91%. These results are consistent with previous studies confirming significant differences in saccadic behaviors for people with ADHD (Lee et al. 2015; Roberts et al. 2011). During the R-SPAN task, the rapid movement of the eye across the scan path from one fixation point to the other yields a more accurate classification of ADHD than the ability to sustain gaze. These preliminary results indicate that detailed and discrete eye gaze metrics during a measure of attention control (i.e. WMC) provide unique indices of ADHD and offer physiological insight regarding cognitive resources underlying WMC, an important cognitive construct responsible for behavioral inhibition and attention monitoring. Moreover, they are consistent with previous investigations finding that adults with ADHD demonstrate similar broad visual attention patterns as adults without ADHD but different scan patterns (Krejtz et al. 2015) and different pupillometry metrics as a function of visual cue type (Michalek and Roche 2017).

FUTURE DIRECTIONS

The results of this feasibility study confirm the utility of eye movement feature set indexing WMC as a predictor of a diagnosis of ADHD in adults. RandomForest classifiers performed best in-terms of predicting a classification of ADHD with 91.14% percent accuracy by combining saccade feature set representing a physiological measure of visual attention during a WMC task. This project is a necessary first step in delineating a feature set of objective physiological biomarkers for important diagnostic criteria, including attention control, in adult ADHD.

In the future, we are interested in expanding the experimental studies to further analyze a fixation as well as saccade features set according to stimulus areas of interest using a larger sample size. Specifically, identifying relationships between sentence units which determine sentence accuracy, the visual point of decision, the item to be remembered, and performance on the WMC measure. Using these areas of interest will generate a more detailed understanding of the relationships between covert measures of visual attention utilized during WMC tasks which also delineate a diagnosis of ADHD in adults.

REFERENCES

Abibullaev, B., & An, J. (2012). Decision support algorithm for diagnosis of adhd using electroencephalograms. *Journal of Medical Systems, 36*(4), 2675–2688. doi:10.100710916-011-9742-x PMID:21671069

Alderson, R. M., Kasper, L. J., Hudec, K. L., & Patros, C. H. (2013). Attention-deficit/hyperactivity disorder (ADHD) and working memory in adults: a meta-analytic review. *Neuropsychology, 27*(3), 287.

Barkley, R. A. (1997). Behavioral inhibition, sustained attention, and executive functions: constructing a unifying theory of adhd. *Psychological Bulletin, 121*(1), 65.

Biederman, J., Hammerness, P., Sadeh, B., Peremen, Z., Amit, A., Or-Ly, H., ... Faraone, S. (2017). Diagnostic utility of brain activity flow patterns analysis in attention deficit hyperactivity disorder. *Psychological Medicine, 47*(7), 1259–1270. doi:10.1017/S0033291716003329 PMID:28065167

Blazey, R. N., Patton, D. L., & Parks, P. A. (2003). *ADHD Detection By Eye Saccades*. US Patent 6,652,458.

Colflesh, G. J., & Conway, A. R. (2007). Individual differences in working memory capacity and divided attention in dichotic listening. *Psychonomic Bulletin & Review, 14*(4), 699–703. doi:10.3758/BF03196824 PMID:17972736

Conway, A., Jarrold, C., & Kane, M. (2008). *Variation in working memory*. Oxford University Press. doi:10.1093/acprof:oso/9780195168648.001.0001

Conway, A. R., Kane, M. J., Bunting, M. F., Hambrick, D. Z., Wilhelm, O., & Engle, R. W. (2005). Working memory span tasks: A methodological review and user's guide. *Psychonomic Bulletin & Review, 12*(5), 769–786. doi:10.3758/BF03196772 PMID:16523997

Daneman, M., & Carpenter, P. A. (1983). Individual differences in integrating information between and within sentences. *Journal of Experimental Psychology: Learning, Memory, and Cognition, 9*(4), 561.

Engle, R. W. (2002). Working memory capacity as executive attention. *Current Directions in Psychological Science, 11*(1), 19–23. doi:10.1111/1467-8721.00160

Engle, R. W., Tuholski, S. W., Laughlin, J. E., & Conway, A. R. (1999). Working memory, short-term memory, and general fluid intelligence: a latent-variable approach. *Journal of Experimental Psychology: General, 128*(3), 309.

Fields, S. A., Johnson, W. M., & Hassig, M. B. (2017). Adult adhd: Addressing a unique set of challenges. *The Journal of Family Practice, 66*(2), 68–74. PMID:28222452

Fostick, L. (2017). The effect of attention-deficit/hyperactivity disorder and methylphenidate treatment on the adult auditory temporal order judgment threshold. *Journal of Speech, Language, and Hearing Research: JSLHR, 60*(7), 2124–2128. doi:10.1044/2017_JSLHR-H-16-0074 PMID:28672285

Greenhill, L. L. (1998). Diagnosing attention-deficit/hyperactivity disorder in children. *The Journal of Clinical Psychiatry, 59*, 31–41. PMID:9680051

Hart, H., Chantiluke, K., Cubillo, A. I., Smith, A. B., Simmons, A., Brammer, M. J., ... Rubia, K. (2014). Pattern classification of response inhibition in adhd: Toward the development of neurobiological markers for adhd. *Human Brain Mapping, 35*(7), 3083–3094. doi:10.1002/hbm.22386 PMID:24123508

Kane, M. J., Bleckley, M. K., Conway, A. R., & Engle, R. W. (2001). A controlled-attention view of working-memory capacity. *Journal of Experimental Psychology: General, 130*(2), 169.

Komogortsev, O., Holland, C., Jayarathna, S., & Karpov, A. (2013). 2d linear oculomotor plant mathematical model: Verification and biometric applications. *ACM Transactions on Applied Perception (TAP), 10*(4), 27.

Komogortsev, O. V., Jayarathna, S., Aragon, C. R., & Mahmoud, M. 2010. Biometric identification via an oculomotor plant mathematical model. In *Proceedings of the 2010 Symposium on Eye-Tracking Research & Applications*. ACM. 10.1145/1743666.1743679

Krejtz, K., Duchowski, A., Szmidt, T., Krejtz, I., González Perilli, F., Pires, A., Vilaro, A., & Villalobos, N. (2015). Gaze transition entropy. *ACM Transactions on Applied Perception (TAP), 13*(1), 4.

Krejtz, K., Duchowski, A. T., Niedzielska, A., Biele, C., & Krejtz, I. (2018). Eye tracking cognitive load using pupil diameter and microsaccades with fixed gaze. *PloS One, 13*(9).

Lee, Y.-J., Lee, S., Chang, M., & Kwak, H.-W. (2015). Saccadic movement deficiencies in adults with adhd tendencies. *ADHD Attention Deficit and Hyperactivity Disorders, 7*(4), 271–280. doi:10.100712402-015-0174-1 PMID:25993912

Leigh, R. J., & Zee, D. S. (2015). The neurology of eye movements. Oxford University Press.

Leigh, R. J., & Kennard, C. (2004). Using saccades as a research tool in the clinical neurosciences. *Brain, 127*(3), 460–477. doi:10.1093/brain/awh035 PMID:14607787

Manevitz, L., & Yousef, M. (2007). One-class document classification via neural networks. *Neurocomputing, 70*(7-9), 7–9, 1466–1481. doi:10.1016/j.neucom.2006.05.013

Marcano, J. L. L., Bell, M. A., & Beex, A. L. (2016). Classification of adhd and non-adhd using ar models. In *Engineering in Medicine and Biology Society (EMBC), 2016 IEEE 38th Annual International Conference of the*. IEEE. 10.1109/EMBC.2016.7590715

Michalek, A. M., Watson, S. M., Ash, I., Ringleb, S., & Raymer, A. (2014). Effects of noise and audiovisual cues on speech processing in adults with and without adhd. *International Journal of Audiology, 53*(3), 145–152. doi :10.3109/14992027.2013.866282 PMID:24456181

Michalek, A. P., & And Roche, J. (2017). Pupil dilation as a measure of attention in adhd: A pilot study. *America, 116*, 2395–2405.

Mostofsky, S. H., Lasker, A., Cutting, L., Denckla, M., & Zee, D. (2001). Oculomotor abnormalities in attention deficit hyperactivity disorder a preliminary study. *Neurology, 57*(3), 423–430. doi:10.1212/WNL.57.3.423 PMID:11502907

Mueller, A., Candrian, G., Kropotov, J. D., Ponomarev, V. A., & Baschera, G.-M. (2010). Classification of adhd patients on the basis of independent erp components using a machine learning system. In Nonlinear biomedical physics (Vol. 4). BioMed Central, S1. doi:10.1186/1753-4631-4-S1-S1

Munoz, D. P., Armstrong, I. T., Hampton, K. A., & Moore, K. D. (2003). Altered control of visual fixation and saccadic eye movements in attention-deficit hyperactivity disorder. *Journal of Neurophysiology*, *90*(1), 503–514. doi:10.1152/jn.00192.2003 PMID:12672781

National Academies Of Sciences. E., Medicine. (2016). Improving diagnosis in health care. National Academies Press.

Peng, X., Lin, P., Zhang, T., & Wang, J. (2013). Extreme learning machine-based classification of adhd using brain structural mri data. *PloS One, 8*(11).

Richmond, J., & Nelson, C. A. (2009). Relational memory during infancy: Evidence from eye tracking. *Developmental Science*, *12*(4), 549–556. doi:10.1111/j.1467-7687.2009.00795.x PMID:19635082

Roberts, W., Fillmore, M. T., & Milich, R. (2011). Separating automatic and intentional inhibitory mechanisms of attention in adults with attention-deficit/hyperactivity disorder. *Journal of Abnormal Psychology, 120*(1), 223.

Rommelse, N., Van Der Stigchel, S., Witlox, J., Geldof, C., Deijen, J.-B., Theeuwes, J., ... Sergeant, J. (2008). Deficits in visuo-spatial working memory, inhibition and oculomotor control in boys with adhd and their non-affected brothers. *Journal of Neural Transmission (Vienna, Austria)*, *115*(2), 249–260. doi:10.100700702-007-0865-7 PMID:18253811

Rönnberg, J., Lunner, T., Zekveld, A., Sörqvist, P., Danielsson, H., Lyxell, B., ... Rudner, M. (2013). The ease of language understanding (elu) model: Theoretical, empirical, and clinical advances. *Frontiers in Systems Neuroscience*, *7*, 31. doi:10.3389/fnsys.2013.00031 PMID:23874273

Rubia, K. (2018). Cognitive neuroscience of attention deficit hyperactivity disorder (adhd) and its clinical translation. *Frontiers in Human Neuroscience*, *12*, 100. doi:10.3389/fnhum.2018.00100 PMID:29651240

Tseng, P.-H., Cameron, I. G., Pari, G., Reynolds, J. N., Munoz, D. P., & Itti, L. (2013). High-throughput classification of clinical populations from natural viewing eye movements. *Journal of Neurology*, *260*(1), 275–284. doi:10.100700415-012-6631-2 PMID:22926163

Van Der Stigchel, S., Rommelse, N., Deijen, J., Geldof, C., Witlox, J., Oosterlaan, J., ... Theeuwes, J. (2007). Oculomotor capture in adhd. *Cognitive Neuropsychology*, *24*(5), 535–549. doi:10.1080/02643290701523546 PMID:18416506

Willcutt, E. G. (2012). The prevalence of dsm-iv attention-deficit/hyperactivity disorder: A meta-analytic review. *Neurotherapeutics; the Journal of the American Society for Experimental NeuroTherapeutics*, *9*(3), 490–499. doi:10.100713311-012-0135-8 PMID:22976615

Xu, G., Strathearn, L., Liu, B., Yang, B., & Bao, W. (2018). Twenty-year trends in diagnosed attentiondeficit/hyperactivity disorder among us children and adolescents, 1997-2016. *JAMA Network Open*, *1*(4), e181471–e181471. doi:10.1001/jamanetworkopen.2018.1471 PMID:30646132

Chapter 4
Computational Healthcare System With Image Analysis

Ramgopal Kashyap

(iD) https://orcid.org/0000-0002-5352-1286
Amity University Chhattisgarh, India

ABSTRACT

The quickly extending field of huge information examination has begun to assume a crucial part in the advancement of human services practices and research. In this chapter, challenges like gathering information from complex heterogeneous patient sources, utilizing the patient/information relationships in longitudinal records, understanding unstructured clinical notes in the correct setting and efficiently dealing with expansive volumes of medicinal imaging information, and removing conceivably valuable data is shown. Healthcare and IoT and machine learning along with data mining are also discussed. Image analysis and segmentation methods comparative study is given for the examination of computer vision, imaging handling, and example acknowledgment has gained considerable ground amid the previous quite a few years. Examiners have distributed an abundance of essential science and information reporting the advance and social insurance application on medicinal imaging.

DOI: 10.4018/978-1-5225-7467-5.ch004

INTRODUCTION

The quickly extending field of image analysis examination has begun to assume a crucial part in the advancement of human services practices and research. It has given devices to amass, oversee, dissect, and absorb substantial volumes of divergent, organized, and unstructured information delivered by current human services frameworks. Enormous information examination has been as of late connected towards supporting the procedure of care conveyance and illness investigation. In any case, the appropriation rate and research improvement in this space is still prevented by some crucial issues characteristic inside the image analysis worldview (Cruz-Cunha, Simoes, Varajão & Miranda, 2014). Potential zones of research inside this field which can give significant effect on medicinal services conveyance are additionally analyzed. The idea of "image analysis" isn't new; however the way it is characterized is continually evolving. Different endeavors at characterizing image analysis basically portray it as a gathering of information components whose size, speed, type keeping in mind the end goal to effectively store, examine, and imagine the information. Human services are a prime case of how the three information, speed of age of information, assortment, and volume are an intrinsic part of the information it produces. This information is spread among various medicinal services frameworks, wellbeing back up plans, analysts.

Notwithstanding the inalienable complexities of social medical information, there is potential and advantage in creating and actualizing image analysis arrangements inside this domain. A report by McKinsey Global Institute recommends that on the off chance that US social insurance were to utilize enormous information imaginatively and adequately, the segment could make more than $300 billion in esteem each year (Mutula, 2009) 66% of the esteem would be through decreasing US human services consumption. Authentic ways to deal with medicinal research have by and large centered on the examination of illness states in light of the adjustments in physiology as a restricted perspective of certain particular methodology of information. In spite of the fact that this way to deal with understanding illnesses is fundamental, inquire about at this level quiets the variety and interconnectedness that characterize the genuine hidden medicinal instruments. Following quite a while of innovative slouch, the field of pharmaceutical has started to adapt to the present computerized information age. New advances make it conceivable to catch huge measures of data about every individual patient over a substantial timescale. In any case, regardless of the coming of therapeutic hardware, the information caught and assembled from these patients has remained immensely underutilized and along these lines squandered. Essential physiological and patho physiological marvels are simultaneously showed as changes over various clinical streams (Gan & Dai, 2014). In this way, understanding and anticipating ailments require a collected approach where organized and unstructured information originating from a heap of clinical and nonclinical modalities are used for a more thorough viewpoint of the illness states. A part of human services inquire about that has as of late picked up footing is in tending to a portion of the developing torments in presenting ideas of image analysis examination to medication. Specialists are examining the mind boggling nature of human services information as far as the two qualities of the information itself and the scientific classification of examination that can be genuinely performed on them.

Restorative images are an essential wellspring of information regularly utilized for finding, treatment evaluation and arranging. Computed tomography (CT), magnetic resonance imaging (MRI), are some of the examples of imaging techniques, therapeutic image information can go anyplace (Cai, Zhou, Liao & Tan, 2017) from a couple of megabytes for a solitary report e.g., histology images to many megabytes per contemplate e.g., thin-cut CT examines involving upto 2500+ outputs for every examination. Such information requires extensive capacity limits if put away for long haul. It additionally requests quick and precise calculations if any choice helping robotization were to be performed utilizing the information. Furthermore, if different wellsprings of information gained for every patient are likewise used amid the determinations, visualization, and treatment forms, at that point the issue of giving durable stockpiling and creating productive techniques fit for epitomizing the wide scope of information turns into a test.

RESTORATIVE IMAGE PROCESSING FROM BIG DATA POINT OF VIEW

Restorative imaging gives imperative data on life systems and organ work notwithstanding recognizing infections states (Miles-Tribble, 2017). Also, it is used for organ depiction, recognizing tumors in lungs, spinal disfigurement finding, corridor stenosis discovery, aneurysm location, et cetera. In these applications, image handling strategies, for example, improvement, division, and denoising notwithstanding machine learning techniques are utilized.

As the size and dimensionality of information increment, understanding the conditions among the information and planning productive, exact, and computationally successful strategies computer vision methods and stages as shown in figure 1. How the requirement of data by radiologist is increasing day by day.

In the accompanying, information created by imaging procedures is checked on and utilizations of therapeutic imaging from a major information perspective are talked about.

Information Produced by Imaging Techniques

Therapeutic imaging envelops a wide range of various image obtaining procedures ordinarily used for an assortment of clinical applications (Chung, 2017). For instance, picturing vein structure can be performed utilizing attractive reverberation imaging (MRI), registered tomography (CT), ultrasound, and photoacoustic imaging. From an information measurement perspective, therapeutic images may have 2, 3, and 4 measurements. PET, CT, 3D ultrasound, and practical MRI (fMRI) are considered as multidimensional medicinal information. Present day therapeutic image advancements can create high-determination images, for example, breath related or "four-dimensional" computed tomography (4D CT). Higher determination and measurements of these images create vast volumes of information requiring superior figuring

Figure 1. Challenges with increasing the size of data

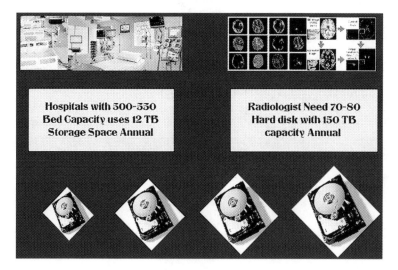

and progressed investigative strategies. For example, minuscule sweeps of a human cerebrum with high determination can require 66TB of storage room. In spite of the fact that the volume and assortment of therapeutic information make its investigation a major test, propels in medicinal imaging could make individualized care more down to earth and give quantitative data in assortment of utilizations, for example, malady stratification, prescient demonstrating, and basic leadership frameworks. In the accompanying we allude to two restorative imaging strategies and one of their related difficulties.

The quick development in the quantity of human services associations and also the quantity of patients has brought about the more prominent utilization of computerized restorative diagnostics and choice emotionally supportive networks in clinical settings. Numerous zones in human services, for example, determination, visualization, and screening can be enhanced by using computational insight (Cresswell & Sheikh, 2012). The combination of computer investigation with suitable care can possibly enable clinicians to enhance symptomatic precision. Figure 2 is showing the combination of therapeutic images with different sorts of electronic human record (EHR) information and genomic information can likewise enhance the exactness and decrease the time taken for a conclusion.

Figure 2. Compositions of medical data

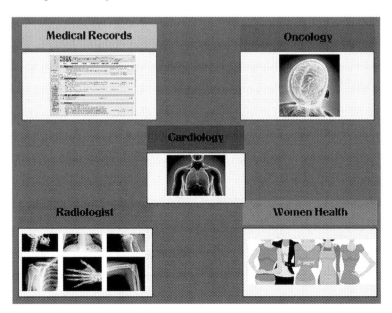

Microwave imaging is a developing technique that could make a guide of electromagnetic wave disseminating emerging from the differentiation in the dielectric properties of various tissues (Fromenteze, Decroze, Abid & Yurduseven, 2018). It has both practical and physiological data encoded in the dielectric properties which can help separate and describe distinctive tissues as well as pathologies. Notwithstanding, microwaves have disseminating conduct that makes recovery of data a testing undertaking. The joining of images from various modalities as well as other clinical and physiological data could enhance the exactness of finding and result forecast of malady. Deferred upgraded MRI has been utilized for correct evaluation of myocardial localized necrosis scar. For this sort of illness, electroanatomic mapping (EAM) can help in distinguishing the subendocardial augmentation of infarct. The part of assessing both MRI and CT images to build the exactness of conclusion in distinguishing the nearness of disintegrations and osteophytes in the temporomandibular joint (TMJ) has been researched ("Fusion of MRI and CT Images of Brain Tumor – Comprehensive Survey", 2018), as per this examination concurrent assessment of all the accessible imaging methods is a neglected need. Other than the colossal space required for putting away every one of the information and their examination, finding the guide and conditions among various information writes are challenges for which there is no ideal arrangement yet.

Strategies

The volume of therapeutic images is developing exponentially for example, Image therapeutic image dataset contained around 66,000 images in the vicinity of 2005 and 2007 while just in the time of 2013 around 300,000 images were put away regular . Notwithstanding the developing volume of images, they vary in methodology, determination, measurement, and quality which present new difficulties, for example, information coordination and mining exceptionally if different datasets are included (Mi, Petitjean, Vera & Ruan, 2015). Contrasted with the volume of research that exists on single modular therapeutic image examination, there is extensively lesser number of research activities on multimodal image investigation. While using information at a neighborhood/institutional level, an imperative part of an exploration venture is on how the created framework is assessed and approved.

PREPARING SUPPLIERS, MEDICAL FACILITIES FOR IMAGE ANALYSIS

The capacity of the social insurance industry to open of the capability of image analysis relies upon the way medicinal services associations execute enormous information arrangements lay out the means essential for the fruitful usage of image analysis answers for suppliers. Following data innovation in different businesses, the human services industry is setting its sights on utilizing enormous information to change quality care through examination that give constant help to give, perceive patterns among populaces, enable research to broaden its compass, and advise basic leadership by government officials and offices. At its most essential, suppliers will profit most altogether from enormous information, yet the degree of this advantage will rely upon how well their associations oversee and incorporate their wellbeing data frameworks. "Once Big Data is overseen and coordinated, associations can apply examination to better comprehend the clinical and operational conditions of their business in light of recorded and current patterns, and anticipate what may happen later on with a confided in level of unwavering quality (Dalessandro, Perlich & Raeder, 2014)," .

As indicated by the creators, the fruitful execution of image analysis arrangements relies upon associations following four critical advances:

1. Set up information administration, characterize information destinations: Implementing major information arrangements starts with setting up the ideal individuals. With an official board of senior individuals set up, an association would then be able to proceed onward to thinking about how and why it will use image analysis. Uncommon thought must be given to the new mechanized procedures, surmising, measurements, and checking apparatuses gave by Big Data arrangements (Hoskins, 2014). Arrangements and systems will likewise be required that administer the utilization of information, characterize the required activities and quality control forms, and streamline, secure, and use data as an endeavor resource by adjusting the destinations of numerous capacities.

2. Distinguish information and data necessities: Big information is about the information contingent upon the measure of an association, its information could be spread out among a variety of frameworks and settings (Kashyap & Piersson, 2018a). Besides, information exist in various structures, and some the most imperative data is unstructured

e.g., free content, imaging. Associations should first perceive the present condition of their information and suspect future changes to the way data is catch (Zhu, Lee & Rosenthal, 2016). "Associations need to comprehend what information they will utilize today, and any potential information that they might need to access later on," the creators clarify. "Associations will likewise need to set up an information procurement guide in light of business and investigation needs."

3. Standardize, incorporate, and arrange enormous information arrangements: Normalizing a database requires wellbeing IT experts to recognize potential redundancies and conditions in their information fields and tables (Rey-del-Castillo & Cardeñosa, 2016). Moving to the size of image analysis will just worsen these wasteful aspects and adversely affect the esteem a major information arrangement going ahead. Flawed data prompts blemished outcomes.

4. Ensure security and protection of image analysis: In the human services industry, the protection and security are significant worries for suppliers and patients. Compiling all the more by and by identifiable data and offering it to a wide range of associations and organizations adds to these worries. The creators prescribe following best practice when moving toward these issues (Recio, 2017). The most ideal approach to address security concerns or necessities is for Big Data answers for help FIPPs. FIPPs are industry-rationalist, fundamental data security rules that can control the prickly dialogs that might be required when systematic tasks cross enterprises, information sources, and information write. Regardless of whether image analysis positively affects human services will boil down to how well social insurance associations and wellbeing IT experts get ready it and what measures they take to shield the security of patients and the respectability of these information.

CHALLENGES IN HEALTHCARE

*   Gathering information from complex heterogeneous patient sources.
*   Utilizing the patient/information relationships in longitudinal records.
*   Understanding unstructured clinical notes in the correct setting (Fatt & Ramadas, 2018).
*   Efficiently dealing with expansive volumes of medicinal imaging information and removing conceivably valuable data and biomarkers.

- Analyzing genomic information is a computationally concentrated undertaking and joining with standard clinical information includes extra layers of many-sided quality, the biggest challenge is to find out insights and evidence as shown in figure 3.
- Capturing the patient's behavioral information through a few sensors; their different social cooperation's and interchanges.

Establishment for Overseeing Image Analysis in Medicinal Services

It is clear in the present human services industry that enormous information is winding up something beyond a popular expression. As indicated by IBM, 90 percent of the information on the planet today has been made over the most recent two years alone. Notwithstanding whether that claim is exact, the measure of information we produce both organized and unstructured is quickening quickly.

The human services industry is in the thick of this information blast. We can trait a portion of the abundance of information to the HITECH Act and EHR

Figure 3. Challenges in healthcare

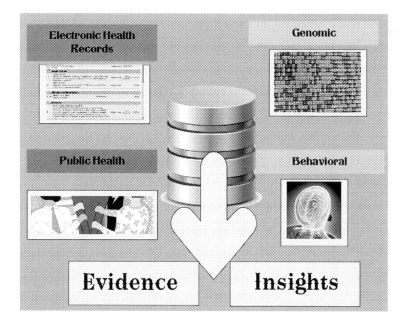

Incentive Programs i.e. important utilize, yet a lot of different components contribute also (Palojoki, Pajunen, Saranto & Lehtonen, 2016). Consider these patterns that should demonstrate to make image analysis considerably all the more a reality in social insurance:

- Increasingly itemized clinical documentation will be required to get exact codification from the extended ICD-10 analysis codes;
- Continued extension of biomedical, bedside and versatile innovation gadgets will bring about expanding measures of gushing information;
- Recent advances in restorative and human hereditary qualities, establishment objects for customized medication and where genomic sequencing will be connected to the therapeutic care of individual patients will bring about enormous measures of sequenced information;
- Natural Language Processing (NLP) and other innovation progressions are bringing about even the talked word being catches as an information resource;
- Secure clinician to clinicians informing and amongst clinicians and patients will keep on producing developing measures of unstructured information.

Feeling overpowered by the potential flood of information? The way to dealing with this tidal wave is to build up an arrangement proactively those changes this heap of information into a reasonable and effective vital resource.

Building an Establishment for Image Analysis

New business insight (BI) instruments are entering the market to enable improve to utilization of the developing rush of information. Be that as it may, instruments alone won't influence a BI to extend fruitful. Achievement lies in the compelling utilization of these instruments to get significant data from the information. Furthermore, this requires culture and process change. One essential basic to propelling a major information activity is the foundation of information driven culture. This regularly requires changes to an association's key objectives and center business forms and in addition the key aptitudes required by its representatives (Skiera & Ringel, 2017). Foundation of such a culture is a "best down" process requiring continuous help from the official group to actualize two critical projects: information administration and ace information administration.

Information Administration

Information Governance sets up the parts, duties, and work process for dealing with an association's undertaking wide information. A compelling information administration system relegates responsibility to singular information for at least one sorts of ace information (Naimur Rahman, Esmailpour & Zhao, 2016). Information stewards are then settled to help information proprietors by planning definitions and measurements used to oversee and measure information quality and execution. Proper information administration guarantees the consistency of an association's information definitions, measurements, and execution markers an imperative prerequisite in the administration of data as a key corporate resource. Information administration gives partners trust in the information that they would then be able to depend on to settle on more educated choices.

Ace Information Administration

Ace information administration is the specialized framework for information administration; It empowers information proprietors and stewards to effortlessly keep up the association's lord information resources. Without ace information administration technique, numerous information administration activities neglect to accomplish their targets. Why? Since without ace information administration the sheer measure of exertion required to keep up the ace information is excessively incredible. It would be ideal if you take note of that enormous information situations are as subject to ace information as big business information stockrooms or information stores (Tian & Peng, 2011). A solitary wellspring of truth for patient and supplier information is just as imperative in a major information condition and information administration and ace information administration give the essential hierarchical structure, work process, and devices in the event that medicinal services in the United States were to utilize image analysis in an imaginative and productive way in their endeavors to drive effectiveness and quality, we could make more than $300 billion in esteem each year. 66% of this esteem would be perceived in an expected 8 percent diminishment in general medicinal services uses.

HEALTHCARE

That is a noteworthy result for the hierarchical exertion required to set up information driven culture.

The human services industry, maybe more than some other, is on the precarious edge of a noteworthy change using progressed examination and image analysis advances.

In this section 5 major information inclines in medicinal services are given

Esteem Based, Patient-Centric Care

An objective of current medicinal services frameworks is to give ideal human services through the significant utilization of wellbeing data innovation with a specific end goal to:

- Improve human services quality and coordination, so results are reliable with current expert information
- Reduce social insurance costs; diminish avoidable abuse
- Provide bolster for improved installment structures

Safety net providers and general wellbeing frameworks e.g., Medicare and Medicaid are in the beginning times of moving from expense for-benefit pay to esteem based information driven motivators that reward brilliant, financially savvy quiet care and exhibit significant utilization of electronic human records (Phone, 2018). This approach requires noteworthy upgrades in announcing, claims handling, information administration, and process computerization. The attention on esteem based care compares with an expanded spotlight on tolerant driven care. By utilizing innovation and concentrating human services forms on quiet results, a continuum of care, specialists, doctor's facilities, and medical coverage need to work with each other to customize mind that is proficient and cost cognizant, straightforward in its conveyance and charging, and estimated in view of patient fulfillment. In this way, the objective now is to start to move all the more conclusively far from the long-standing charge for-benefit hone by which installments are made to suppliers. Fundamentally, suppliers get paid for seeing and treating patients. As of now, there is next to zero reward when and if suppliers enhance nature of administrations, help tolerant results, or decrease costs. Charge for-benefit has been a noteworthy barrier in plans or wants to put resources into computerized answers for, say, enhance persistent results if the suppliers can't recover their ventures. As one senior official at KPMG put it, "Rather than remunerating pioneers for changing social insurance, our frameworks compensate pioneers for making restricted upgrades inside them." Current reasoning around long-standing, significant installment hones is starting to change, making ready for a hearty advanced change of human services.

The Healthcare Internet of Things (IOT)

Likewise called the Industrial Internet, these terms allude to the quickly expanding number of shrewd, interconnected gadgets and sensors and the tidal volumes of information they will produce and move amongst gadgets, and at last to individuals. Spending on human services IoT could top $120 billion in only four years, by a few evaluations (Blake, 2015). What's more, the greater part of the information made by the medicinal services IoT is of the unstructured assortment, making a noteworthy part for Hadoop and progressed enormous information investigation working inside the Hadoop system. Today, an assortment of gadgets screens each kind of patient conduct from glucose screens to fetal screens to electrocardiograms to pulse. A large number of these estimations require a subsequent visit with a doctor. In any case, more quick witted observing gadgets speaking with other patient gadgets could extraordinarily refine this procedure, conceivably diminishing the requirements for coordinate doctor mediation and perhaps supplanting it with a telephone call from a medical caretaker. Other keen gadgets as of now set up can recognize if pharmaceuticals are being taken consistently at home from savvy distributors. If not, they can start a call or other contact from suppliers to get patients appropriately cured. The conceivable outcomes offered by the social insurance IoT to bring down expenses and enhance tolerant care are relatively boundless.

Prescient Analytics to Improve Outcomes

Activities, for example, significant utilize are quickening the appropriation of Electronic Health Records (EHR), and the volume and detail of patient data is developing quickly. The surge in the creation and expanding utilization of EHR was driven to some degree by a $30 billion government jolt, provided by the Health Information Technology for Economic and Clinical Health (HITECH) Act. The Act was composed particularly to give motivations to receive EHR and after that energize the sharing of patient data by clinicians wherever trying to bring down costs, speed finding, and enhance persistent results (Fife & Eckert, 2017). Having the capacity to consolidate and dissect an assortment of organized and unstructured information over different information sources helps in the exactness of diagnosing understanding conditions, coordinating medicines with results, and foreseeing patients in danger for sickness or readmission. Prescient displaying over information got from EHRs is being utilized for early determination and is decreasing death rates from issues, for example, congestive heart disappointment and sepsis. Congestive Heart Failure (CHF) represents the most human services spending. The prior it is analyzed, the better it can be dealt with, keeping away from costly difficulties, however early indications can be barely noticeable by doctors. A machine taking in case from Georgia Tech exhibited that machine learning calculations could take a gander at numerous a greater number of elements in patients' outlines than specialists, and by including extra highlights, there was a significant increment in the capacity of the model to recognize individuals who have CHF from individuals who don't. Prescient demonstrating and machine learning on vast example sizes, with more patient information, can reveal subtleties and examples that couldn't be already uncovered. Optum Labs has gathered EHRs of more than 30 million patients to make a database for prescient investigation devices that will enable specialists to settle on enormous information educated choices to enhance patients' treatment.

Constant Monitoring of Patients

Medicinal services offices are hoping to give more proactive care to their patients by continually observing patient fundamental signs. The information from these different screens can be investigated continuously and send cautions to mind suppliers so they know in a split second about changes in a patient's condition. Preparing constant occasions with machine learning calculations can give doctors bits of knowledge to enable them to settle on lifesaving choices and take into consideration successful mediations. Wearable sensors and gadgets show the open door for guardians to interface with patients in completely new ways, making human services more helpful and determined. Constant checking changes the very idea of the relationship in that up close and personal care isn't generally a need. For instance, applications are being utilized for remote or in-home checking of patients with constant obstructive pneumonic infection. Different screens track the heaviness of patients doing combating obstructive coronary illness to identify liquid maintenance before hospitalization is required. Still others track a kid's asthma solution use to make certain home parental figures and relatives know about what should be directed, decreasing visits to the ER (Kashyap & Piersson, 2018b). As is so frequently the case with new information volumes in human services, sensor information from wearable screens is unstructured information that respects the information procurement and capacity abilities of Hadoop, and additionally to the power and adaptability of cutting edge enormous information examination.

HOW MACHINE LEARNING COULD REVOLUTIONIZE HEALTHCARE DIAGNOSTICS

Machine learning could be the way to altogether enhancing social insurance diagnostics, particularly with regards to extricating most extreme incentive from imaging ponders. In the event that you are in human services, you may have heard the expression "machine learning" without extremely comprehending what it implies. It is anything but another innovation, however it is one that has taken gigantic jumps forward finished the recent years and is turned out to be precious in social insurance. Basically, machine learning is a type of counterfeit consciousness that alludes to the capacity of a PC to distinguish and "recollect" already experienced examples and to gain from new information about those examples and any new examples that are recognized (Chalmers, Altman, McHaffie, Owens & Cooke, 2013). It's a valuable innovation in circumstances that require investigation of a lot of information or in assignments that require the capacity to respond to evolving information. It's utilized as a part of a wide cluster of businesses, enabling PCs to drive autos, run sequential construction systems, contend on Jeopardy and give new experiences from filed information. In medicinal services, machine learning enables a PC to break down huge measures of information and distinguish designs in the information. It can be utilized to enable us to find a wide range of new data. Consider utilizing your medicinal history and related curios to connect the likelihood of a wellbeing episode later on. That would be worth knowing, wouldn't it? New bits of knowledge about patient wellbeing from filed images (R Mingle, 2017).

Advanced images are included examples of pixels a computer vision can perceive and respond to those examples and utilize calculations to figure or measure the information contained in the examples. Basically, it can distinguish the example of pixels in a image of your spine, for instance, measure the physical characteristics spoke to, and ascertain whether you are in danger for osteoporosis, it doesn't really need to be an image that was made to inspect your danger of osteoporosis (Kashyap & Tiwari, 2018). On the off chance that you have had a chest x-ray, maybe preceding surgery, the image was utilized to take a gander at your lungs. Be that as it may, it additionally will contain information about your spine. A computer vision with the privilege examination programming can audit that image and recognize your hazard, assuming any, for osteoporosis.

Imagine a scenario where the greater part of your symptomatic images could be utilized for various screening investigation notwithstanding the infection express that provoked the test. That would increase the value of each demonstrative investigation. Watching considerably farther, consider the possibility that the utilization of this optional imaging examination could incite your parental figure to arrange a genomic concentrate to upgrade the information got from the image, or if a genomic study could be improved by investigation of past images (Kashyap & Gautam, 2017). This could decide whether you have an inclination to a therapeutic hazard or even recognize a potential medication to address the hazard. While this is a modern situation, the building hinders for the vision are happening today.

Mining and Image Information for Bring Down Cost

How about we take a gander at how indicative images could build chance screening to distinguish individuals who could profit by preventive treatment. This is a helpful thought, in light of the fact that, while everybody that hazard screening can be valuable; it is additionally an additional cost and is frequently an additional burden for patients. Subsequently, general adherence to numerous screening programs is low. On the off chance that we can examine understanding images without requiring extra activity by the patient, we can enormously expand our capacity to foresee wellbeing dangers. In most indicative images, there is a life structure outside the bit of the image that the radiologist is assessing (Kashyap, Gautam & Tiwari,

2018). This life structures may contain information that can be accessible for auxiliary discoveries prompting distinguishing proof of asymptomatic sickness, for example, osteoporosis as I noted previously. The normal healing facility imaging office has terabytes of information away, and the measure of information is developing exponentially. In the event that we can mine this information, it would help distinguish malady considerably prior, better match treatment with patients who could profit by it, and through early discovery decrease the effect of an incessant sickness or counteract hospitalization because of the infection.

Machine Vision Can Enable Make to Utilization of Enormous Information Files

This is the place machine vision and machine learning winds up important. When you have gigantic informational collections like this, it takes complex programming and computational energy to examine thousands, even millions, of images and "see" the examples. It's not something a human could do in a convenient or financially savvy way. There is basically a lot of information there to be valuable without examination. While a prepared radiologist could locate these same examples, it is more compelling to spare the radiologist's the ideal opportunity for other work, for example, making considered symptomatic judgments of intense infection forms, in view of a top to bottom comprehension of a patient. There are organizations starting to run machine vision calculations programming that searches for designs against the pixels in early X-rays, CT and MRI sweeps to recognize auxiliary abnormalities that connect to wellbeing dangers (Kashyap & Gautam, 2016). For instance, in a CT sweep of the guts, the broadness of the life systems in the image offers the chance to recognize numerous discoveries that demonstrate a proclivity for heart malady. At the point when this examination is joined with other clinical information related with the patient, the blend would more be able to obviously characterize the patient's hazard for instance, the blend of blood work with greasy liver discoveries could likewise distinguish qualities that are related with later advancement of cardiovascular malady, permitting a notice flag that could help recognize patients who require preventive treatment. The innovation to examine image information exists now, and we are simply starting to see new bits of knowledge from it.

Restorative Technologies, Robotics Improves Radiology Imaging

As designers make more perplexing and refined restorative advances, social insurance suppliers actualize remote checking instruments, versatile wellbeing applications, wearable gadgets, telemedicine highlights, and patient entrances with an end goal to enhance the nature of medicinal services administrations and populace wellbeing results. Alongside the wide assortment of medicinal innovations, mechanical autonomy is assuming a part in influencing understanding consideration. For example, some unpredictable surgeries are currently utilizing mechanical autonomy nearby the surgical group. One fascinating robot that has been having an effect on the social insurance industry is IBM's Watson. The organization declared a week ago that Watson will pick up a type of vision by joining its image examination and psychological capacities with data and images from Merge Healthcare Incorporated's restorative imaging administration framework, as indicated by an official statement from IBM.

As a demonstrated pioneer in conveying medicinal services answers for more than 20 years, Merge is a colossal expansion to the Watson Health stage. Medicinal services will be one of IBM's greatest development zones throughout the following 10 years, which is the reason we are making a noteworthy speculation to drive industry change and to encourage a higher nature of care. Giving Watson 'eyes' on therapeutic images open altogether new conceivable outcomes for the business. IBM is hoping to procure Merge keeping in mind the end goal to better serve social insurance associations by offering a more grounded an incentive to restorative images that would help doctors with clinical basic leadership. At present, Merge is putting forth administrations and therapeutic advancements to in excess of 7,500 social insurance associations over the United States including pharmaceuticals and clinical research organizations (Kashyap & Gautam, 2015). The arrangement is for these restorative foundations to use Watson's abilities to oversee therapeutic images and gain new bits of knowledge from electronic patient records, images, medicinal information, and data from wearable gadgets. "As Watson advances, we are handling more mind boggling and significant issues by continually assessing greater and additionally difficult informational indexes," Kelly proceeded. "Therapeutic images are the absolute most confused informational indexes conceivable, and there is maybe not any more vital territory in which specialists can apply machine learning and psychological figuring. That is the genuine guarantee of psychological figuring and its counterfeit consciousness segments making us more advantageous and to enhance the nature of our lives." With the extensive volumes of images that numerous human services experts must deal with on an everyday premise, Watson's capacities could demonstrate basic in lessening medicinal mistakes and enhancing the nature of care among the patient base. A few radiologists in clinic crisis rooms may need to oversee upwards of 100,000 therapeutic images for every day.

Machine Learning, Imaging Analytics Predict Kidney Function

Imaging investigation supported by machine learning can precisely anticipate renal survival time in patients with ceaseless kidney malady. Machine taking in and imaging examination from renal biopsies can anticipate to what extent a kidney will work satisfactorily in patients with incessant kidney harm, says an investigation distributed in Kidney International Reports. Utilizing profound learning and neural systems, a type of machine discovering that imitates the basic leadership examples of the human personality, scientists found that a progression of new convolutional neural system (CNN) calculations was more exact and precise than customary pathologist-evaluated scoring frameworks while computing kidney decrease. Unending kidney harm is routinely surveyed semi-quantitatively by scoring the measure of fibrosis and tubular decay in a renal biopsy test, clarifies the exploration group from Boston University.

In spite of the fact that according to master pathologists can measure the seriousness of infection and to recognize subtleties of histopathology with momentous precision, such skill isn't accessible in all areas, particularly at a worldwide level. In the United States, roughly 14 percent of the populace experiences unending kidney infection, as per the National Institutes of Health. The condition habitually delivers couple of indications until the point that it is extremely best in class, uplifting the significance of standard checking and exact distinguishing proof of how the sickness is advancing. Besides, there is an earnest need to institutionalize the evaluation of obsessive infection seriousness, to such an extent that the adequacy of treatments built up in clinical trials can be connected to treat patients with similarly extreme ailment in routine practice, the group included (Manlhiot, 2018). Manmade brainpower and imaging investigation are promising advances for helping pathologists with these undertakings. With the capacity to perceive designs down to the pixel in multi-gigabyte images, AI offers a level of itemized investigation for fantastically extensive volumes of information that human clinicians may essentially be notable match. Early outcomes joining machine learning and imaging information have been empowering and how healthcare data is collected as shown in figure 4.

A few pilots have just demonstrated that AI devices can be about as precise as human pathologists while fundamentally lessening the time it takes to dissect substantial amounts of information. The calculation was prepared to distinguish patients with likely renal survival rates of 1, 3, and 5 years. Since the investigation utilized review information, the group could coordinate the calculation's forecasts with real results. The outcomes showed that the CNN demonstrate was quantifiably superior to anything the pathologist-assessed scoring framework while foreseeing renal survival rates over the three target time frames. The calculation was additionally ready to all the more precisely recognize the condition of kidney ailment for the people.

Figure 4. Healthcare Data and Sources

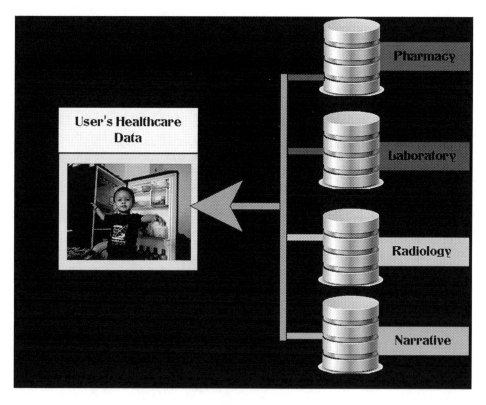

What's more, independent therapeutic assignments of screening, observing, and endless malady administration can be characterized. Flat administrative undertakings, for example, asset advancement, quality control, adherence to the conventions and treatment designs are likewise to be considered. Summing up both methodologies, the goals of Data Mining (DM) utilization in pharmaceutical can be summed up into two principle gatherings: treatment assets enhancement (social insurance administration area), and treatment quality change (restorative treatment and research areas). We show destinations of DM applications in the medicinal space assembled by the objectives in Table 1.

Exploit the huge measures of information and give right mediation to the correct patient at the opportune time. Conceivably advantage every one of the segments of a social insurance system Personalized care to the patient. i.e.supplier, payer, patient, and administration.

SPECIALIZED DIFFICULTIES

In the accompanying, specialized difficulties and openings are talked about with respect to the utilization of Big Information innovations in human services.

Table 1. Objectives and destinations of DM in prescription Goals Objectives

Advancement of treatment assets	• Identification of chances for potential cost diminishment and income upgrade • Dependence of length of stay (LOS) at a healing facility on the patient's statistic information, anamnesis, chose technique for treatment, and different components • Prediction of rehospitalisation • Prediction of postoperative difficulties and their probabilities; • Prediction of medicinal staff effectiveness pointers • Identification of pointless restorative intercessions; • Identification of uncalled for remedies
Change of treatment quality	• Early determination of infections (screening) • Evaluation of plausible entanglements; • Modelling the advance of ailment • Determining relationship of particular clinical ascribes to modify the analysis or select an arrangement of treatment; • Generalizing multidimensional biomedical information recorded progressively keeping in mind the end goal to encourage basic leadership • Analysis of the nature of biomedical datasets • Determination of dataset fulfillment; • Determination of dataset fracture; • Diagnosis setting or alteration of analysis; • Formation of medicinal master frameworks database; • Prediction of solution viability; • Micro-exhibit investigation for undertaking fathoming; • Early conclusion of sicknesses; • Selection of individual treatment • Determination of the likelihood of infection event.

Information Quality

There is a need solid and reproducible outcomes especially in therapeutic and pharmaceutical examine where information gathering is to a great degree costly. Information provenance gives a comprehension of the wellspring of the information how it was gathered, under which conditions, yet in addition how it was prepared furthermore, changed before being put away. This is imperative not just for reproducibility of examination and tests yet in addition for understanding the dependability of the information that can influence results in clinical also, pharmacological research (Waoo, Kashyap and Jaiswal, 2010). As the many-sided quality of activities develops, with new investigation strategies being created quickly, it winds up key to record and comprehend the cause of information which in turn can altogether impact the conclusion from the examination.

Information Amount

The wellbeing division is an information concentrated industry relying upon information and investigation to make strides treatments and practices. There has been colossal development in the scope of data being gathered, including clinical, hereditary, behavioral, ecological, budgetary, and operational data. Social insurance information is developing at stunning rates that have not been found before. There is a need to manage this vast volume and speed of information to determine significant bits of knowledge to enhance social insurance quality and productivity. Associations today are gathering a vast volume of information from both exclusive information sources and open sources, for example, online networking and open information. Through better examination of these enormous Data sets, there is a noteworthy potential to better comprehend partner (e.g., persistent, clinician) needs, streamline existing items and administrations, and additionally grow new incentives.

Multi-Modular Information

In medicinal services, distinctive kinds of data are accessible from various sources, for example, electronic social insurance records, tolerant synopses, genomic and pharmaceutical information, clinical test outcomes, imaging (e.g. x-ray, MRI, and so forth.), protection claims, imperative signs from e.g., telemedicine, versatile applications, home checking, on-going clinical trials, ongoing sensors, and data on prosperity. This information can be both organized and unstructured. The combination of human services information from numerous sources could exploit existing cooperative energies between information to enhance clinical choices and to uncover totally new ways to deal with treating diseases. For example, the combination of various wellbeing information sources could make the investigation and connection of various phenotypes e.g. watched articulation of illnesses or hazard factors conceivable that have demonstrated hard to precisely portray from a genomic perspective just, and in this manner empower the advancement of programmed demonstrative apparatuses and customized drug (Melin & Sánchez, 2017). The mix and investigation of multi-modular information postures a few specialized difficulties identified with interoperability, machine learning and mining.

Information to Get

In spite of the fact that there is a feeling of incredible open doors with respect to the examination of wellbeing information for progressing human services, there are critical hindrances that point of confinement the entrance and sharing of wellbeing information among distinctive organizations and nations. Other than the political concerns, morals and passionate viewpoints have a huge weight around there since individuals try not to like others benefitting from their sicknesses. Security concerns are an imperative viewpoint that requirements to be overcome also and image analysis process is given in figure 5.

There is a high level of fracture in the wellbeing division: gathered information is not shared among organizations, even not inside divisions. This prompts the presence and spread of distinctive separated information storehouses that are not completely abused. Bits of knowledge can't be gotten from datasets that are disengaged. Top-down Big Data activities have not gained much ground up until now and afterward a few endeavors are presently concentrating on a base up approach. By changing the point of view to be persistent situated, this gives patients responsibility for information. Patients should in this way have the capacity to get to their own information, choose whom to impart it to, and for what reason. Cases are the informal organization which not just enables patients to cooperate and gain from other individuals with similar conditions, however likewise gives a confirmation base of individual information for examination and a stage for connecting patients with clinical trials.

Figure 5. Effectively data collection and integrating healthcare data

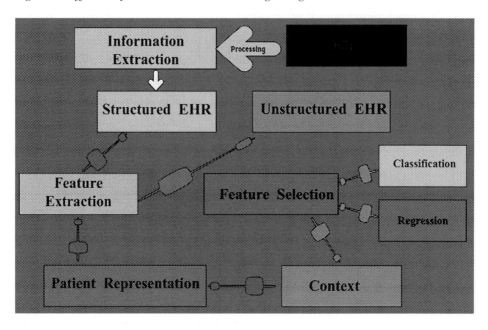

Understanding Image Segmentation in Healthcare

Image segmentation suffers with incorrect results, many methods have been developed for correct results, but some methods take so much time for computation and some method gives over segmented results. The globally optimal geodesic active contour (GOGAC) is one if the best method based on energy, but it stuck in local minima and gives incorrect results (Juneja and Kashyap 2016). Here microarray images have attracted much attention because of the inability of creating correctly segmented spots. Figure 6 shows comparative analysis of image segmentation methods. Experimental results demonstrated that model possesses better performance than the CV model and LIF model. They confirmed its effectiveness in various synthetic images and actual images, and promising experimental results display its advantages regarding accuracy, proficiency, and robustness.

An automated lung extraction as well as the edge modification method written by Changli Feng includes CV model, LBF model, the throughout the world convex segmentation approach. The diagnostic accuracy of the new border detection operates is much more accurate than the traditional border detection operate presents the actual segmentation result image obtained when using the GOGAC. If segmented result will be incorrect and it will be

Figure 6. Result comparisons of image segmentation methods

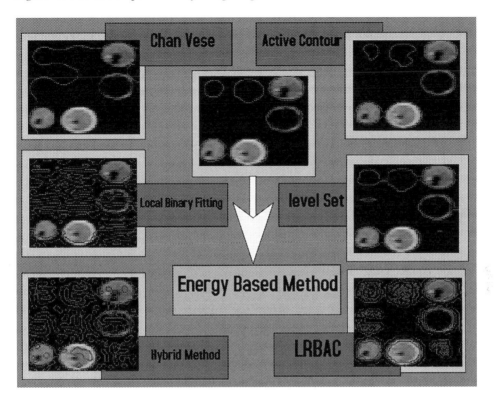

given for further analysis of the image, then surely it will give wrong results because it will affect the whole process like information extraction, analysis, quantification and evaluation the aim is to get better and accurate result so that correct analysis must be generated through segmentation.

Information Analytics

Therapeutic research has dependably been information driven science, with randomized clinical trials being a gold standard by and large summary of data is given in the table 2. Be that as it may, because of late advances in therapeutic imaging, far reaching electronic human records, and shrewd gadgets, restorative research and additionally clinical rehearse are rapidly changing into Big Data-driven fields. Accordingly, the medicinal services space overall specialists, patients, administration, protection, and governmental issues can fundamentally benefit from current advances in Big Data advancements, and specifically from investigation.

Table 2. Summary of HER Data

	ICD (%)	CPT (%)	Lab (%)	Medication (%)	Clinical Notes (%)
Availability	100	100	100	50	50
Recall	50	5	50	90-95	45-55
Precision	50	100	90-95	45-50	100

There are sure difficulties and prerequisites to create particular techniques and methodologies for Big Information investigation in human services. These include:

- **Multi-Modular Information:** Optimally in information investigation there is an arrangement of all around curated, institutionalized, and organized information for instance as now and then found in electronic wellbeing records. Be that as it may, a high level of wellbeing information is an assortment of unstructured information. A lot of it comes in types of ongoing sensor readings, for example, ECG estimations in concentrated care, content information in clinical reports by specialists, restorative writing in characteristic dialect, imaging information, or omics information in customized drug. It is imperative to pick up learning from that data. The objective ought to be to acquire important data from such heterogeneous information, make such data accessible to clinicians, and join learning into the clinical history of patients.

- **Complex Foundation Learning:** Medical information needs to depict extremely complex marvels; from multi-level patient information on medicinal treatment and methodology, way of life data, the tremendous measure of accessible medicinal information in the writing, bio banks, or trial stores. Subsequently, medicinal information normally accompanies complex metadata that should be taken into account with a specific end goal to ideally break down the information, make determinations, and find suitable theories, what's more, bolster clinical choices.

- **Highly Qualified End-Clients:** End-clients of explanatory instruments in pharmaceutical for example, specialists, clinical analysts and bioinformaticians are profoundly qualified. They additionally have a high duty, from which take after exclusive requirements on the nature of examination instruments before believing them in the treatment of patients. Thus, an ideal scientific approach should, however much as could reasonably be expected, create reasonable examples keeping in mind the end goal to take into account cross-checking comes about and empowering confide in the arrangements. It should likewise empower master driven self-benefit investigation to permit the master to control the examination procedure.

- **Supporting Complex Choice:** The examination of imaging information, pathology, serious care checking, or the treatment of multi-morbidities are cases of regions in which restorative choices must be taken from loud information, in complex circumstances, and with conceivably absent data (Liu, Liang & Xu, 2011). Neither people nor calculations might be ensured to dependably convey an ideal arrangement, yet they might be required to take imperative choices or indicate alternatives in insignificant time. Another zone of medicinal choice help with possibly high future effect are keen aides for patients that make utilization of cell phones and new wearable gadgets and sensor advancements to enable patients to oversee ailments and have more beneficial existences.
- **Security:** Medical information is exceptionally touchy data that is ensured by solid lawful shields at the European level. A sufficient legitimate system to empower the investigation of such information, and the advancement of satisfactory security protecting logical devices to execute this structure, is of high significance for the pragmatic pertinence and effect of information driven pharmaceutical and medicinal services. Ways to deal with address information investigation under the up to specified difficulties will be displayed in the following.

Certain time-basic human services applications require moves to be made comfortable moment that a specific occasion is distinguished (e.g. cautions in ICU). Various floods of heterogeneous information offer the plausibility to remove bits of knowledge progressively.

A few applicable, interconnected methodologies exist:

- Real-time examination alludes to investigation strategies, which can dissect and make experiences from every accessible datum and assets remarkably into a framework.
- Data stream mining alludes to the capacity to break down and process spilling information in the present or on the other hand as it arrives, as opposed to putting away the information and recovering it eventually.

- Complex occasion recognition alludes to the revelation and administration of examples over various information streams, where designs are abnormal state, semantically rich, and are made at last justifiable to the client.

"An essential quality of the investigation is that the machine learning innovation was connected to trichrome-recolored histologic images of routine kidney biopsy tests with no exceptional preparing or control other than advanced examining," the group noted, "which enabled us to specifically think about the aftereffects of the machine taking in examination with those got from the clinical neurotic provide details regarding similar examples (Miyagi, 2009)." The utilization of profound learning strategies likewise made a more mind boggling assessment structure than the pathologist-evaluated score, which basically depends on the level of fibrosis show in a specific example. "Utilizing administrators, for example, convolution, initiation, and pooling, preparing a CNN show includes playing out these tasks numerous circumstances in a deliberate manner to change pixel-level data to abnormal state highlights of the info image," says the investigation.

AS IMAGING ANALYTICS GROWS, HEALTHCARE ORGS SHOULD PROCEED CAUTIOUSLY

Imaging examination is a quickly developing piece of wellbeing IT, yet suppliers should insightfully pick the best instruments and procedures that will enable them to enhance care and cut expenses. Imaging examination helped by manmade brainpower is quickly growing inside the wellbeing IT circle, however suppliers must evaluate their associations and see precisely how this innovation will upgrade the patient experience and decrease human services costs before making any ventures. As indicated by a current report from ReportBuyer, the worldwide medicinal imaging examination market will increment to $4.26 billion by 2025 as suppliers embrace instruments to separate important bits of knowledge from singular images and additionally bigger scale information resources. The rising interest for examination programming mirrors the business' day of work to esteem based care. A current Frost and Sullivan investigation expresses that the US medicinal imaging market is turning into an industry driven by quality as opposed to amount, with partners progressively centered around enhancing wellbeing, cutting expenses, and improving work process proficiency. Nonetheless, finishing this change is no simple undertaking. Actualizing new framework is expensive, and it is regularly hard to know whether new devices will deliver an arrival on speculation. Medicinal imaging tests represent $10 billion of Medicare spending yearly, and rehashed restorative imaging tests considerably add to yearly social insurance costs, A recent report from RAND Corporation included that imaging for back torment and cerebral pains were among the best performed low-esteem benefits in medicinal services, costing the business $3.1 million and $3.6 million every year, separately.

The impact of both interior and outside difficulties has officially inflicted significant damage on the business. The path for partners to address these difficulties as well as succeed will be to reasonably utilize items, administrations, and arrangements that enhance the proficiency of the imaging procedure, decrease costs, and enhance effectiveness without trading off quality. To change from amount to quality in restorative imaging, social insurance suppliers must consider what mechanical arrangements will most precisely examine images while lessening costs. Computerized reasoning, especially profound learning, has demonstrated noteworthy guarantee in enhancing image examination. Profound taking in, a machine learning system, copies the basic leadership rationale of the human cerebrum and offers an inexorably precise approach to order messages, images, and other clinical information. Engineers and scientists have been displaying these abilities through pilots, studies, and utilize cases that are creating amazing outcomes.

Regardless of seller eagerness, AI is still particularly in its early stages, and suppliers should think about these instruments as clinical help capacities instead of machines that can settle on therapeutic choices totally all alone. What's more, associations shouldn't bounce into concurrences with merchants before knowing precisely what they're putting forth, and all the more significantly, how the innovation will be utilized to tackle issues. That wasn't the offering point. His pitch was taking care of the issue, and I believe that frequently gets missed in the buildup about AI and machine learning. Suppliers ought to likewise evaluate where their association remains as far as information trustworthiness and clinical work processes before conveying new wellbeing IT apparatuses. Associations that make a point by point guide delineating their significant objectives will guarantee that their innovative speculations will have important outcomes. Staying away from discovery, AI instruments ought to likewise be a basic worry for associations. When utilizing AI to settle on clinical choices, suppliers must ensure that they comprehend why and how these frameworks are influencing specific proposals and relationship, to regardless of whether it is troublesome for clinicians to see precisely how a calculation capacities.

DISCUSSION

AI-based medicinal applications can be ordered into either information serious or information driven. The information serious methodologies mean to get computational models, extricated from the clinical writing and specialists' understanding, to speak to ideas, their relations, and the instruments to empower programmed thinking to help medicinal choices. Not at all like information escalated, information driven methodologies, at the focal point of the vision of learning wellbeing frameworks, concentrate such learning specifically from the gathered clinical information and this learning is generally used to clarify a patient's ebb and flow indications/imperative signs and to anticipate future malady movement of the patient. While an expanding measure of information is being created by different biomedical and medicinal services frameworks, they have not yet completely gained by the transformative open doors that these information give. Applying information driven strategies to huge wellbeing information can be of extraordinary advantage in the biomedical and human services space, permitting ID and extraction of pertinent data and decreasing the time spent by biomedical and medicinal services experts and specialists who are attempting to discover significant examples and new strings of learning. As one of the world's biggest and quickest developing businesses, medicinal services designing alludes to all parts of the anticipation, analysis, treatment, and administration of sickness, and in addition the conservation and change of physical and psychological well-being and prosperity through restorative administrations.

Today, the usage of restorative advances has been inadequate with regards to with regards to imaging examination in the radiology field and a great part of the investigation must be done physically. IBM is hoping to utilize the Watson Health Cloud to gauge therapeutic images among a lot of information including lab comes about, wellbeing records, clinical examinations, hereditary tests, and other medicinal data. Human services suppliers would have the capacity to think about any current medicinal images against a patient's past images and over a patient base of comparable restorative conditions and side effects to decide any progressions or divergences. "Consolidating Merge's driving medicinal imaging arrangements with the world-class machine learning and investigation abilities of IBM's Watson Health is the eventual fate of social insurance innovation," Michael W. Ferro, Jr., Merge's director, said in an open proclamation. "Consolidation's driving innovation and demonstrated aptitude speak to a one of a kind mix of advantages that will convey unparalleled incentive to Watson Health customers. Together, we will open phenomenal new chances to enhance understanding diagnostics and convey upgraded mind.

Medicinal imaging innovations play an ever increasing number of essential parts not just in the analysis and treatment of sicknesses yet in addition in ailment aversion, wellbeing checkup, significant malady screening, wellbeing administration, early conclusion, and infection seriousness assessment, decision of treatment techniques, treatment impact assessment, and restoration. The status of restorative imaging advancements has expanded ceaselessly in social insurance applications. Because of its capacity to influence the finding and treatment of illness, to image guided surgery and other therapeutic connections all the more convenient, exact, and effective, medicinal image improvement has turned into a normal errand. Through delivering incredible tissue consistency, advanced complexity, edge improvement, relic end, keen commotion decrease, et cetera, front line image upgrade helps specialists precisely decipher medicinal images, an urgent establishment for better analysis and treatment.

CONCLUSION

Enormous information examination which uses armies of different, organized, and unstructured information sources will assume a crucial part in how social insurance is drilled later on. One would already be able to see a range of examination being used, helping in the basic leadership and execution of social insurance work force and patients. Here we concentrated on three territories of intrigue: restorative image examination, physiological flag preparing, and genomic information handling. The exponential development of the volume of medicinal images powers computational researchers to think of imaginative answers for process this substantial volume of information in tractable timescales. The pattern of selection of computational frameworks for physiological flag preparing from both research and honing restorative experts is developing relentlessly with the improvement of some extremely innovative and unbelievable frameworks that assistance spare life. Restorative image investigation covers numerous zones, for example, image procurement, development/recreation, improvement, transmission, and pressure. New mechanical advances have brought about higher determination, measurement, and accessibility of multimodal images which prompt the expansion in precision of finding and change of treatment. In any case, incorporating restorative images with various modalities or with other medicinal information is a potential opportunity. New scientific systems and strategies are required to dissect this information in a clinical setting. These techniques address a few concerns, openings, and difficulties, for example, highlights from images which can enhance the precision of finding and the capacity to use divergent wellsprings of information to expand the exactness of determination and lessening cost and enhance the precision of preparing strategies, for example, therapeutic image upgrade, enrollment, and division to convey better proposals at the clinical level. In spite of the fact that there are some genuine difficulties for flag preparing of physiological information to manage, given the ebb and flow condition of information competency and non standardized structure, there are openings in each progression of the procedure towards giving foundational changes inside the medicinal services research and practice groups. Aside from the conspicuous requirement for additionally look into in the zone of information wrangling, amassing, and orchestrating ceaseless and discrete therapeutic information positions, there is likewise an equivalent requirement for creating novel flag handling procedures particular towards physiological signs. Research relating to digging for biomarkers and undercover examples inside biosignals to comprehend and anticipate a malady case has indicated potential in giving noteworthy data. Be that as it may, there are open doors for creating calculations to address information separating, addition, change, highlight extraction, include determination, et cetera. Besides, with the reputation and change of machine learning calculations, there are openings in enhancing and creating hearty CDSS for clinical expectation, medicine, and diagnostics.

Incorporation of physiological information and high-throughput "- omics" methods to convey clinical suggestions is the amazing test for frameworks scientists. Despite the fact that partner utilitarian impacts with changes in quality articulation has advanced, the consistent increment in accessible genomic information and its relating impacts of comment of qualities and blunders from test and scientific practices make examining useful impact from high-throughput sequencing procedures a testing undertaking. Remaking of systems on the genome-scale is a not well postured issue. Vigorous applications have been created for remaking of metabolic systems and quality administrative systems. Restricted accessibility of dynamic constants is a bottleneck and consequently different models endeavor to defeat this confinement. There is a fragmented comprehension for this extensive scale issue as quality control, impact of various system designs, and developmental consequences for these systems are as yet being broke down. To address these worries, the blend of watchful plan of analyses and model improvement for remaking of systems will help in sparing time and assets spent in building comprehension of direction in genome-scale systems. The chance of tending to the stupendous test requires close participation among experimentalists, computational researchers, and clinicians.

The examination of computer vision, imaging handling and example acknowledgment has gained considerable ground amid the previous quite a few years. Additionally, therapeutic imaging has pulled in expanding consideration as of late because of its fundamental part in social insurance applications. Examiners have distributed an abundance of essential science and information reporting the advance and social insurance application on medicinal imaging. Since the improvement of these examination fields has set the clinicians to progress from the seat to the bedside, the Journal of Healthcare Engineering set out to distribute this uncommon issue committed to the theme of cutting edge computer vision techniques for social insurance building, and in addition audit articles that will animate the proceeding with endeavors to comprehend the issues for the most part experienced in this field. The outcome is an accumulation of fifteen remarkable articles put together by agents. There is a push toward confirm based medication, which includes making utilization of every single clinical datum accessible and considering that into clinical and progressed examination. Catching and bringing the majority of the data about a patient together gives a more total view for understanding into mind coordination and results based repayment, populace wellbeing administration, and patient commitment and effort. Picking up this 360-degree perspective of the patient can likewise wipe out repetitive and costly testing, lessen blunders in regulating and recommending drugs, and even maintain a strategic distance from preventable passings. Likewise, it is surely critical that in the present human services condition, an unmistakable dominant part of the information created and in this way accessible for utilizes at least 75% of the information by a few assessments is unstructured information. It rises up out of sources like the quickly developing number of computerized gadgets and sensors, messages, specialists' and medical caretakers' notes, lab tests, and outsider sources outside the doctor's facility.

REFERENCES

Blake, M. (2015). An Internet of Things for Healthcare. *IEEE Internet Computing, 19*(4), 4–6. doi:10.1109/MIC.2015.89

Cai, S., Zhou, B., Liao, H., & Tan, C. (2017). Imaging Diagnosis of Chronic Encapsulated Intracerebral Hematoma, a Comparison of Computed Tomography (CT) and Magnetic Resonance Imaging (MRI) characteristics. *Polish Journal of Radiology / Polish Medical Society of Radiology, 82*, 578–582. doi:10.12659/PJR.902417 PMID:29662588

Chalmers, I., Altman, D., McHaffie, H., Owens, N., & Cooke, R. (2013). Data sharing among data monitoring committees and responsibilities to patients and science. *Trials, 14*(1), 102. doi:10.1186/1745-6215-14-102 PMID:23782486

Chung, H. (2017). Endoscopic Accessories Used for More Advanced Endoluminal Therapeutic Procedures. *Clinical Endoscopy, 50*(3), 234–241. doi:10.5946/ce.2017.079 PMID:28609821

Cresswell, K., & Sheikh, A. (2012). Electronic Health Record Technology. *Journal of the American Medical Association, 307*(21). doi:10.1001/jama.2012.3520 PMID:22706825

Cruz-Cunha, M., Simoes, R., Varajão, J., & Miranda, I. (2014). Information Technology Supporting Healthcare and Social Care Services. *Journal of Information Technology Research, 7*(1), 41–58. doi:10.4018/jitr.2014010104

Dalessandro, B., Perlich, C., & Raeder, T. (2014). Bigger is Better, but at What Cost?Estimating the Economic Value of Incremental Data Assets. *Big Data, 2*(2), 87–96. doi:10.1089/big.2014.0010 PMID:27442302

Fatt, Q., & Ramadas, A. (2018). The Usefulness and Challenges of Big Data in Healthcare. *Journal of Health Communication, 3*(2). doi:10.4172/2472-1654.100131

Fife, C., & Eckert, K. (2017). Harnessing electronic healthcare data for wound care research: Standards for reporting observational registry data obtained directly from electronic health records. *Wound Repair and Regeneration, 25*(2), 192–209. doi:10.1111/wrr.12523 PMID:28370796

Fromenteze, T., Decroze, C., Abid, S., & Yurduseven, O. (2018). Sparsity-Driven Reconstruction Technique for Microwave/Millimeter-Wave Computational Imaging. *Sensors (Basel)*, *18*(5), 1536. doi:10.339018051536 PMID:29757241

Gan, M., & Dai, H. (2014). Detecting and monitoring abrupt emergences and submergences of episodes over data streams. *Information Systems*, *39*, 277–289. doi:10.1016/j.is.2012.05.009

Hoskins, M. (2014). Common Big Data Challenges and How to Overcome Them. *Big Data*, *2*(3), 142–143. doi:10.1089/big.2014.0030 PMID:27442494

Juneja, P., & Kashyap, R. (2016). Optimal approach for CT image segmentation using improved energy based method. *International Journal of Control Theory and Applications*, *9*(41), 599–608.

Kashyap, R., & Gautam, P. (2015). Modified region based segmentation of medical images. In *International Conference on Communication Networks (ICCN)*. IEEE. 10.1109/ICCN.2015.41

Kashyap, R., & Gautam, P. (2016). Fast level set method for segmentation of medical images. In *Proceedings of the International Conference on Informatics and Analytics (ICIA-16)*. ACM. 10.1145/2980258.2980302

Kashyap, R., & Gautam, P. (2017). Fast Medical Image Segmentation Using Energy-Based Method. *Biometrics. Concepts, Methodologies, Tools, and Applications*, *3*(1), 1017–1042. doi:10.4018/978-1-5225-0983-7.ch040

Kashyap, R., Gautam, P., & Tiwari, V. (2018). Management and Monitoring Patterns and Future Scope. In Handbook of Research on Pattern Engineering System Development for Big Data Analytics. IGI Global. doi:10.4018/978-1-5225-3870-7.ch014

Kashyap, R., & Piersson, A. (2018a). *Impact of Big Data on Security. In Handbook of Research on Network Forensics and Analysis Techniques* (pp. 283–299). IGI Global. doi:10.4018/978-1-5225-4100-4.ch015

Kashyap, R., & Piersson, A. (2018b). Big Data Challenges and Solutions in the Medical Industries. In Handbook of Research on Pattern Engineering System Development for Big Data Analytics. IGI Global. doi:10.4018/978-1-5225-3870-7.ch001

Kashyap, R., & Tiwari, V. (2018). Active contours using global models for medical image segmentation. *International Journal of Computational Systems Engineering*, *4*(2/3), 195. doi:10.1504/IJCSYSE.2018.091404

Liu, W., Liang, W., & Xu, S. (2011). More information in imaging examination. *European Journal of Radiology*, *80*(2), 325. doi:10.1016/j.ejrad.2010.12.026 PMID:21255954

Manlhiot, C. (2018). Machine learning for predictive analytics in medicine: Real opportunity or overblown hype? *European Heart Journal Cardiovascular Imaging*, *19*(7), 727–728. doi:10.1093/ehjci/jey041 PMID:29538756

McPhail, G. (2017). Constructivism: Clearing up the confusion between a theory of learning and "constructing" knowledge. *Set: Research Information for Teachers*, (2), 30-22. doi:10.18296et.0081

Melin, P., & Sánchez, D. (2017). Multi-objective optimization for modular granular neural networks applied to pattern recognition. *Information Sciences*. doi:10.1016/j.ins.2017.09.031

Mi, H., Petitjean, C., Vera, P., & Ruan, S. (2015). Joint tumor growth prediction and tumor segmentation on therapeutic follow-up PET images. *Medical Image Analysis*, *23*(1), 84–91. doi:10.1016/j.media.2015.04.016 PMID:25988489

Miles-Tribble, V. (2017). Restorative justice as a public theology imperative. *Review & Expositor*, *114*(3), 366–379. doi:10.1177/0034637317721704

Mingle, R. (2017). Machine Learning Techniques on Microbiome -Based Diagnostics. *Advances In Biotechnology & Microbiology*, *6*(4). doi:10.19080/AIBM.2017.06.555695

Miyagi, T. (2009). Estimation of Inter-regional Trade Coefficients Using Nueral Network Models. *Studies In Regional Science*, *39*(3), 519–538. doi:10.2457rs.39.519

Mutula, S. (2009). Ethical, Legal, and Social Issues in Medical Informatics. Online Information Review, 33(5), 1009-1010. doi:10.1108/14684520911001981

Naimur Rahman, M., Esmailpour, A., & Zhao, J. (2016). Machine Learning with Big Data An Efficient Electricity Generation Forecasting System. *Big Data Research*, *5*, 9–15. doi:10.1016/j.bdr.2016.02.002

Palojoki, S., Pajunen, T., Saranto, K., & Lehtonen, L. (2016). Electronic Health Record-Related Safety Concerns: A Cross-Sectional Survey of Electronic Health Record Users. *JMIR Medical Informatics*, *4*(2), e13. doi:10.2196/medinform.5238 PMID:27154599

Phone, D. (2018). Proactive medicines management supports more patient centric services. *International Journal of Integrated Care*, *18*(s1), 31. doi:10.5334/ijic.s1031

Recio, M. (2017). Practitioner's Corner • Data Protection Officer: The Key Figure to Ensure Data Protection and Accountability. *European Data Protection Law Review*, *3*(1), 114–118. doi:10.21552/edpl/2017/1/18

Rey-del-Castillo, P., & Cardeñosa, J. (2016). An Exercise in Exploring Big Data for Producing Reliable Statistical Information. *Big Data*, *4*(2), 120–128. doi:10.1089/big.2015.0045 PMID:27441716

Ruan, G., & Zhang, H. (2017). Closed-loop Big Data Analysis with Visualization and Scalable Computing. *Big Data Research*, *8*, 12–26. doi:10.1016/j.bdr.2017.01.002

Skiera, B., & Ringel, D. (2017). Using Big Search Data to Map Your Market: Marketing in a Digital Age. *IESE Insight*, (32), 31-37. doi:10.15581/002.art-2982

Tian, Y., & Peng, Y. (2011). Study on Communication of Massive 3D Spatial Data Based on ACE. *Geo-Information Science*, *12*(6), 819–827. doi:10.3724/SP.J.1047.2010.00819

Waoo, N., Kashyap, R., & Jaiswal, A. (2010). DNA nano array analysis using hierarchical quality threshold clustering. In *2010 2nd IEEE International Conference on Information Management and Engineering*. IEEE. 10.1109/ICIME.2010.5477579

Zhu, H., Lee, Y., & Rosenthal, A. (2016). Data Standards Challenges for Interoperable and Quality Data. *Journal Of Data And Information Quality*, *7*(1-2), 1–3. doi:10.1145/2903723

KEY TERMS AND DEFINITIONS

DM: Data mining is the way toward finding designs in expansive informational indexes including techniques at the crossing point of machine learning, insights, and database systems. It is a basic procedure where canny strategies are connected to extricate information patterns. It is an interdisciplinary subfield of PC science. The general objective of the information mining process is to remove data from an informational collection and change it into a justifiable structure for assist use. Aside from the crude investigation step, it includes database and information administration viewpoints, information pre-preparing, model and derivation contemplations, intriguing quality measurements, many-sided quality contemplations, post-handling of found structures, representation, and online updating Data mining is the examination venture of the "learning disclosure in databases" process, or KDD.

EHR: An electronic human record (EHR), or electronic restorative record (EMR), is the systematized accumulation of patient and populace electronically-put away wellbeing data in an advanced format. These records can be shared crosswise over various human services settings. Records are shared through system associated, endeavor wide data frameworks or other data systems and trades. EHRs may incorporate a scope of information, including socioeconomics, therapeutic history, solution and hypersensitivities, vaccination status, research facility test comes about, radiology pictures, fundamental signs, individual measurements like age and weight, and charging information. EHR frameworks are intended to store information precisely and to catch the condition of a patient crosswise over time. It takes out the need to find a patient's past paper medicinal records and helps with guaranteeing information is precise and neat. It can lessen danger of information replication as there is just a single modifiable document, which implies the record is more probable forward, and diminishes danger of lost printed material. Because of the advanced data being accessible and in a solitary document, EMRs are more successful while extricating restorative information for the examination of conceivable patterns and long-haul changes in a patient. Populace based investigations of therapeutic records may likewise be encouraged by the across the board selection of EHRs and EMRs.

NLP: Natural language processing is a zone of software engineering and computerized reasoning worried about the connections amongst PCs and human (characteristic) dialects, specifically how to program PCs to productively process a lot of regular dialect information. Difficulties in common dialect preparing as often as possible include discourse acknowledgment, normal dialect comprehension, and regular dialect age.

Chapter 5
Deep Learning Models for Biomedical Image Analysis

Bo Ji
Nanjing Tech University Pujiang Institute, China

Wenlu Zhang
California State University – Long Beach, USA

Rongjian Li
KeyBank, USA

Hao Ji
California State Polytechnic University – Pomona, USA

ABSTRACT

Biomedical image analysis has become critically important to the public health and welfare. However, analyzing biomedical images is time-consuming and labor-intensive, and has long been performed manually by highly trained human experts. As a result, there has been an increasing interest in applying machine learning to automate biomedical image analysis. Recent progress in deep learning research has catalyzed the development of machine learning in learning discriminative features from data with minimum human intervention. Many deep learning models have been designed and achieved superior performance in various data analysis applications. This chapter starts with the basic of deep learning models and some practical strategies for handling biomedical image applications with limited data. After that, case studies of deep feature extraction for gene expression pattern image annotations, imaging data completion for brain disease diagnosis, and segmentation of infant brain tissue images are discussed to demonstrate the effectiveness of deep learning in biomedical image analysis.

DOI: 10.4018/978-1-5225-7467-5.ch005

INTRODUCTION

Biomedical image analysis is critically important to the public health and welfare. The advancements in imaging devices such as Computed Tomography (CT) scans, Magnetic Resonance Imaging (MRI), and X-ray, have made biomedical images readily available to the public for early diagnosis and medical treatment of diseases. On the other hand, analyzing biomedical images is a complex task that has long been performed manually by highly-trained experts such as radiologists and pathologists. This manual process is time-consuming and laborious which may involve wrong interpretation due to fatigue or stress in human experts. Hence, machine learning approaches have been used to assist in biomedical image analysis.

In machine learning, finding informative features for data representation is the key step in learning from data. Over the past several decades, task-specific features have been handcrafted by human experts based on their domain expertise and engineering skills. The barrier to designing appropriate features was generally high for non-experts in their own applications. Recent breakthroughs in deep learning research overcome this barrier by moving feature extraction from the human side to the computer side (LeCun et al., 2015; Goodfellow et al., 2016). Inspired by biological neural systems, deep learning models consist of deep neuromorphic processing layers to take into account both feature extraction and domain-specific learning at the same time. Thus deep learning is capable of obtaining a hierarchy of increasingly complex features directly from data with minimum human intervention, which greatly helps to achieve accurate models for various data analysis applications.

Regarding image-related tasks, Convolution Neural Network (CNN) is one particular architecture of deep learning. A typical CNN architecture incorporates convolutional layers and pooling layers to reduce the number of network parameters while learning from spatial image information. Motivated by the efficacy of the deep CNN architecture, many CNN-based deep learning models have been designed and achieved superior performance in image-related tasks. For example, (Krizhevsky et al., 2012) presented a CNN-based model (denoted as AlexNet) which won the ImageNet Large Scale Visual Recognition Challenge (ILSVRC) 2012 with a Top-5 test accuracy of 84.6% in its image classification task. It is worth noting that AlexNet significantly outperformed the 2nd place using the traditional bag of words approach with the accuracy of 73.8%. Later, (He et al., 2016) proposed a

CNN model (denoted as ResNet) achieved the accuracy of 96.43% which surpassed human-level performance on the same ImageNet data. The CNN architecture has now become a prominent approach to analyzing image data.

Although the deep CNN architecture has achieved remarkable results, training effective deep learning models usually requires a large number of training data samples. For example, the CNN models like AlexNet and ResNet were trained on the ImageNet dataset, which contains more than 14 million of natural images with 1,000 classes (Deng et al., 2009). However, biomedical image applications usually have very limited training data available in practice. To tackle this challenge, many practical strategies have been developed to facilitate the training process of deep learning models under small data, i.e., transfer learning, which transfers the knowledge learned from large-scale natural images to domain-specific tasks, and data augmentation, which enlarges the training dataset by performing geometric or photometric transformations on images.

In this chapter, we start with the basic of deep learning models and some training strategies for applications with limited data in Section 2. Section 3 presents some recent work that applies deep learning to biomedical image analysis, including deep feature extraction for gene expression pattern image annotations (Zhang et al., 2016), imaging data completion for brain disease diagnosis (Li et al., 2014), and segmentation of infant brain tissue images (Zhang et al., 2015). Finally, Section 4 summarizes the chapter.

THE BASIC OF DEEP LEARNING MODELS

Deep learning is a subset of the machine learning algorithms derived from neural networks. In this section, we review the basic of neural networks and one particular deep learning architecture, convolutional neural network. Transfer learning and data augmentation are discussed for training deep learning models in scenarios with insufficient data.

Neural Networks

Neural networks consist of multiple layers of neurons to constitute a cognitive function between the input signals and the associated targets (Bishop, 2006; Ji et al., 2015, 2016; Zhang et al., 2018). Figure 1 presents an N-layer neural network which has one input layer, $N - 1$ hidden layers, and one output layer.

Figure 1. An N-layer fully connected feed-forward neural network

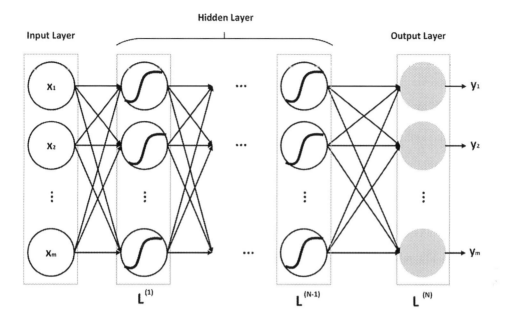

The leftmost layer is called the input layer which takes the input signals. The rightmost layer is called the output layer, where the generated output prediction is evaluated with the given targets to measure the prediction error. The intermediate layers between the input layer and the output layer are called the hidden layers, which transform the input signals and transmit to the output layer. In Figure 1, we use $L^{(i)}$ to denote the i th hidden layer, $L^{(N)}$ to be the output layer, and circles to indicate the input units and the neurons in the network. As each neuron is connected to every neuron in the next layer without going backward, this type of neural networks is also called a fully connected feed-forward neural network.

In neural networks, each neuron is the basic computational unit that receives a set of weighted signals from the neurons (or the inputs) in the previous layer and applies an activation function to generate a signal. In turn, the generated signal of the neuron is transmitted as an input signal to the connected neurons in the next layer. Figure 2 shows a single neuron in the first hidden layer as an example. Given an input vector x with m elements, the generated signal of a neuron $o(x)$ in the first hidden layer can be expressed as

Figure 2. A simple neuron model in the first hidden layer

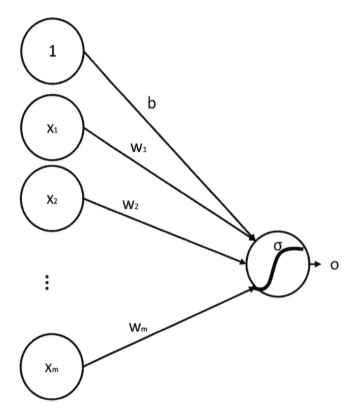

$$o\left(x\right) = \sigma\left(w^{T}x + b\right) = \sigma\left(\sum_{j=1}^{m} w_{j}x_{j} + b\right)$$

where $w = \left[w_{1}, w_{2}, \ldots, w_{m}\right]^{T}$ is the weight vector of weights (or parameters) associated with the connections to the input elements, b is the bias term associated with the neuron, and $\sigma\left(x\right)$ is an activation function. The activation functions such as tanh, sigmoid, and rectified linear unit (ReLU) are often used to introduce nonlinear behaviors into neurons. Note that the choice of the activation function for the rightmost output layer depends on the target task. For example, the linear activation function is often used in regression tasks, the sigmoid activation function is used in binary classification tasks, and the softmax activation function is performed in multi-class classification tasks.

Based on this basic neuron model, the computation performed by each layer of the general N-layer neural network can be formed, such that

$$o^{(1)} = \sigma\left(W^{(1)}x + b^{(1)}\right)$$

$$o^{(2)} = \sigma\left(W^{(2)}o^{(1)} + b^{(2)}\right)$$

$$\vdots$$

$$o^{(N)} = \sigma\left(W^{(N-1)}o^{(N-1)} + b^{(N-1)}\right)$$

where $o^{(i)}$ is a vector of the signals generated by the neurons in the ith hidden layer, $W^{(i)}$ is the weight matrix that stores the weights associated with the connections from the neurons of $(i-1)$th layer to that of the ith layer, and $b^{(i)}$ is the bias vector of biases associated with the neurons in the ith layer. Thus the N-layer neural network involves the parameter $\theta = \left(W^{(1)}, b^{(1)}, \ldots, W^{(N-1)}, b^{(N-1)}\right)$ to estimate a nonlinear mapping between the inputs and the given targets.

Theoretically, neural networks with at least one hidden layer have proven to be universal approximators to any nonlinear function (Cybenko, 1989). The goal of training a neural network is to find the optimal parameter values that minimize the prediction error between the neural network's predictions (the outputs) and the given targets. Let's take a multi-class classification as an example. Suppose the training dataset $\left\{\left(x^{(i)}, t^{(i)}\right)\right\}, i = 1 \ldots, n$, where $x^{(i)}$s and $t^{(i)}$s are the inputs and one-hot encoded targets, the following cross-entry loss function is often used to measure the prediction error,

$$\ell(\theta) = -\sum_{i=1}^{n}\sum_{j=1}^{m} t_j^{(i)} \log\left(y_j^{(i)}\right).$$

For simplicity, we let $y^{(i)}$ denote the neural network output vector for the data sample $x^{(i)}$, and the variables $y_j^{(i)}$ and $t_j^{(i)}$ denote the jth element of the output $y^{(i)}$ and the corresponding target $t^{(i)}$, respectively. To minimize the loss function, the gradient descent technique is often used to find a satisfactory parameter values (Goodfellow, et al., 2016; Bishop, 2006). Especially, as the negative gradient gives the direction where the loss function decreases most locally, the gradient descent technique optimizes the parameter values by using the following parameter update iteratively until a satisfactory accuracy is achieved,

$$\theta = \theta - \epsilon \nabla_\theta \ell \left(\theta \right)$$

where ϵ denotes learning rate and $\nabla_\theta \ell \left(\theta \right)$ the gradient vector. To be computationally efficient, the gradient vector $\nabla_\theta \ell \left(\theta \right)$ of the loss function with respect to the parameters is calculated via backpropagation in neural networks.

In deep learning, the depth of neural networks continues to increase to enhance its learning capability. However, the layers of the deep learning architecture can be roughly viewed as two function steps: feature extraction and domain-specific learning. The lower hidden layers function as a feature extractor to extract meaningful features to represent data, while higher hidden layers and the output layer use the explored features to make the prediction decision. Powered by this deep architecture, feature extraction and learning are trained together in the same model, which allows deep learning to learn a hierarchy of increasingly complex features directly from data and to achieve significant performance improvements in learning from data.

Convolutional Neural Networks

Fully connected neural networks have a huge number of parameters to be estimated. For example, given a simple 2-layer neural network with 1,000 neurons in each layer, this model has about a million of parameters due to connections between neurons. Convolution neural network (CNN), one particular architecture of deep learning, solves this problem by incorporating convolutional layers and pooling layers to dramatically reduce the number of network parameters.

Unlike a general fully connected neural network, the CNN architecture receives images as input and introduces local connections by applying convolution operation. Figure 3 takes the generation of neurons in the first

Figure 3. The first convolutional layer with multiple activation maps

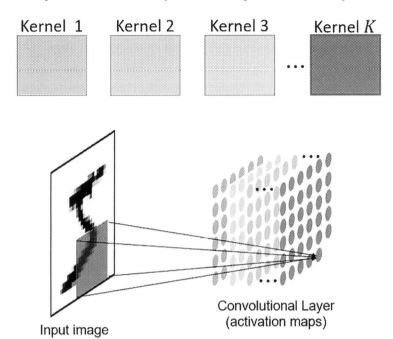

convolutional layer as an example. Given an image I and a convolution kernel F, the convolution operation is defined to work with a small area of pixels in the image I (Gonzalez, 2016), such that

$$G(i,j) = \sum_{u=-k}^{k} \sum_{v=-k}^{k} F(u,v) I(i-u, j-v)$$

where $G(i,j)$ denotes the signal generated by the neuron (i,j) in the first convolutional layer.

Each neuron in the convolutional layer is connected only to the neurons (or inputs in the input layer) located within a small rectangular area in the previous layer. By sliding the convolution kernel over the previous layers, it generates a 2D activation map of neurons within the convolution layer. Since the weights associated with the connections are stored in the convolution kernel, the neurons in one feature map are sharing the same parameters. Consequently, it helps to reduce the total number of network parameters in CNN models. More importantly, sliding behavior of convolution kernels

Figure 4. A max-pooling layer

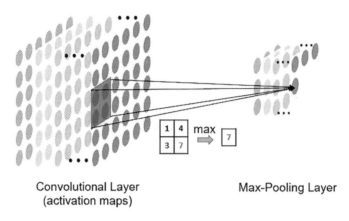

Convolutional Layer   Max-Pooling Layer
(activation maps)

enables the convolution layer to detect translation invariant feature patterns. When K kernels are applied, the convolutional layer has K activation maps at the same time, as shown in Figure 3.

A pooling layer is designed to subsample the activation maps of a convolutional layer and generate a new layer with new activation maps of smaller size. This is based on the observation that appropriate subsampling on the image pixels may not significantly alter the appearance of objects in images, but could help to reduce image size. In the CNN architecture, the pooling layer treats each activation map separately and uses a value to represent the neurons within each small rectangular area of the activation maps in the previous layer. There are many choices to determine the representative value to each small neighborhood. For example, Figure 4 shows the max-pooling layer which represents each small neighborhood of activation maps by using max value of its neuron signals.

Some Practical Strategies

Training a deep learning model usually requires a large number of data samples. However, labeled image data is very limited in many biomedical image applications. This challenge greatly limits the application of deep learning models to biomedical image analysis. In practice, transfer learning and data augmentation are often used to tackle this challenge.

Transfer Learning

Transfer learning is to build a new effective deep learning model on the basis of a pre-trained model that has been trained with millions of labeled natural images with thousands of categories (Bengio, 2012). Many state-of-the-art pre-trained models pertaining to general image classification tasks have been made available to the public, such as AlexNet (Krizhevsky, et al., 2012), VGG (Simonyan, et al., 2014), GoogLeNet (Szegedy, et al., 2015), and Resnet (He et al., 2016).

As aforementioned, the lower hidden layers tend to extract more features for data representation. Reusing lower hidden layers in a new model could help to explore meaningful features and reduce the number of data sample needed in the training process. While the upper hidden layers and the output layer are apt to domain-dependent, these layers are usually replaced by new custom layers, as shown in Figure 5. To train the new model, it is helpful to initialize the lower hidden layers by using the weights already learned from the pre-trained model instead of random ones, and then continuing the training process to fine-tune the weights for the target tasks.

Figure 5. A new deep learning model via transfer learning

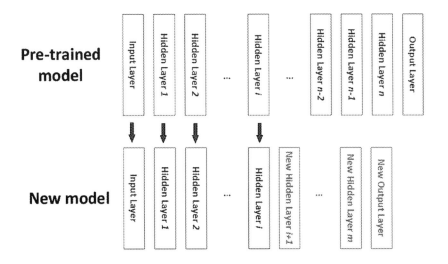

Figure 6. New training images examples generated via data augmentation

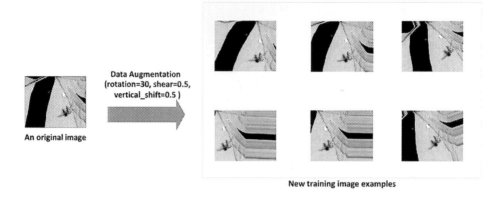

Data Augmentation

Data augmentation is to artificially enlarge the training dataset by applying geometric or photometric transformations on images (Krizhevsky et al., 2012). For example, geometric transforms such as flipping, rotation, shearing, and scaling, as well as crop operations are often used to generate new images to include shape variations of the real objects. Figure 6 shows some new training images created by applying rotation, shearing, and vertical shift to an original image. Additionally, photometric transforms are often used to generate new images by introducing changes to color, contrast, as well as random noise to the training images. With the enlarged new training data, it is expected that the trained deep learning model could achieve the enhanced generalization capability.

APPLICATION EXAMPLES OF DEEP LEARNING IN BIOMEDICAL IMAGE ANALYSIS

In this section, we present several application examples as case studies of applying deep learning models to biomedical image analysis. These case studies include deep feature extraction for gene expression pattern image annotations (Zhang et al., 2016), imaging data completion for brain disease diagnosis (Li et al., 2014), and segmentation of infant brain tissue images (Zhang et al., 2015).

Case Study 1: Deep Feature Extraction for Gene Expression Pattern Annotation

Problem Formulation

An important step in biomedical image analysis is extraction of appropriate feature for image representation. In this case study, we discuss the use of deep learning models in extracting the hierarchy of increasing level of abstraction features to achieve the performance improvements in Drosophila gene expression pattern annotation.

Table 1. Gene expression image examples and their associated controlled vocabularies in BDGP

Stages	Images	CV annotations
1-3		maternal
4-6		ubiquitous
7-8		trunk mesoderm PR vent nerve cord A ant endoderm A head mesoderm PR post endoderm PR ubiquitous
9-10		post endoderm PR procephalic ectoderm PR ubiquitous trunk mesoderm PR vent nerve cord PR P3 ant endoderm PR head mesoderm PR
11-12		ant midgut PR vent nerve cord PR post midgut PR brain PR
13-16		central brain glia vent nerve cord lateral cord glia brain central brain surface glia central nervous sys lateral cord neuron gonad cat_term:any_neural central brain neuron

(Retrieved from http://insitu.fruitfly.org/cgi-bin/ex/report.pl?ftype=3&ftext=LD38718-dg)

The Drosophila melanogaster, a species of fly in the family of Drosophila, has been widely used to study the spatiotemporal gene expression patterns during Drosophila embryogenesis. To facilitate this analysis, the Berkeley Drosophila Genome Project (BDGP) has collected sets of gene expression pattern images of Drosophila melanogaster (Stapleton et. al., 2002, Tomancak et. al., 2002, 2007). These images are categorized into six groups such as stage 1-3, stage 4-6, stage 7-8, stage 9-10, stage 11-12, and stage 13-16, based on the different development stages of the embryogenesis of Drosophila. Each gene expression image is manually annotated using controlled vocabularies (CVs) to identify its anatomical structures in embryogenesis. Table 1 shows an example of gene expression groups and the associated controlled vocabulary annotations.

The process of manual annotation to gene expression images is time-consuming. As the number of available gene expression images is increasing year-by-year, it is imperative to develop an automated annotation approach to gene expression images. Prior studies employed traditional computer vision techniques with hand-crafted features to accomplish this task. However, since Drosophila gene expression patterns exhibit high variation in size, shape, and position, hand-crafted features appear to be insufficient for recognizing all kinds of patterns in gene expression images. To develop more accurate annotation, there is a growing interest in applying deep CNN models to automatically learn discriminative features from Drosophila gene expression pattern images.

Figure 7. A CNN model based on transfer learning
(Zhang et. al., 2016)

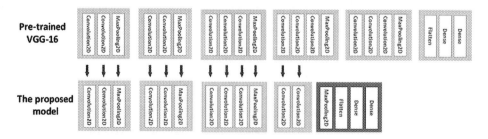

Deep Models

To extract informative features from the limited Drosophila gene expression pattern images, (Zhang et. al., 2016) proposed a deep learning model by applying transfer learning technique to the pre-trained VGG-16 model, as shown in Figure 7.

In particular, the proposed new CNN model was created by truncating the pre-trained VGG-16 model and stacking one new max pooling layer and two fully connected layers. Then, the weights of this CNN model were fine-tuned with the labeled gene expression images from BDGP. Since each gene expression image may have different controlled vocabulary annotations, the following loss function was designed to perform multi-task learning.

$$loss\left(y,\hat{y}\right) = -\sum\sum\left(y_i^j \log f\left(\hat{y}_i^j\right) + \left(1 - y_i^j\right)\log\left(1 - f\left(\hat{y}_i^j\right)\right)\right)$$

where

$$y_i^j = \begin{cases} 1 & \textit{if the ith training example is annotated with the jth CV term} \\ 0 & \textit{otherwise} \end{cases}$$

It is worth noting that in order to identify the most informative features, (Zhang et. al., 2016) evaluated several different CNN models using the

Table 2. Comparisons between the proposed deep learning model and sparse coding method

	The Proposed Deep Learning Model		Traditional Sparse Coding Method	
	Accuracy	AUC	Accuracy	AUC
Stage 4-6	0.8197±0.0279	0.8607±0.0415	0.7217±0.0352	0.7687±0.0432
Stage 7-8	0.8471±0.0225	0.8671±0.0341	0.7401±0.0351	0.7834±0.0358
Stage 9-10	0.8307±0.0291	0.8736±0.0302	0.7549±0.0303	0.7921±0.0294
Stage 11-12	0.8099±0.0318	0.8913±0.0246	0.7659±0.0326	0.8061±0.0342
Stage 13-16	0.8591±0.0301	0.8972±0.0231	0.7681±0.0231	0.8105±0.0280

(Zhang et. al., 2016)

features learned from the lower hidden layers 17, 21, 24, and 30 and found that the layer 21 outperformed all other layers. Moreover, as the Drosophila gene expression pattern images dataset is highly imbalanced with much more negative samples than the positive ones, subsampling on the majority class was carried out (Sun et. al., 2013; Zhang et. al., 2016) to obtain the same number of samples as the minority class. After that, classifier ensembles based on majority voting was further performed to determine the final prediction. For more details on this deep models, we refer to (Zhang et. al., 2016).

Results

Table 2 showed the experimental comparison between the proposed deep learning model and the prior work based on sparse coding image representation method (Sun et al., 2013), in terms of accuracy and area under the ROC curve (AUC). One could find that the deep features generated by deep learning model achieved significantly higher accuracy and AUC than the traditional method by using sparse coding in all cases.

Case Study 2: Imaging Data Completion for Brain Disease Diagnosis

Problem Formulation

Alzheimer's disease (AD) is a common brain disorder that is still unsolved. Advances in neuroimaging techniques, magnetic resonance imaging (MRI) and positron emission tomography (PET), have made possible early detection and intervention at its prodromal stage, such as the mild cognitive impairment (MCI) stage, which greatly helps to delay the onset of AD. However, the neuroimaging data often contain incomplete data modalities. Completing data modality in neuroimaging data could lead to significant improvements in disease diagnosis accuracy. In this case study, we discuss the use of deep learning models in completing and integrating multi-modality neuroimaging data.

Deep Models

The data modalities of MRI images and PET images from Alzheimer's Disease Neuroimaging Initiative (ADNI) database are 3D format (Mueller et al.,

Figure 8. The proposed CNN model for 3D imaging data completion
(Li et. al., 2014)

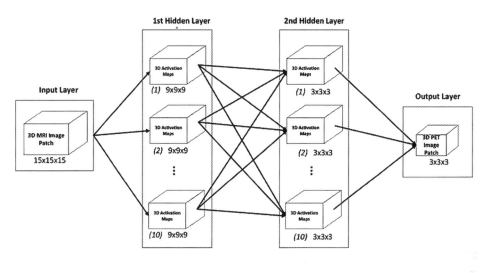

2005). To learn the nonlinear relationship between MRI image patches and PET image patches, (Li et al., 2014) presented a 3-dimensional (3-D) CNN model which uses an MRI data modality patch of $15 \times 15 \times 15$ as input and PET data modality patch of $3 \times 3 \times 3$ volumetric data modality as the output. Being trained in an end-to-end manner, the proposed model allows to predict and estimate the output data modality given any input modality. Figure 8 illustrates the proposed 3D CNN model.

The proposed 3D CNN model has two hidden convolutional layers. Similar to the CNN models presented in Section 2.2, the convolutional layer are generated via convolution operations but working with 3-D formatted kernels. Each hidden layer contains ten 3D activation maps. Let v_{ij}^{xyz} denote the value

Table 3. Comparisons between Ground Truth, KNN method, Zero method, and the proposed 3-D CNN model

Classification Tasks		MCI vs. NC	pMCI vs. sMCI	AD vs. NC
PET	Ground Truth	0.7014±0.0212	0.6823±0.0241	0.8982±0.0224
	3-D CNN Model	0.6947±0.0281	0.6804±0.0267	0.8868±0.0208
	KNN Method	0.6304±0.0248	0.6278±0.0326	0.7421±0.0282
	Zero Method	0.6175±0.0213	0.6124±0.0243	0.6928±0.0225

(Li et. al., 2014)

at position (x, y, z) on the jth activation map in the ith layer. The signal generated by a neuron in the resulting 3-D convolution can be expressed as

$$v_{ij}^{xyz} = \sigma\left(b_{ij} + \sum_{m}\sum_{p=0}^{P_i-1}\sum_{q=0}^{Q_i-1}\sum_{r=0}^{R_i-1} w_{ij}^{pqr} v_{(i-1)m}^{(x+p)(y+q)(z+r)}\right)$$

where $\sigma(.)$ denotes the activation function, b_{ij} is the bias associated with each neuron, m is the index of feature maps in the $(i-1)$th layer connected to the current feature map, P_i, Q_i and R_i are the dimensions of the 3-D kernel, respectively, and w_{ij}^{pqr} denotes the weight value located at (p, q, r) in the mth activation map. For more details on this deep models, we refer to (Li et. al., 2014).

Results

Table 3 showed the experimental comparison between the proposed 3-D CNN model, K-Nearest Neighbors (KNN) method, and Zero method (Yuan et. al, 2012) in completing PET data for the three classification tasks, i.e., MCI vs NC, pMCI vs. sMCI, and AD. The ground truth of PET data is also presented. One can find that the predictions by 3-D CNN model outperformed the KNN model and Zero method significantly in all three classification tasks, which demonstrates that the deep learning model is able to extract the complex, nonlinear relationship between the MRI and PET images. We also

Figure 9. The proposed CNN model for patch-based image segmentation (Zhang et. al., 2015).

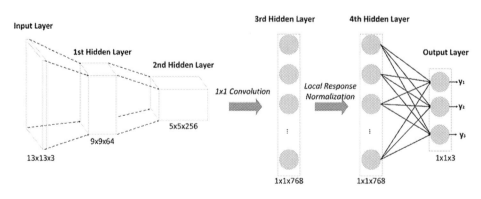

Table 4. Comparisons between the proposed CNN model, Random Forest, and Support Vector Machine

	The Proposed CNN Model	**Random Forest**	**Support Vector Machine**
CSF	0.8323	0.8192	0.7409
GM	0.8531	0.8288	0.7933
WM	0.8798	0.8612	0.8172

(Zhang et al., 2015).

can observe that the prediction of the 3-D CNN model is comparable with those of the ground truth of PET images.

Case Study 3: Segmentation of Infant Brain Tissue Images

Problem Formulation

The segmentation of White Matter (WM), Gray Matter (GM), and Cerebrospinal Fluid (CSF) in infant brain tissues plays an important role in studying early brain development in health and disease. In the isointense stage (approximately 6-8 months of age), WM and GM show similar levels of intensity in both T1 and T2 MR Images. It is still very challenging to accurate segment tissues. In this case study, we discuss the use of deep learning models in segmenting isointense stage brain tissues based on multi-modality MR images.

Deep Models

(Zhang et al., 2015) proposed a new CNN model to segment infant brains tissues by taking into account multi-modality T1, T2 and FA images simultaneously. Figure 9 showed the proposed CNN model, which contains three input feature maps corresponding to T1, T2, and FA image in patches of 13×13, followed by three convolutional layers and one fully connected layer. Note that the local response normalization was designed to enhance features correlations at the same spatial location across different activation maps. Moreover, (Zhang et al., 2015) also evaluated three other CNN models with input patch sizes of 9×9, 17×17, and 22×22. These CNN models consist of different numbers of convolutional layers and feature maps. For more details on this deep models, we refer to (Zhang et al., 2015).

Results

Table 4 showed the experimental comparison between the proposed CNN models, Random Forest, and Support Vector Machine (Zhang et al., 2015) for three different tissue types, i.e., CSF, GM, and WM. The segmentation performance is measured by the Dice Ratio (DR), and a larger Dice Ratio value indicates a higher segmentation accuracy. One can find that the proposed CNN model outperformed the two traditional approaches in all the three tissue types.

SUMMARY

Deep learning models have become powerful tools used in biomedical image analysis. We review the basic of deep learning models and some training strategies to handle applications with limited data. Some application examples of using deep learning to biomedical image analysis are presented as case studies, including deep feature extraction for gene expression pattern image annotations (Zhang et al., 2016), imaging data completion for brain disease diagnosis (Li et al., 2014), and segmentation of infant brain tissue images (Zhang et al., 2015).

REFERENCES

Bengio, Y. (2012, June). Deep learning of representations for unsupervised and transfer learning. In *Proceedings of ICML Workshop on Unsupervised and Transfer Learning* (pp. 17-36). Academic Press.

Bishop, C. M. (2006). *Pattern recognition and machine learning*. Springer.

Cybenko, G. (1989). Approximation by superpositions of a sigmoidal function. *Mathematics of Control, Signals, and Systems, 2*(4), 303–314. doi:10.1007/BF02551274

Deng, J., Dong, W., Socher, R., Li, L. J., Li, K., & Fei-Fei, L. (2009, June). Imagenet: A large-scale hierarchical image database. In *Computer Vision and Pattern Recognition, 2009. CVPR 2009. IEEE Conference on* (pp. 248-255). IEEE. 10.1109/CVPR.2009.5206848

Gonzalez, R. C. (2016). *Digital image processing*. Pearson.

Goodfellow, I., Bengio, Y., Courville, A., & Bengio, Y. (2016). *Deep learning* (Vol. 1). Cambridge, MA: MIT Press.

He, K., Zhang, X., Ren, S., & Sun, J. (2016). Deep residual learning for image recognition. In *Proceedings of the IEEE conference on computer vision and pattern recognition* (pp. 770-778). IEEE.

Ji, H., O'saben, E., Boudion, A., & Li, Y. (2015). March madness prediction: A matrix completion approach. *Proceedings of Modeling, Simulation, and Visualization Student Capstone Conference.*

Ji, H., O'Saben, E., Lambi, R., & Li, Y. (2016). Matrix completion based model V2. 0: Predicting the winning probabilities of march madness matches. *Proceedings of Modeling, Simulation, and Visualization Student Capstone Conference.*

Krizhevsky, A., Sutskever, I., & Hinton, G. E. (2012). Imagenet classification with deep convolutional neural networks. In Advances in neural information processing systems (pp. 1097-1105). Academic Press.

LeCun, Y., Bengio, Y., & Hinton, G. (2015). Deep learning. *Nature, 521*(7553), 436.

Li, R., Zhang, W., Suk, H. I., Wang, L., Li, J., Shen, D., & Ji, S. (2014, September). Deep learning based imaging data completion for improved brain disease diagnosis. In *International Conference on Medical Image Computing and Computer-Assisted Intervention* (pp. 305-312). Springer. 10.1007/978-3-319-10443-0_39

Mueller, S. G., Weiner, M. W., Thal, L. J., Petersen, R. C., Jack, C., Jagust, W., ... Beckett, L. (2005). The Alzheimer's disease neuroimaging initiative. *Neuroimaging Clinics, 15*(4), 869–877. doi:10.1016/j.nic.2005.09.008 PMID:16443497

Simonyan, K., & Zisserman, A. (2014). *Very deep convolutional networks for large-scale image recognition.* arXiv preprint arXiv:1409.1556.

Stapleton, M., Liao, G., Brokstein, P., Hong, L., Carninci, P., Shiraki, T., ... Yu, C. (2002). The Drosophila gene collection: Identification of putative full-length cDNAs for 70% of D. melanogaster genes. *Genome Research, 12*(8), 1294–1300. doi:10.1101/gr.269102 PMID:12176937

Sun, Q., Muckatira, S., Yuan, L., Ji, S., Newfeld, S., Kumar, S., & Ye, J. (2013). Image-level and group-level models for Drosophila gene expression pattern annotation. *BMC Bioinformatics, 14*(1), 350. doi:10.1186/1471-2105-14-350 PMID:24299119

Szegedy, C., Liu, W., Jia, Y., Sermanet, P., Reed, S., Anguelov, D., ... Rabinovich, A. (2015, June). *Going deeper with convolutions.* CVPR.

Tomancak, P., Beaton, A., Weiszmann, R., Kwan, E., Shu, S., Lewis, S. E., ... Rubin, G. M. (2002). Systematic determination of patterns of gene expression during Drosophila embryogenesis. *Genome Biology, 3*(12).

Tomancak, P., Berman, B. P., Beaton, A., Weiszmann, R., Kwan, E., Hartenstein, V., ... Rubin, G. M. (2007). Global analysis of patterns of gene expression during Drosophila embryogenesis. *Genome Biology, 8*(7), R145. doi:10.1186/gb-2007-8-7-r145 PMID:17645804

Yuan, L., Wang, Y., Thompson, P. M., Narayan, V. A., & Ye, J. (2012). Multi-source feature learning for joint analysis of incomplete multiple heterogeneous neuroimaging data. *NeuroImage, 61*(3), 622–632. doi:10.1016/j.neuroimage.2012.03.059 PMID:22498655

Zhang, L., Saleh, I., Thapaliya, S., Louie, J., Figueroa-Hernandez, J., & Ji, H. (2018). An Empirical Evaluation of Machine Learning Approaches for Species Identification through Bioacoustics. *Proceedings of the 2017 International Conference on Computational Science and Computational Intelligence.*

Zhang, W., Li, R., Deng, H., Wang, L., Lin, W., Ji, S., & Shen, D. (2015). Deep convolutional neural networks for multi-modality isointense infant brain image segmentation. *NeuroImage, 108*, 214–224. doi:10.1016/j.neuroimage.2014.12.061 PMID:25562829

Zhang, W., Li, R., Zeng, T., Sun, Q., Kumar, S., Ye, J., & Ji, S. (2016). *Deep model based transfer and multi-task learning for biological image analysis. IEEE Transactions on Big Data.* doi:10.1109/TBDATA.2016.2573280

Chapter 6

Development of a Classification Model for CD4 Count of HIV Patients Using Supervised Machine Learning Algorithms:
A Comparative Analysis

Peter Adebayo Idowu

(iD) https://orcid.org/0000-0002-3883-3310
Obafemi Awolowo University, Nigeria

Jeremiah Ademola Balogun
Obafemi Awolowo University, Nigeria

ABSTRACT

This chapter was developed with a view to present a predictive model for the classification of the level of CD4 count of HIV patients receiving ART/HAART treatment in Nigeria. Following the review of literature, the pre-determining factors for determining CD4 count were identified and validated by experts while historical data explaining the relationship between the factors and CD4 count level was collected. The predictive model for CD4 count level was formulated using C4.5 decision trees (DT), support vector machines (SVM), and the multi-layer perceptron (MLP) classifiers based on the identified factors which were formulated using WEKA software and validated. The results showed that decision trees algorithm revealed five (5) important variables, namely age group, white blood cell count, viral load, time of diagnosing HIV, and age of the patient. The MLP had the best performance with a value of 100% followed by the SVM with an accuracy of 91.1%, and both were observed to outperform the DT algorithm used.

DOI: 10.4018/978-1-5225-7467-5.ch006

INTRODUCTION

HIV is a human immunodeficiency virus. It is the virus that can lead to acquired immunodeficiency syndrome or AIDS if not treated (Lakshmi and Isakki, 2017). HIV is spread primarily by unprotected sex, contaminated blood transmission, hypodermic, and from mother during pregnancy, delivery, or breastfeeding. HIV attacks the body's immune system, specifically the CD4 cells (T cells), a type of white blood cell, which help the immune system fight off infections. Untreated, HIV reduces the number of CD4 cells (T cells) in the body, making the person more likely to get other infections or infection-related cancers. Anti-retro viral treatment is one of the best treatment for HIV patients. Anti-retroviral treatment can slow the course of the disease, and may lead to a near-normal life expectancy (Kama and Prem, 2013).

There is no cure for HIV but it is being managed with antiretroviral drugs (ARV) and Highly Active Antiretroviral drugs (HAART) which is the optimal combination of ARV (Rosma et al., 2012). ARV does not kill the virus but slow down the growth of the virus (Ojunga *et al.*, 2014). Antiretroviral therapy (ART) and highly antiretroviral therapy (HAART) are the mechanisms for treating retroviral infections with drugs. (Brain *et al.*, 2006). Monitoring of the progression of the disease is made even more important due to the emergence of HIV drug resistance, especially in developing countries with limited resource. HIV drug resistance refers to the inability of the ARV drug to reduce the viral reproduction rate sufficiently. Poor management of HIV drug resistance will lead to opportunistic infections that make treatment of HIV more difficult and even may lead to fatalities.

Common clinical markers of disease progression are weight loss, mucocutaneous manifestations, bacterial infections, chronic fever, chronic diarrhea, herpes zoster, oral candidiasis, and pulmonary tuberculosis (Morgan et al., 2002). One of the best available surrogate markers for HIV progression is the use of CD4 cell count information (Post *et al.*, 1996). Although this is also standard of care in developing countries, the measurement of CD4 cell count requires many complex and expensive flow cytometric procedures which burden the minimal resources available. There have been previous attempts to predict CD4 cell count information using cheaper chemical assays and even correlating a patient's total lymphocyte count (TLC) with CD4 cell counts using logistic and linear regression (Schechter *et al.,* 1994; Mwamburi *et al.*, 2005).

The CD4 cell count remains the strongest predictor of HIV related complications, even after the initiation of therapy. The baseline pretreatment value is informative: lower CD4 counts are associated with smaller and slower improvements in counts. However, precise thresholds that define treatment failure in patients starting at various CD4 levels are not yet established. As a general rule, new and progressive severe immunodeficiency is demonstrated by declining longitudinal CD4 cell counts which should trigger a switch in therapy. Another problem associated with CD4 count is, frequent failure happening on the CD4 counting machine which creates a great challenge in taking CD4 counts regularly in the scheduled time.

Machine learning algorithms provide a means of obtaining objective unseen patterns from evidence-based information especially in the public health care sector. These techniques have allowed for not only substantial improvements to existing clinical decision support systems, but also a platform for improved patient-centered outcomes through the development of personalized prediction models tailored to a patient's medical history and current condition (Moudani *et al.*, 2011a). Predictive research aims at predicting future events or an outcome based on patterns within a set of variables and has become increasingly popular in medical research (Olayemi *et al.*, 2016). Accurate predictive models can inform patients and physicians about the future course of an illness or the risk of developing illness and thereby help guide decisions on screening and/or treatment (Waijee *et al.*, 2013).

The aim of this study is to apply machine learning to the identification of the relevant variables that are important for developing a predictive model for the classification of the level of CD4 count. The model will provide decision support to healthcare providers regarding alternate therapy to patients thereby improving HIV survival. There is a need for the development of a predictive model for the classification of the CD4 count of HIV patients receiving ART treatment using machine learning techniques needed for providing clinical decision support and improving the survival of HIV patients receiving ART treatment.

RELATED WORKS

Singh *et al.* (2013) applied machine learning algorithms to the prediction of patient-specific current CD4 cell count in order to determine the progression of human immunodeficiency virus (HIV) infections. This work shows the application of machine learning to predict current CD4 cell count of an HIV-positive patient using genome sequences, viral load and time. A regression model predicting actual CD4 cell counts and a classification model predicting if a patient's CD4 cell count is less than 200 was built using a support vector machine and neural network. The most accurate regression and classification model took as input the viral load, time, and genome and produced a correlation of co-efficient of 0.9 and an accuracy of 95%, respectively, proving that a CD4 cell count measure may be accurately predicted using machine learning on genotype, viral load and time.

Ojunga *et al.* (2014) applied logistic regression in modeling of survival chances of HIV -positive patients on highly active antiretroviral therapy (HAART) in Nyakach District, Kenya. The aim of this study was to outline the various social and economic factors affecting survival of HIV patients on highly active antiretroviral therapy (HAART). The study was expected to provide suitable model for predicting the chances of survival among the HIV positive patients attending ART clinic in Nyakachi District and also provide information for policy makers on the factors affecting survival of HIV positive individual on ARV drugs. The strength shows that the survival of infected patient under study can be improved if their access to socio-economic factors is considered. The outcome may only be obtained in services that have smaller numbers of patients. Socioeconomic factors are not enough to predict survival as CD4, viral load; opportunistic infections and nutritional status were added to the existing study in this thesis as predictive factors.

Idowu *et al.* (2016) developed a predictive model for the survival of HIV/AIDS in pediatric patients in Nigeria. The study identified survival variables for HIV/AIDS Peadiatric patients, developed predictive model for determining the survival of the patients who were receiving antiretroviral drug in the Southwestern Nigeria based on identified variables, compared and validate the developed model. Interviews were conducted with the virologists and Pediatricians at two health institutions from the study area in order to identify survival variables for HIV/AIDS Peadiatric patients. 216 Peadiatric HIV/AIDS patients' data were also collected, preprocessed and the 10-fold cross validation technique was used to partition the datasets into training and testing data. Predictive model was developed using supervised learning technique and WEKA was used to simulate the models in which CD4 count, Viral Load, Opportunistic infections and Nutritional status were used as the independent variables for the prediction. The result showed that The Multi-layer Perception (MLP) was suitable for carrying out the task of forecasting the survival of Peadiatric HIV/AIDS patients with an accuracy of 99.07%. Additional study involved the use of naïve Bayes' classifier

(Idowu *et al.*, 2017a) and C4.5 decision trees classifier (Idowu *et al.*, 2017b) for the development of a predictive model for the survival of HIV/AIDS among pediatrics. However, the study by Idowu *et al.* (2017b) revealed that the variables viral load and CD4 count were redundant and recommended instead of using both variables only one of them should be used for classifying survival of HIV/AIDS among pediatrics.

Tarekegn and Sreenivasaro (2016) applied data mining techniques on Pre ART data. The dataset for the study contains pre ART records of the year 2005 and 2006 produced by the ART office of patients Felege Hiwot Referral Hospital. The dataset has been utilized for the purpose of predicting clients' eligibility for ART. Before these data has been used for the purpose of classification a number of pre-processing steps such as data cleaning, data reduction and data transformation have been effectively used which helped in achieving the objective finally or to increase the speed and efficiency of mining process. The final goal of this paper is to build ART eligibility predictive model that helps to deciding whether HIV positive individual should start Anti-retroviral treatment or not. For building ART eligibility predictive model, Naive Bayesian Classifier and J48 Decision Tree Classifier are used. After experimenting J48 decision tree and Naive Bayesian classifier using both 10-fold cross validation and percentage split (66%) test modes, J48 classifier using 10-fold cross validation (95.83%) that performs well and can be used as a best predicting model algorithm than Naive Bayesian classifier (93.64%%) in predicting clients' eligibility for ART was created.

Lakshmi and Isakki (2017) performed a comparative study of data mining classification techniques using HIV/AIDS and STD data. The performance of classifiers is actively dependent on the data set used for learning. It leads to better performance of the classification models in terms of their predictive or descriptive accuracy and computing time needed to build models as they learn faster and better understanding of the models. The paper performed a comparative analysis of data mining, classification techniques, Decision Tree, Support Vector Machine (SVM), and Naïve Bayes' Classification algorithms. The total of 800 medical data set having many attributes with Boolean value in addition to age and sex. The proposed algorithm uses four data sets called – Symptoms, Virus type, Cd4 count type of white blood cell and STD cell for Chlamydia count. There are numerical values allocated to each cell count and severe. The aim is to classify the diseases and predict the presence of HIV infection. The decision trees algorithm outperformed SVM and naïve Bayes classification with an accuracy of 90.07% compared to 77.5% and 85.05% for naïve Bayes and SVM respectively.

METHODS

The methodological approach of this study composes of a number of methods, namely: the identification of the required variables for CD4 count classification, the collection of historical datasets about CD4 count measures, formulation of the predictive models using the supervised machine learning algorithms proposed, the simulation of the predictive models using the WEKA simulation environment and the performance evaluation metrics applied during model validation for the evaluation of the performance of the predictive models. The model for the classification of CD4 count was formulated using decision trees, support vector machines and multi-layer perceptron algorithms with their performance compared.

Data Identification and Collection

For the purpose of this study, data was collected following the identification of the factors for determining CD4 count level from 45 patients located in the south-western part of Nigeria using structured questionnaires that consisted of two (2) main sections, namely: demographic section which included: gender, age, ethnicity, religion, educational qualification, occupation, weight, height and body mass index (BMI) while the clinical factors for determining CD4, namely: date of HIV diagnosis, baseline CD4 count measure, time since baseline CD4 count, opportunistic infection, total lymphocyte count, patient on ART, patient HAART, white blood cell count, level of hematocrit, platelets level, viral load, last recorded CD4 count level and the time since the last CD4 count level. The information collected consisted of the variables used to identify the CD4 count level risk factors associated with the osteoporosis for each patient as proposed by the medical expert. The variables that were identified following the review of related works regarding the CD4 count level are stated in Table 1.

Data-Preprocessing

Following the collection of data from the 45 patients alongside the attributes (22 factors in all) alongside the CD4 count level, the data collected was checked for the presence of error in data entry including misspellings and missing data. Following this process, there was no error in misspellings nor missing data in the cells describing the records for the identified factors. The

Table 1. Identified variables for the classification of CD4 count level

Categories	Risk Factors	Labels
Demographic Factors	Gender	Male, Female
	Age (years)	Numeric
	Age Group	Youth, Adult, Aged, Teenager
	Ethnicity	Yoruba, Hausa, Ibo, Idoma
	Religion	Christian, Islam, Traditional
	Education	Primary, Secondary, Polytechnic, University
	Occupation	Nil, Trader, Teacher, Artisan, Student, Clerical
	Weight (Kg)	Numeric
	Height (m)	Numeric
	Body Mass Index (Kg/m)	Numeric
	BMI Class	Normal, Underweight, Overweight, Obese
Clinical Factors	Time of HIV Diagnosis	Numeric
	Baseline CD4 count	Numeric
	Time of Baseline count	Numeric
	Opportunistic Infection	Protozoa, Typhoid, Nil, Virus, Malaria, Bacteria, Gonorrhea, Ulcer, Asthma, Fungi
	Total Lymphocyte count	Numeric
	On ART Treatment	Yes, No
	On HAART	Yes, No
	White Blood Cell Count	Numeric
	Hematocrit Level	Numeric
	Platelets Level	Numeric
	Viral Load	Numeric
	Last recorded CD4 count	Numeric
	Time since last CD$ count	Numeric
Target	CD4 Count Level	Low, Moderate, High

data was stored in an .arff file format, the most acceptable file format for the simulation environment chosen for this study. The arff file is composed of three parts, namely:

1. The relation name section which contains the tag @relation CD4CountTrainingData, used to identify the name of the relation (or file) that contains the data needed for simulation. This section is located at the first line of the file and the tag 'name' following @relation must

always be the same as the file name else the file loader of the simulation environment will cease to open the file. This section is followed in the next line by the attribute names section;

2.   The attribute names section which contains the tag @attribute attribute_ name label was used to identify the attributes that describe the dataset stored in the .arff file needed for simulation. Each attribute name alongside its labels is stated following the @relation tag on each line. The label can be a set of values inserted between brackets or a descriptor (e.g. date, numeric etc.). The last attribute is identified as the target class (CD4 count class) while the previous attributes are the input variables. This section is followed in the next line by the data section; and

3.   The data section which contains the tag @data followed in the next line by the values of the attributes for each record of the HIV patients collected separated by a comma. Each value was listed on a row for each record in the same order as the attributes were listed in the attribute names section. The values inserted into each record must be the same values defined in each respective attribute; if there is an error in spelling or a label not defined is inserted then the file loader of the simulation environment will fail to load the file.

The dataset collected for the purpose of the development of the predictive model for the quality of service was stored in .arff in the name CD4CountTrainingData.arff while the number of attributes listed in the attribute section were 23 including the target attribute. Following this, the values of the input variables for the record of the 45 records recorded form the sites for this study was provided.

Model Formulation

Following the identification and validation of variables relevant to the CD4 count level in HIV patients and the collection of historical explaining the relationship between the identified risk factors and their respective class for each record of individuals, the predictive model for the CD4 count level in HIV patients was formulated using the decision trees algorithm, support vector machines and artificial neural networks. Supervised machine learning algorithms make it possible to assign a set of records (CD4 count indicators) to a target class – the CD4 count level. Equation 1 shows the mapping function that describes the relationship between the risk factors and the target class – CD4 count level.

$$\varphi : X \rightarrow Y \tag{1}$$

defined as: $\varphi(X) = Y$

The equation shows the relationship between the set of identified factors represented by a vector, X consisting of the values of i factors and the label Y which defines the CD4 count level – low, moderate and high level as expressed in equation 3.2. Assuming the values of the set of risk factors for an individual is represented as $X = \{X_1, X_2, X_3, \ldots\ldots, X_i\}$ where X_i is the value of each risk factor, i = 1 to i; then the mapping φ used to represent the predictive model for osteoporosis risk maps the identified factors of each individual to their respective CD4 count level according to equation 2.

$$\varphi(X) = \begin{cases} Low\ Level \\ Moderate\ Level \\ High\ Level \end{cases} \tag{2}$$

Decision Trees Algorithm

The theory of a decision tree has the following parts: a root node is the starting point of the tree; branches connect nodes showing the flow from question to answer. Nodes that have child nodes are called interior nodes. Leaf or terminal nodes are nodes that do not have child nodes and represent a possible value of target variable given the variables represented by the path from the root. The rules are inducted by definition from each respective node to branch to leaf. Given a set X_{ij} of j number of cases, the decision trees algorithm grows an initial tree using the divide-and-conquer algorithm as follows:

- If all the cases in X_{ij} belong to the same class or X_{ij} is small, the tree is a leaf labeled with the most frequent class in X_{ij}.

- Otherwise, choose a test based on a single attribute X_i with two or more outcomes. Make this test the root of the tree with one branch for each outcome of the test, partition X_{ij} into corresponding subsets according to the outcome for each case, and apply the same procedure recursively to each subset.

The C4.5 decision trees algorithm builds decision trees from a set of training dataset, X_{ij} the same way as ID3, using the information entropy. For this study, the C4.5 decision trees algorithm was used for the formulation of the predictive model for the diagnosis of hypertension due to its advantages over the ID3 decision trees algorithm due to its ability to: handle continuous and discrete attributes, handle missing values, handle attributes with differing costs and prune trees after creation. The two criteria used by the C4.5 decision trees in developing its decision trees are presented in equations (3) and (4) defined as the information gain and the split criteria respectively. Equation (3) is used in determining which attribute is used to split the dataset at every iteration while equation (4) is used to determine which of the selected attribute split is most effective in splitting the dataset after attribute selection by equation (3).

$$IG(X_i) = H(X_i) - \sum_{t \in T} \frac{|t|}{|X_{ij}|} \cdot H(X_i) \tag{3}$$

where:

$$H(X_i) = -\sum_{t \in T} \frac{|t, X_i|}{|X_{ij}|} \cdot \log_2 \frac{|t, X_i|}{|X_{ij}|}$$

$$Split(T) = -\sum_{t \in T} \frac{|t|}{|X_{ij}|} \cdot \log_2 \frac{|t|}{|X_{ij}|} \tag{4}$$

T is the set of values for a given attribute X_i.

Perceptron-Based Networks

The support vector machines and the artificial neural networks both fall under the class of machine learning algorithms called the perceptron network systems since input values are fired into nodes using synaptic weights attached to the nodes – inputs are sum of products of weights w_i and input x_i, equation (5) shows the expression. The variables selected by the decision trees algorithm in tree construction will also be used in the formulation of the predictive model for CD4 count level of HIV patients using support vector machines and the artificial neural networks' multi-layer perceptron architecture.

$$\sum_{k=1}^{i} w_k x_k = w_1 x_1 + w_2 x_2 + \ldots + w_i x_i = \langle w.x \rangle \tag{5}$$

Support Vector Machines

An SVM model is a representation of the examples as points in space, mapped so that the examples of the separate categories are divided by a clear gap that is as wide as possible. New examples are then mapped into that same space and predicted to belong to a category based on which side of the gap they fall on. In formal terms, SVM constructs a hyper-plane or set of hyper-planes in a high-dimensional space, which can be applied for classification, regression or any other task. A good separation is achieved by the hyperplane that has the largest distance to the nearest training data points x called the support vectors since in general the larger the margin the lower the generalization error of the classifier. Therefore, the SVM during model formulation attempts to minimize the cost by maximizing the distance between hyper-planes. A good separation is achieved by the hyperplane $\langle w, x \rangle + b = 0$ that has the largest distance $\dfrac{2}{\|w\|}$ to the neighbouring data points of either classes at opposite ends, since in general the larger the margin the lower the generalization error of the SVM classifier. Figure 1 shows the separation of the different classes of CD4 count level in the dataset. Figure 1 (left) shows how two hyper-planes were used to separate the dataset into three classes, such that hyperplane 1 was used to extract the low CD4 level records after which hyperplane2 was used to separate the moderate CD4 level records and the

Figure 1. Separation of Support Vectors Using Hyper-planes

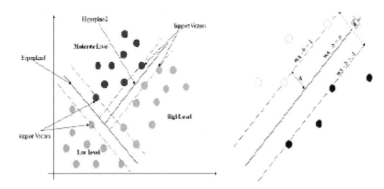

high CD4 level records. Figure 1 (right) shows a clear description of the relationship between the parameters and the hyper-plane and separating margins from the support vectors *x*.

A hyperplane created is defined as $\langle w, x \rangle + b = 0$ where $w \in \mathbb{R}^p$ and $b \in \mathbb{R}$ while $\langle w, x \rangle + b = -1$ and $\langle w, x \rangle + b = 1$ are the margins required for the separation *w* of support vectors *x* within the *n* variables. Therefore, equation (6) was defined for a linearly separable function for which the decision function in equation (7) was used to propagate the output of equation (6) using a sigmoid function with interval {-1, 1}. The aim of the SVM is to maximize the separation of the hyper-planes in equation (8) subject to the decision function defined in equation (7).

$$CD4\_Count_i = f\left(x_i\right) = \left(\langle w, x_i \rangle + b\right) > 0, \forall i \in \left[1, n\right] \tag{6}$$

$$f_d\left(x_i\right) = sign\left(CD4\_count_i\right) = \left(\langle w, x_i \rangle + b\right) > 0, \forall i \in \left[1, n\right] \tag{7}$$

$$maximize \frac{1}{2}\|w\|^2 \tag{8}$$

Artificial Neural Network

An artificial neural network (ANN) is an interconnected group of nodes, akin to the vast network of neurons in a human brain. Multi-layer perceptron are

ANNs which are generally presented as systems of interconnected neurons (containing activation functions) which send messages to each other such that each connection have numeric weights that can be tuned based on experience, making neural nets adaptive to inputs and capable of learning using the back-propagation algorithm. The word network refers to the inter-connections between the neurons in the different layers of each system. Figure 2 shows an MLP with 3 hidden layers having 2, 3 and 2 nodes located in each layer, in all there are $j=7$ nodes.

Therefore, the MLP propagates the sum of product of the weights and the inputs through nodes at multiple inner layers to the output layer. Using the back-propagation algorithm, the MLP compares the output calculated with the actual in order to compute an error-function. Gradient descent was then used to feed the error back to the system from output nodes through the nodes in the hidden layers to the nodes at the input layer while adjusting the weights as a function of the error determined at each node. The process was repeated for a number of training cycles for which the MLP network converged to a state where the error determined is small enough, then the MLP network was able to learn the target function.

The back-propagation learning algorithm can be divided into two phases: propagation and weight update.

1. **Phase 1 – Propagation:** Each propagation involves the following steps:
    a. Forward propagation of training pattern's input through each node j in the neural network in order to generate the propagation's output activations;

$$output\ O_j = \varphi\left(\sum_{k=1}^{i} w_{kj}x_k + b_k\right) = \varphi(z) = \frac{1}{1+e^{-z}} \tag{9}$$

Figure 2. Multi-Layer Perceptron Architecture

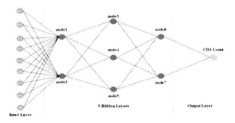

b. Backward propagation of the propagation's output activations through the neural network using the training pattern target in order to generate deltas δ_j of all output and hidden neurons.

$$\delta_j = \frac{\partial E}{\partial O_j}\frac{\partial O_j}{\partial net_j} = \begin{cases} \left(O_j - p_j\right)\varphi\left(net_j\right)\left(1 - \varphi\left(net_j\right)\right) j \text{ is output neuron,} \\ \left(\sum_{l \text{ / } L}\delta_j w_{jl}\right)\varphi\left(net_j\right)\left(1 - \varphi\left(net_j\right)\right) j \text{ is inner neuron} \end{cases} \tag{10}$$

2. **Phase 2 – Weight Update:** For each weight-synapse, hence the following:
    a. Multiply its output delta and input activation to get the gradient of the weight

$$\frac{\partial E}{\partial w_{ij}} = \delta_j x_i \tag{11}$$

b. Subtract a ratio (percentage α) of the gradient from the weight.

$$\Delta w_{ij} = -\alpha\frac{\partial E}{\partial w_{ij}} \tag{12}$$

Performance Evaluation

In order to evaluate the performance of the supervised machine learning algorithms used for the classification of CD4 count level, there was the need to plot the results of the classification on a confusion matrix as shown in Figure 3. A confusion matrix is a square which shows the actual classification along the vertical and the predicted along the horizontal. Correct classifications were plotted along the diagonal from the north-west position for the low cases predicted as Low (A), Moderate (E) and High (I) on the south-east corner (also called true positives and negatives). The incorrect classifications were plotted in the remaining cells of the confusion matrix (also called false positives). These results are presented on confusion matrix – for this study the confusion matrix is a 3 x 3 matrix table owing to the three (3) labels of the output class.

Figure 3. Diagram of a Confusion Matrix

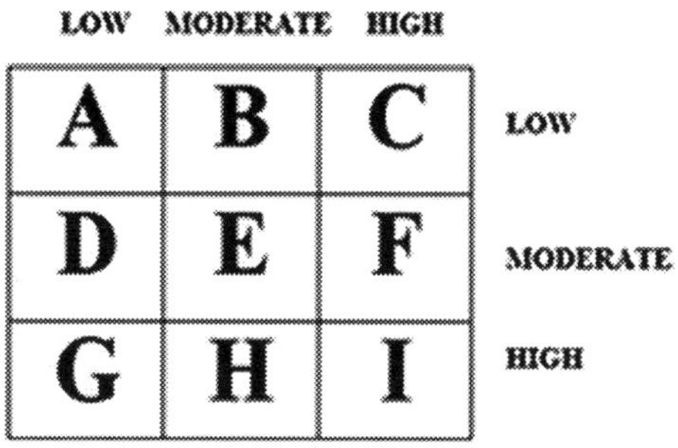

Also, the actual Low cases are A+B+C, actual Moderate cases are D+E+F and the actual High cases are G+H+I while the predicted Low are A+D+G, predicted Moderate are B+E+H and predicted High are C+F+I. The developed model was validated using a number of performance metrics based on the values of $A - I$ in the confusion matrix for each predictive model. They are presented as follows.

1. **Accuracy:** The total number of correct classification

$$Accuracy = \frac{A + E + I}{total\_cases} \tag{13}$$

2. **True Positive Rate (Recall/Sensitivity):** The proportion of actual cases correctly classified

$$TP_{low} = \frac{A}{A + B + C} \tag{14}$$

$$TP_{moderate} = \frac{E}{D + E + F} \tag{15}$$

$$TP_{high} = \frac{I}{G + H + I} \tag{16}$$

3. **False Positive (False Alarm/1-Specificity):** The proportion of negative cases incorrectly classified as positive

$$FP_{low} = \frac{D+G}{actual_{high} + actual_{moderate}} \tag{17}$$

$$FP_{moderate} = \frac{B+H}{actual_{low} + actual_{high}} \tag{18}$$

$$FP_{high} = \frac{C+F}{actual_{moderate} + actual_{low}} \tag{19}$$

4. **Precision:** The proportion of predictions that are correct

$$Precision_{low} = \frac{A}{A+D+G} \tag{20}$$

$$Precision_{moderate} = \frac{F}{B+E+H} \tag{21}$$

$$Precision_{high} = \frac{K}{C+F+I} \tag{22}$$

RESULTS

This section presents the results of the methods that were applied for the development of the predictive model for the classification of CD4 count level. The results presented were that of the data collection, model formulation and simulation results using the WEKA software following the results of the model validation of the predictive model for osteoporosis.

Results of Data Description

For this study, data was collected from 45 patients using the questionnaires constructed for this study among which; the CD4 count of Nigerian HIV patients was identified for 45 patients. Table 2 gives a description of the number of patients with respect to their level of CD4 counts which shows that majority of the patients selected had moderate CD4 count levels with a proportion of 40% composing of 15.6% female and 24.4% male followed by the patients with low CD4 count levels with a proportion of 31.1% composing of 17.8% male and 13.3% female with minority of the patients with high CD4 count levels with a proportion of 28.9% composing of 13.3% male and 15.7% female.

Table results showed that among the adults, majority of the patients were male moderate CD4 count cases and female high CD4 count cases followed by female moderate CD4 count cases with the least patients selected from female low CD4 count and male high CD4 count levels while among the youths, an equal number of patients were selected from male moderate and female low CD4 count levels while none was selected for female moderate and high CD4 count levels. The results showed that among the Hausa, majority of the patients were selected from male low and moderate CD4 count levels followed by female low and moderate CD4 count levels and a minority selected from male high and female low CD4 count levels.

Table 2. Distribution of Level of CD4 Count among Patients' Dataset

CD4 Count Class	Gender	Total	
		Frequency	Percentage (%)
High	Female	7	15.56
	Male	6	13.33
Sub-Total		13	28.89
Low	Female	6	13.33
	Male	8	17.78
Sub-Total		14	31.11
Moderate	Female	7	15.56
	Male	11	24.44
Sub-Total		18	40.00
TOTAL		45	100.00

The results showed that among the Christian patients, none was selected among the male low CD4 count levels and none selected from female moderate and lowCD4 count levels while among the Islamic patients, an equal proportion of male and female high CD4 count levels were selected while majority were selected from male low CD4 count level cases and minority from female low and moderate CD4 count level cases. The results showed that majority of the patients were normal representing 42.2% followed by underweight representing 26.7% and obese representing 20% with minority been overweight representing 11.1% of patients selected while majority of the patients selected were male moderate CD4 count cases among normal, female low and female high CD4 count levels among obese, male high and low CD4 count levels among overweight patients and male low CD4 count levels among underweight patients. No patients were selected from male high CD4 count levels among normal patients, female low CD4 count levels among obese patients, female high, and low and moderate CD4 count levels among overweight patients.

Tables 3, 4 and 5 show the descriptive statistics of the numeric variables among the dataset selected from the patients receiving HIV treatment in

Table 3. Descriptive Statistics across High CD4 Count Patients

Variables	Descriptive Statistics			
	Minimum	Maximum	Mean	Deviation
Age (years)	19	69	43	12
Weight (Kg)	39	70	54	10
Height (m)	1.08	1.95	1.55	0.27
BMI (Kg/m2)	12.35	40.29	24.10	7.70
Time since HIV diagnosis (weeks)	8	18	13	4
Baseline CD4 count (cell/mm3)	340	1200	685	240
Time since baseline CD4 count (in weeks)	3	15	10	4
Total Lymphocyte Count (cell/mm3)	5	9	7	1
White Blood Cell	4000	8000	5546	1083
Level of Hematocrit (%)	27	51	39	7
Platelets	152000	600000	355154	120997
Viral Load	3	55	11	13
Time since last count CD4 (weeks)	10	19	13.85	2.764
Relative Time since Last CD4 count	.526	1.000	.729	.145
Last CD4 Count (cell/mm3)	13	24	18	3
Relative Last CD4 Count	10	18	13	3

Table 4. Descriptive Statistics across Moderate CD4 Count Patients

Variables	Descriptive Statistics			
	Minimum	Maximum	Mean	Deviation
Age (years)	25	61	38	9
Weight (Kg)	35	75	59	10
Height (m)	.96	1.80	1.55	.29
BMI (Kg/m2)	16.36	70.53	27.05	13.28
Time since HIV diagnosis (weeks)	4	19	13	5
Baseline CD4 count (cell/mm3)	350	1000	705	239
Time since baseline CD4 count (in weeks)	7	18	10	3
Total Lymphocyte Count (cell/mm3)	5	10	8	1
White Blood Cell	3000	7000	4679	1436
Level of Hematocrit (%)	20	60	37	12
Platelets	45000	500000	351722	162486
Viral Load	3	12	7	2
Time since last count CD4 (weeks)	6	15	9	2
Relative Time since Last CD4 count	.316	.789	.471	.119
Last CD4 Count (cell/mm3)	10	20	15	3
Relative Last CD4 Count	5	9	7	1

Nigeria. The descriptive statistics used included the minimum which returns the lowest recorded value from the 45 records for each numeric variable; the maximum returns the greatest recorded value from the 45 records for each numeric variable; the mean returns the average recorded value from the 45 records for each numeric variable identified while the standard deviation gives the deviation with respect to the mean, minimum and maximum for a 95% confidence interval from the 45 records for each numeric variable identified for this study.

Simulation Results

Two different supervised machine learning algorithms were used to formulate the predictive model for the classification CD4 count level, namely: decision trees, support vector machines and the multi-layer perceptron classifiers. They were used to train the development of the prediction model using the dataset containing 45 patients' records. The simulation of the prediction models was done using the Waikato Environment for Knowledge Analysis (WEKA). The

Table 5. Descriptive Statistics across Low CD4 Count Patients

Variables	Descriptive Statistics			
	Minimum	Maximum	Mean	Deviation
Age (years)	12	55	33	11
Weight (Kg)	20	70	54	14
Height (m)	1.20	1.80	1.60	0.21
BMI (Kg/m2)	10.21	38.54	21.72	7.46
Time since HIV diagnosis (weeks)	4	15	9	4
Baseline CD4 count (cell/mm3)	320	2800	808	604
Time since baseline CD4 count (in weeks)	5	15	9	2
Total Lymphocyte Count (cell/mm3)	5	10	8	1
White Blood Cell	4000	46200	8479	10901
Level of Hematocrit (%)	26	65	37	11
Platelets	5000	700000	357500	168874
Viral Load	3	19	9	5
Time since last count CD4 (weeks)	5	10	7	2
Relative Time since Last CD4 count	.263	.526	.383	.091
Last CD4 Count (cell/mm3)	6	18	10	3
Relative Last CD4 Count	2	5	4	1

models were trained using the 10-fold cross validation method which splits the dataset into 10 subsets of data – while 9 parts are used for training the remaining one is used for testing; this process is repeated until the remaining 9 parts take their turn for testing the model.

C4.5 Decision Trees Classifier

The J4.8 decision trees algorithm was used to implement the C4.5 decision trees algorithm for the formulation of the predictive model using the simulation environment. The results of the formulation of the predictive model for the CD4 count levels of HIV patients using the C4.5 decision trees algorithm showed that five (5) variables were the most important factors for determining the level of CD4 count and were used by the algorithm to develop the tree that was used in formulating the predictive model for level of CD4 count using the C4.5 decision trees algorithm. The variables identified in the order of their importance were: age group, white blood cell (WBC) count, age, time HIV was diagnosed and viral load of patient. Based on the five (5) variables identified by the C4.5 decision tees algorithm, the predictive model for the CD4 count levels of HIV patients was using the J48 decision trees algorithm on the WEKA simulation environment. Figure 4 shows the decision trees that was formulated based on the variables that were proposed by the algorithm.

The tree was used to deduce the set of rules that are used for determining the CD4 count levels of HIV patients based on the values of the 5 variables identified by the algorithm. The rules extracted from the tree were 9 and are stated as follows:

1. If (Age Group = Youth) AND (White Blood Cell Count <= 4620 cell/mm3) Then (CD4 count level = Moderate);
2. If (Age Group = Youth) AND (White Blood Cell Count > 4620 cell/mm3) Then (CD4 count level = Low);
3. If (Age Group = Adult) AND (Age <= 38 years) AND (Viral Load <= 12 cell/mm3) Then (CD4 count level = Moderate);
4. If (Age Group = Adult) AND (Age <= 38 years) AND (Viral Load > 12 cell/mm3) Then (CD4 count level = Low);
5. If (Age Group = Adult) AND (Age > 38 years) AND (White Blood Cell Count <= 6000 cell/mm^3) AND (Time of HIV diagnosis <= 7 weeks) THEN (CD4 count level = Low);
6. If (Age Group = Adult) AND (Age > 38 years) AND (White Blood Cell Count <= 6000 cell/mm^3) AND (Time of HIV diagnosis > 7 weeks) THEN (CD4 count level = High);

Figure 4. Decision Tree formulated using C4.5 for CD4 Count in HIV Patients

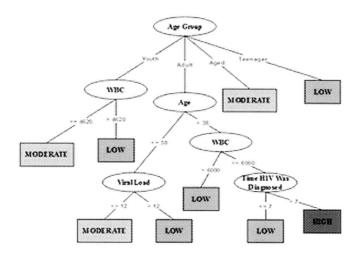

7.   If (Age Group = Adult) AND (Age > 38 years) AND (White Blood Cell Count > 6000 cell/mm^3) THEN (CD4 count level = Low);
8.   If (Age Group = Aged) THEN (CD4 Count level = Moderate); and
9.   If (Age Group = Teenager) THEN (CD4 Count Level = Low).

The results presented in Figure 4 was used to evaluate the performance of the C4.5 decision trees algorithm and thus, the confusion matrix determined. Figure 5 shows the confusion matrix that was used to interpret the results of the true positive and negative alongside the false positive and negatives of the validation results.

From the confusion matrix shown in Figure 5, the following sections present the results of the model's performance. Out of the 14 actual low cases, 13 were correctly classified as low while 1 was misclassified as moderate, out of the 18 actual moderate cases, there were 12 correct classifications with 1 misclassified as low and 5 misclassified as high and out of the 13 high, there were 9 correct classifications with 3 misclassified as low and 1 misclassified as moderate. Therefore, there were 34 correct classifications out of the 45 records considered for the model development owing for an accuracy of 75.56%.

Results of the Support Vector Machines (SVM)

Following the simulation of the predictive model for CD4 count level using the SVM algorithm, the evaluation of the performance of the model following validation using the 10-fold cross validation method was recorded. The results were used to evaluate the performance of the SVM algorithm and thus, the

Figure 5. Confusion matrix of performance evaluation using C4.5

Low	Moderate	High	<-- Predicted as
13	1	0	Low
1	12	5	Moderate
3	1	9	High

confusion matrix determined. Figure 6 shows the confusion matrix that was used to interpret the results of the true positive and negative alongside the false positive and negatives of the validation results. The confusion matrix shown in Figure 6 was used to evaluate the performance of the predictive model for CD4 count level of HIV patients. From the confusion matrix shown in Figure 6, the results of the model's performance were presented. Out of the 14 actual low cases, 12 were correctly classified as low while 2 was misclassified as moderate, out of the 18 actual moderate cases, all were correctly classified with no misclassifications and out of the 13 high, there were 11 correct classifications with 2 misclassified as low. Therefore, there were 41 correct classifications out of the 45 records considered for the model development owing for an accuracy of 91.11%.

Results of the Multi-Layer Perceptron (MLP)

Following the simulation of the predictive model for CD4 count level using the MLP algorithm, the evaluation of the performance of the model following validation using the 10-fold cross validation method was recorded. The results presented were used to evaluate the performance of the MLP algorithm and thus, the confusion matrix determined. Figure 7 shows the confusion matrix that was used to interpret the results of the true positive and negative alongside the false positive and negatives of the validation results. The confusion matrix shown in Figure 7 was used to evaluate the performance of the predictive model for CD4 count level of HIV patients. From the confusion matrix shown in Figure 7, the results of the model's performance were presented. Out of the 14 actual low cases, all were correctly classified with no misclassifications,

Figure 6. Confusion matrix of performance evaluation using SVM

Low	Moderate	High	<-- Predicted as
12	2	0	Low
0	18	0	Moderate
2	0	11	High

Figure 7. Confusion matrix of performance evaluation using MLP

Low   Moderate   High   <.. Predicted as

14	0	0	Low
0	18	0	Moderate
0	0	13	High

out of the 18 actual moderate cases, all were correctly classified with no misclassifications and out of the 13 high, all were correctly classified with no misclassifications. Therefore, all 45 records considered for the model development were correctly classified owing for an accuracy of 100%.

Discussion

The result of the performance evaluation of the machine learning algorithms are presented in Table 6 which presents the average values of each performance evaluation metrics considered for this study. For the C4.5 decision trees algorithm, the results showed that the TP rate which gave a description of the proportion of actual cases that was correctly predicted was 0.763 which implied that 76.3% of the actual cases were correctly predicted; the FP rate which gave a description of the proportion of actual cases misclassified was

Table 6. Summary of Validation Results for C4.5, naïve Bayes' and MLP classifiers

Machine Learning Algorithm Used	Performance Evaluation Metrics				
	Correct Classification (Out of 45)	Accuracy (%)	TP Rate (Recall or Sensitivity)	FP Rate (False Positive)	Precision
C4.5 Decision Trees (DT) Algorithm	34	75.56	0.763	0.120	0.755
Support Vector Machines (SVM)	41	91.11	0.901	0.046	0.919
Multi-Layer Perceptron Algorithm (MLP)	45	100.00	1.000	0.000	1.000

0.120 which implied that 12% of actual cases were misclassified while the precision which gave a description of the proportion of predictions that were correctly classified was 0.755 which implied that 75.5% of the predictions made by the classifier were correct.

For the support vector machine (SVM) algorithm, the results showed that the TP rate which gave a description of the proportion of actual cases that was correctly predicted was 0.901 which implied that 90.1% of the actual cases were correctly predicted; the FP rate which gave a description of the proportion of actual cases misclassified was 0.046 which implied that 4.6% of actual cases were misclassified while the precision which gave a description of the proportion of predictions that were correctly classified was 0.919 which implied that 91.9% of the predictions made by the classifier were correct.

For the multi-layer perceptron algorithm, the results showed that the TP rate which gave a description of the proportion of actual cases that was correctly predicted was 1 which implied that all of the actual cases were correctly predicted; the FP rate which gave a description of the proportion of actual cases misclassified was 0 which implied that none of actual cases were misclassified while the precision which gave a description of the proportion of predictions that were correctly classified was 1 which implied that all of the predictions made by the classifier were correct.

In general, the MLP and SVM algorithms were able to predict the CD4 count level better than the C4.5 decision trees algorithm. Although, the difference between the performance of the SVM and the MLP classifiers was 4 misclassification. Overall, the multi-layer perceptron was able to accurately classify all cases of CD4 count level with a value of 100% showing that it had the capacity to identify the complex patterns that existed within the dataset than the SVM and C4.5 DT algorithms. The variables identified by the C4.5 decision trees algorithm can also be given very close attention and observed in order to better understand the level of CD4 count in Nigerian HIV patients receiving treatment.

CONCLUSION

This study focused on the development of a prediction model for the classification of the level of CD4 count of patients receiving treatment in a Nigerian hospital. Historical dataset on the distribution of the classes of CD4 count among HIV patients was collected using questionnaires following the identification of associated factors needed for the classification of CD4 count level from physicians. The dataset containing information about the factors identified and collected from the respondents was used to formulate predictive models for the classification of the level of CD4 count using decision trees, support vector machine sand multi-layer perceptron algorithms. The predictive model development using the algorithms were formulated and simulated using the WEKA software.

Using the decision trees algorithm, the study was also able to identify 5 important variables among the initially identified 21 variables as most relevant for the classification of CD4 count level, namely: age group, white blood cell count, viral load, date of diagnosis of HIV and the age of the patient in addition to 9 rules that were formulated by using a combination of the 5 identified variables for the classification of the level of CD4 count of patients based on the values of the variables identified. The performance of the models developed using decision trees, support vector machines and multi-layer perceptron was done.

Following the comparison of the performance of the machine learning algorithms used in this study, it was observed that the multi-layer perceptron had the best capability to identify the unseen patterns existing within the variables used to classify CD4 count level while decision trees was able to identify the most relevant variables with an accuracy of 75.6%. Following the development of the prediction model for osteoporosis risk classification, a better understanding of the relationship between the attributes relevant to osteoporosis risk was proposed. The model can also be integrated into existing Health Information System (HIS) which captures and manages clinical information which can be fed to the CD4 count level classification prediction model thus improving the clinical decisions affecting the measurement of CD4 count levels and the real-time assessment of clinical information affecting CD4 count level from remote locations.

REFERENCES

Brain, L., Tshilidzi, M., Taryn, T., & Monica, L. (2006). Prediction of HIV Status from Demographic Data using Neural Networks. IEEE Conference on Systems Man and Cybernetics, Taipei, Taiwan.

Idowu, P. A., Aladekomo, T. A., & Agbelusi, O. (2016). Prediction of Pediatrics HIV/AIDS Patient's Survival in Nigeria: A Data Mining Approach. *Journal of Research in Science, Technology, Engineering and Management, 2*(2), 40–45.

Idowu, P. A., Aladekomo, T. A., Agbelusi, O., Alaba, O. B., & Balogun, J. A. (2017a). Prediction of Pediatric HIV/AIDS Survival in Nigeria using Naïve Bayes' Approach. *International Journal of Child Health and Human Development*, *10*(2), 1–12.

Idowu, P. A., Aladekomo, T. A., Agbelusi, O., Alaba, O. B., & Balogun, J. A. (2017b). Prediction of Pediatric HIV/AIDS Survival in Nigeria using C4.5 Decision Trees Algorithm. *International Journal of Child Health and Human Development*, *10*(2), 1–12.

Kama, K., & Prem, S. (2013). Utilization of Data Mining Techniques for Prediction and Diagnosis of Major Life Threatening Diseases Survivability-Review. *International Journal of Scientific & Engineering Research*, *4*(6), 923–932.

Lakshmi, G. S., & Isakki, P. (2017). A Comparative Study of Data Mining Classification Technique Using HIV/AIDS and STD Data. *International Journal of Innovative Research in Computer and Communication Engineering*, *5*(1), 134–139.

Morgan, D., Mahe, C., Mayanja, B., Whitworth, J. A. G., & Kilmarx, P. H. (2002). Progression to symptomatic disease in people infected with HIV-1 in rural Uganda: Prospective cohort study. *Biomedical Journal*, *324*, 193–197. PMID:11809639

Mwamburi, D. M., Ghosh, M., Fauntleroy, J., Gorbach, S. L., & Wanke, C. A. (2005). Predicting CD4 count using total lymphocyte count: A sustainable tool for clinical decisions during HAART use. *The American Journal of Tropical Medicine and Hygiene*, *73*(1), 58–62. doi:10.4269/ajtmh.2005.73.58 PMID:16014833

Ojunga, N., Peter, M., Otulo, W., Omollo, O., & Edgar, O. (2014). The Application of Logistic Regression in Modeling of Survival Chances of HIV-Positive Patients under Highly Active Antiretroviral Therapy (HAART): A Case of Nyakach District, Kenya. *Journal of Medicine and Clinical Sciences*, *3*(3), 14–20.

Olayemi, O. C., Olasehinde, O. O., & Agbelusi, O. (2016). Predictive Model of Pediatric HIV/AIDS Survival in Nigeria using Support Vector Machines. *Communications on Applied Electronics*, *5*(8), 29–36. doi:10.5120/cae2016652349

Post, F. A., Wood, R., & Maartens, G. (1996). CD4 and total lymphocyte counts as predictors of HIV disease progression. *The Quarterly Journal of Medicine, 89*(7), 505–508. doi:10.1093/qjmed/89.7.505 PMID:8759490

Rosma, M. D., Sameem, A. K., Basir, A., Adeeba, K., & Annapurni, K. (2012). The Prediction of AIDS Survival: A Data Mining Approach. *Proceedings of the 2nd WSEAS International Conference on Multivariate Analysis and Its Application in Science and Engineering*, 48 – 53.

Schechter, M., Zajdenverg, R., Machado, L. L., Pinto, M. E., Lima, L. A., & Perez, M. A. (1994). Predicting CD4 Counts in HIV-infected Brazilian Individuals: A Model Based on the World Health Organization Staging System. *Journal of Acquired Immune Deficiency Syndromes, 7*(2), 163–168. PMID:7905525

Singh, Y., Narsai, N., & Mars, M. (2013). Applying Machine Learning to predict Patient-Specific Current CD4 Cell Count in order to determine the Progression of Human Immunodeficiency Virus (HIV) Infection. *African Journal of Biotechnology, 12*(23), 3724–3750.

Tarekegn, G. B., & Sreenivasarao, V. (2016). Application of Data Mining Techniques on Pre ART Data: The Case of Felege Hiwot Referral Hospital. *International Journal of Research Studies in Computer Science and Engineering, 3*(2), 1–9.

Chapter 7

The Importance of Anthraquinone and Its Analogues and Molecular Docking Calculation

Sefa Celik
*Istanbul University – Cerrahpasa,
Turkey*

Sevim Akyuz
Istanbul Kultur University, Turkey

Aysen E. Ozel
Istanbul University, Turkey

Funda Ozkok
*Istanbul University – Cerrahpasa,
Turkey*

ABSTRACT

In drug-delivery systems containing nano-drug structures, targeting the tumorous tissue by anthraquinone molecules with high biological activity, and reaching and destroying tumors by their tumor-killing effect reveals remarkable results for the treatment of tumors. The various biological activities of anthraquinones and their derivatives depend on molecular conformation; hence, their intra-cell interaction mechanisms including deoxyribonucleic acid (DNA), ribonucleic acid (RNA), enzymes, and hormones. Computer-based drug design plays an important role in the design of drugs and the determination of goals for them. Molecular docking has been widely used in structure-based drug design. The effects of anthraquinone analogues in tumor cells as a result of their interaction with DNA strand has increased the number of studies done on them, and they have been shown to have a wide range of applications in chemistry, medicine, pharmacy, materials, and especially in the field of biomolecules.

DOI: 10.4018/978-1-5225-7467-5.ch007

INTRODUCTION

Anthraquinone and its Common Uses

The anthraquinone molecule, which has a synthetically yellow color and has the molecular formula $C_{14}H_8O_2$, is an important organic aromatic compound with a quinone skeleton. These compounds can be obtained naturally from various plants and can also be synthesized in the laboratory environment. Anthraquinone compounds are widely used in dye production and have various applications in textile chemistry. Due to the structure of the main skeleton of the molecule, the electrochemical properties of these dyes ensure that they are resistant to sunlight, and, as a result of this property, they can be safely used for marine transportation and marine vehicles.

Anthraquinones are known to have antifungal (Agarwal et. al., 2000; Manojlovic et. al., 2005; Singh et. al., 2006; Rath et. al., 1995), anti-inflammatory (Cota et. al., 2004; Goel et. al., 1991; Chang et. al., 1996; Choi et. al., 2013), antioxidant (Chen et. al., 2004; Yen et. al., 2000; Zhang et. al., 2005), antibacterial (Demirezer et. al., 2001; Chukwujekwu et. al., 2006; Comini et. al., 2011; Yang et. al., 2012), anticancer (Zhang et. al., 2011; Abu et. al., 2013; Huang et. al., 2007; Fisher et. al., 1990; Perchellet et. al., 2000; Ge et. al., 1997), and antiviral (Lown, 1993; Schinazi et. al., 1990; Barnard et. al., 1992; Ali et. al., 2000; Cohen et. al., 1996) properties. Apart from the synthetically obtained ones, in nature, anthraquinone compounds mostly are found in many different plants, especially in Yellow Centaury and *Aloe vera*. The former, which has an active anthraquinone derivative, is considered to be a natural antidepressant. Yellow Centaury has a therapeutic effect on urinary tract infections, gastritis and ulcer-like stomach ailments, and colds and bronchitis. Moreover, various studies on these active anthraquinone derivatives have reported that the active agents are effective in prostate and breast cancers (Huang et. al., 2010).These active plants from which the anthraquinone groups are obtained by isolation, are used as alternative therapeutic agents in the treatment of ulcers, skin infections, and antidiabetic, antitumor, and immunosuppressive medications. The antioxidant properties of the anthraquinones obtained from the *Cassia* species have a therapeutic effect for many diseases and prevent degradation in food systems. These anthraquinone analogues can be used as cancer therapy drugs in important viral diseases, including polio and acquired immune deficiency syndrome (AIDS) (Dave et. al., 2012). *In vitro* studies were carried out on anthraquinone glycosides, obtained through isolation from *Lasianthus acuminatissimus*, and their antitumor and anticancer effects were examined (Li et. al., 2006).

Synthesis

To obtain selective substitution reactions, various nucleophilic reactions of 1,5-dichloro anthraquinones were examined. These 1,5-dichloro anthraquinones are the preferred starting compounds for the synthesis of more complex molecules. This is due to the activity of the carbonyl groups in the center ring and being easily displaceable position of the chlorine groups. Ruediger *et al.* obtained the 1-amino-5-chloroanthraquinone compound from a 1,5-dichloroanthraquinone starting material by reflux in a sodium azide dimethyl sulfoxide medium. Purification was achieved by chromatographic methods, since isolation and purification of the aminoanthraquinone compounds used in the study were difficult. In the study carried out and patented by Hahn *et al.*, amination of hydroxyl anthraquinones, which are highly active compounds, in an ammonia environment was performed. A new process for the preparation of aminoanthraquinone derivatives was developed by Erwin Hahn, Heike Kilburg and Manfred Patsch, in a study which has been patented under US5424461A (Hahn et. al., 1995). The 1,4-dihydroxyanthraquinone molecule was treated with ammonia in aqueous media at various ratios. In the reaction medium, alkali metal dithionites including lithium dithionide, sodium dithionide, potassium dithionide, hydroxyacetone, thiourea S, S-dioxide, and alkali metal sulfites including lithium sulfide, sodium sulfite or potassium sulfite were used as reducing agents. At the same time, a base was used in the reaction medium; alkali metal hydroxides, alkali metal carbonates, or metal bicarbonates are suitable bases for this purpose. This newly developed process has enabled pure samples of 1-amino-4-hydroxyanthraquinone to be obtained with high efficiency. The 1-amino-4-hydroxy- anthraquinone compound can act as a by-product in the synthesis of many anthraquinone dyes and thus is a particularly reactive molecule. Furthermore, 9,10-anthraquinone derivatives have important areas of use due to their dye and pigment properties. Fluorine-containing dyes, in particular, are important in the field of material chemistry. In fluorine-derived anthraquinones, fluorine atoms can easily be separated from the ring and be substituted by various active substituents during nucleophilic-substitution reactions. In a study by Matsui *et al.*, 1-fluoro-9,10 anthraquinone molecules were used to synthesize 1-mono and 1,4-diaminoanthraquinone derivatives in the presence of dimethylformamide and triethylamine. It is known that electron-donor amino groups at the 1, 4, 5, and 8 positions in the anthraquinone skeleton have a bathochromic effect (Matsui et. al., 2005). The researchers also obtained a molecule with other interesting properties, which has a bathochromic effect (**3**). A 24-hour reflux was carried out on 11H,18H-13,16-dichloro-11,18-diaza-5,6-dithiatrinaphthylene-12,17-dione (**1**) and para-anisidine (p-anisidine) (**2**) in the presence of sodium acetate at 150°C, with the result that the 11H,18H-13,16-bis[4-(methoxyphenyl) amino]-11,18-diaza-5,6-dithiatrinaphthylene-12,17-dione molecule (**3**) was obtained (Figure 1) (Matsui et. al., 2005).

The molecular product (3) shown in Figure 1 has bathochromic effects, with the peak wavelength (λ_{max}) occurring in the region of 800 nanometers (nm). These molecules are regarded as anthraquinone dyes, due to their bathochromic and spectroscopic properties.

Huang *et al.* synthesized anthraquinones containing 1,5-disubstited sulfur bonds and investigated their ability to inhibit the growth of suspended rat glioma C6 cells and human hepatoma G2 cells and their redox properties based on the inhibition of lipid peroxidation in model membranes (Huang et. al., 2002). In a study by Ozkok and Sahin, a practical, economical, and one-step specific synthesis methodology, for the acquisition of amino and thio-substituents of anthraquinones, was established (Ozkok et. al., 2016). This patented process is applied as a one-pot synthesis, without the need for costly chemicals and catalysts. Ethylene glycol is used as the organic solvent in the reaction medium, and this procedure is carried out in the heat

Figure 1. The Synthesis of the 11H,18H-13,16-bis[4-(methoxyphenyl)amino]-11,18-diaza-5,6-dithiatrinaphthylene-12,17-dione Molecule
(Matsui et. al., 2005)

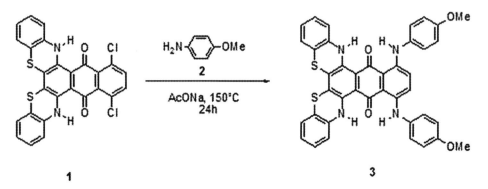

environment. This innovative method is facilitated by the ready availability of this non-volatile and cost-effective solvent.

Electrochemical Properties

Quinones, a class of biologically-important compounds, are found in plants, and both living and dead organisms. Most derivatives containing a quinone fragment in their structure are biologically active. Quinone derivatives in respiratory enzymes form a part of the electron-transfer chain (Patai, 1988). In addition, they exhibit antitermitic activity and are used as protective compounds by some plants during respiration (Pankiewicz et. al., 2007; Ganapathy et. al., 2004). A number of previous studies have shown that the reduction-oxidation (redox) properties of anthraquinones directly depend on their acid-base properties (Figure 2) (Gupta et. al., 1997). Under protic conditions, quinones are reduced to hydroquinones.

However, in an aprotic environment, reduction of quinones occurs in two steps. In the first of these, quinone takes an electron and transforms into the Q radical anion. In the second step, the Q radical anion takes one more electron and turns into an even more negative Q^{2-} anion. In a study by Zarzeczanska *et al.*, the reaction of ethylamine with 1-chloroanthraquinone was carried out by refluxing in the presence of cesium carbonate and under argon gas at 80 °C, for 48 hours, to obtain 1-ethylamino-9,10-anthraquinone (Zarzeczanska et. al., 2014). The reaction of diethylamine with 1-chloroanthraquinone was carried out by refluxing in the presence of toluene at 100 °C, for 24 hours, to obtain 1-(diethylamino)anthraquinone. The synthesized molecules were characterized by ultraviolet-visible (UV-Vis) spectroscopy, acid-base titration, electrochemical methods, and quantum chemical calculations. As a result of these studies, the structure and electrochemical behaviors of 1-aminoanthraquinone and its ethyl derivatives, in acetonitrile solution, were determined. It has been observed that the basicity of the amino derivatives linked to the anthraquinone structure is different.

Figure 2. Electrochemical Reactions of Quinones
(Zarzeczanska et. al., 2014)

$$Q + 2H^+ + 2e^- = H_2Q$$

Figure 3. Aminoanthraquinone Analogue (AQNEt₂)
(Zarzeczanska et. al., 2014)

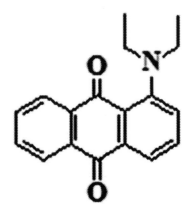

The highest basicity value was observed in AQNEt2 molecule (Figure 3) which contains an amino and two ethyl group substitutions in the anthraquinone ring of the structure. This compound is a strong base which reacts with water, and, during chemical processes, it forms a hydroxyl radical that forms gem-diol-type derivation with neutral AQNEt2 (Figure 3).

Studies on Antimicrobial and Antifungal Activity

The *Senna alata* plant, of the leguminosae family, has been used as a source of powdered anthraquinone extract, and this species is also known as Christmas candles, the candle bush, or candelabra bush. For many years, scientific studies have shown that this plant has important biological properties that can be used in various medical applications. Examples of its uses include the treatment of important health problems, such as constipation relief, anemia prevention, laxative effects, antidote, inhibition of leukemia cells, and the treatment of infections caused by fungi, bacteria and viruses (Ekpo et. al., 2008; Clement et. al., 2007; Pieme et. al., 2009; Benjamin et. al., 1981; Magassouba et. al., 2007; Pasewu et. al., 2008; Wuthi-Udomlert et. al., 2001). In addition, the antimicrobial activities of the anthraquinone glycosides, which are obtained from this plant, are well proven. These include active pharmacological compounds, including rhein, emodin, and chrysophanol, which have also laxative properties. Due to its scientific applications and its traditional use in medicine, this plant is not only recognized by the World Health Organization (WHO) as essential to basic treatment programs, but also, according to Drug Act 2510, as a herbal medicine by the Thai National List of Essential Drugs. Although many studies have examined different properties of these plants, they are classified as herbal remedies for constipation. In a study by Wuthi-Udomlert *et al.*, the active form of anthraquinone, as derived from the *Senna alata* plant, was identified and the effects of its antifungal activity on dermatophytes were investigated (Wuthi-udomlert et. al., 2010). The resulting findings proved that the anthraquinone fraction showed a high degree of biological activity. Qualitative and quantitative studies have also shown that this substance is effective on skin fungi.

Beta-lactams (β-lactams) are another important class of compounds which are highly active and are included in the class of antibiotic drugs. They are widely used as chemotherapeutic agents for the treatment of microbial disorders. These molecules also exhibit important properties which enable their use to counter the effects of human immunodeficiency virus (HIV) and malaria, while they are also suitable for use as thrombin inhibitors and ant-inflammatory agents (Han et. al., 1995; Sperka et. al., 2005; Saturnino et. al., 2000; Jarrahpour et. al., 2011). A major disadvantage of antibiotic drugs is that microorganisms become resistant to β-lactam antibiotics when they are used excessively. In the treatment of diseases, it is important to discover drug molecules that can counteract this resistance. Therefore, the discovery of β-lactam antibiotics has attracted much attention (Han et. al., 1995; Sperka et. al., 2005; Saturnino et. al., 2000; Jarrahpour et. al., 2011). In a study by Jarrahpour *et al.*, β-lactam derivatives of anthraquinones were synthesized and the antimicrobial, antifungal, and antimalarial activities of the obtained molecules were investigated (Jarrahpour et. al., 2012). Although the products did not show a significant effect on Gram-positive and Gram-negative bacteria and antifungal activity tests, they yielded very effective results in antimalarial activity tests. During the latter, they showed resistance to *Plasmodium falciparum* K14, and the half maximal inhibitory concentration (IC$_{50}$) dose determined in these studies varied f between 9 and 50 µM.

Balachandran *et al.* investigated the antimicrobial and antiproliferative effects of the 2-hydroxy-9,10-anthraquinone molecule when isolated from *Streptomyces olivochromogenes* (ERINLG-261). *Streptomyces olivochromogenes* (ERINLG-261) is an important production source of antibiotics. The metabolite and the isolation product 2-Hydroxy-9,10-anthraquinone had a pronounced effect on Gram-positive and Gram-negative bacteria and also on fungi (Balachandran et. al., 2016). However, the 2-hydroxy-9,10-anthraquinone molecule showed a moderate antiproliferative effect on lung adenocarcinoma (A549) and COLO320 cells, whereby anthraquinones were found to bind to cellular DNA and to act as inhibitory anticancer agents through various mechanisms.

In Vitro and *In Vivo* Studies

Quinones are the most important antitumor compounds. The anticancer effects of synthetically obtained anthraquinone derivatives are well documented (McKenzie et. al., 2012; Li et. al., 2016; Lee et. al., 2008; Almutairi et. al., 2014; Zheng et. al., 2017; Huang et. al., 2014; Chen et. al., 2014; Tsang et. al., 2013; Johnson et. al., 1997). Emodin, aloin, and aloe-emodin, which are the most important components of the *Aloe vera* plant, are the most effective of these derivatives (Hsu et. al., 2012). Many *in vitro* and *in vivo* studies have determined the anti-inflammatory, antineoplastic, anti-angiogenesis, and, in the drug chemistry field, toxicological effects of these derivatives.

Emodin (1,3,8-trihydroxy-6-methylanthraquinone) (Figure 4) shows a particularly high cytotoxic effect and initiates apoptosis in cancer cells. In a study conducted by Hsu *et al.*, it was determined that emodin, which is an active anthraquinone derivative, caused apoptosis in -in human hepatoma HepG2 / C3A, PLC / PRF / 5 and SK-HEP-1 cells. In both *in vitro* and *in vivo* studies, emodin showed positive effects against myelomonocytic leukemia WEHI-3 cells in mice (Hsu et. al., 2012). It is known that anticancer drugs target DNA in the mechanism of functioning. However, the mechanism by which these drugs interact with DNA is not yet fully understood, although it is thought that the charge-transfer bonds are effective during this interaction. It is known that quinone compounds contain large quinoid systems that link to DNA molecules. This link can be named as electrostatic interaction,

Figure 4. Molecular Structure of Emodin (1,3,8-Trihydroxy-6-methylanthraquinone)
(Hsu et. al., 2012)

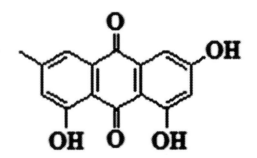

polarization, repelling, charge distribution, and charge transfer. A study was carried out by El-Gogary *et al.* (Figure 5) aimed to find the occurred charge transfer. For the purposes of this investigation, aminoanthraquinone derivative anticancer drugs were chosen (El-Gogary, 2003).

Studies have been carried out on the ability of known donors to convert to charge-transfer form in the presence of pyrene and hexamethylbenzene. The interaction of electron-acceptor and electron-donor molecules allows the formation of new molecular types which are called charge-transfer or molecular complexes.

Various anthraquinone derivatives can be isolated from the common *Morinda elliptica* plant, which grows in Malaysia, and these are used for the treatment of serious illnesses, such as fever, loss of appetite, and cholera (Ali et. al., 2000). Ali *et al.* investigated the anti-HIV, cytotoxic and antimicrobial activites of various isolated anthraquinones, including 2-Formyl-1-hydroxyanthraquinone, 1-Hydroxy-2-methylanthraquinone, damnacanthal and morindone, and tested their cytotoxicity against various tumor cell lines (Ali et. al., 2000).. Among these products, only damnacanthal showed moderate activity against HIV (Ali et. al., 2000).. It was found to be cytotoxic towards the Michigan Cancer Foundation-7 (MCF-7) (breast carcinoma) and CEM-SS (T-lymphoblastic leukemia) cell lines. In addition, the isolated anthraquinones were tested against HeLa (cervical carcinoma) cells and most of these molecules showed low cytotoxicity, whereas damnacanthal and morindone were seen to be more effective. All anthraquinone analogues in the study showed strong antimicrobial activity. Particularly, molecules

Figure 5. (a) The Structure of the 1,4-Bis([2-(dimethylamino)ethyl]amino)anthracene-9,10-dione Molecule (b) The Structure of the 1,4-Bis([2-(dimethylamino)ethyl]amino)-5,8-dihydroxyanthracene-9,10-dione Molecule
(El-Gogary, 2003)

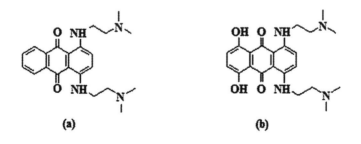

with formyl and hydroxyl groups (nordamnacanthal and damnacanthal) were found to be more active in this respect (Ali et. al., 2000).

The cytotoxicity and anticancer properties of aminoanthraquinones and their thio derivatives have been well documented. In a study by Huang *et al.*, 1,5-bis-thio-substituted anthraquinones were synthesized and their cytotoxicity, effect on cancer cells, and contribution to lipid peroxidation were investigated (Huang et. al., 2002). These molecules were seen to inhibit C6 cells in mice and hepatoma G2 cells in humans. Furthermore, these compounds are effective in redox reactions due to their structure, and have been found to inhibit lipid peroxidation in model membranes due to their redox potential. Therefore, thio derivatives of anthraquinones are active compounds which are suitable for the treatment of many diseases. Mitoxantrone(1,4-dihydroxy-5,8-bis [2-(2-hydroxyethylamino)ethyl-amino]-anthracene-9,10-dione) (Fig.6), which is in the class of antibiotic drugs, is an anticancer analogue of this drug group.

This active analogue (Mitoxantrone) is known to have important effects in the treatment of malignancies in humans (Brück et. al., 2011). In a study by Brück *et al.*, various mitoxantrone metabolites, obtained from mitoxantrone oxidation with different peroxidase enzymes, were investigated (Brück et. al., 2011). Due to the various anti-tumor effects (on breast carcinomas, etc.) of these metabolites, their active use in clinical trials is possible.

Some medicines containing anthraquinone derivatives and their uses are given in Table 1.

Figure 6. The Structure of the Mitoxantrone (1,4-Dihydroxy-5,8-bis[2-(2-hydroxyethylamino)ethyl-amino]-anthracene-9,10-dione) Molecule
(Brück et. al., 2011)

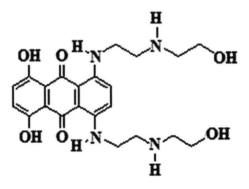

Table 1. Some drugs containing anthraquinone derivatives and their therapeutic effects

Drug	Therapeutic Area	Pharmaceutical Company
Stimucart	Osteoarthritis	Novartis India Ltd.
Sennalax	Diarrhoea	Lennon Limited
Prunelax (Ciruelax)	Bowel regularity	Garden House
Senokot	Constipation and bloating	Reckitt Benckiser Healthcare (UK) Ltd.
Eucarbon	Digestive system	Bio Pharma
Lukin	Osteoarthritis	Gold Line Pharma Ltd.
Danthron	Post-operative nausea and vomiting	Whitehall Robins Inc.
Flexaid-D	Rheumatoid arthritis	Sun Pharmaceutical Industries Ltd
Salivex L Paint	Aphthous stomatitis	Chemical Industries Development "CID" - Giza - A.R.E.

MOLECULAR DOCKING ANALYSIS

Docking Procedure and Its Importance

It is important to determine the most stable conformation of the anthraquinone molecule and its analogues in the cells, which have a large number of biological activities and properties and understand the mechanisms by which they interact in the cell. Depending on the interactions with DNA, enzymes, hormones, proteins, etc., the conformation in which the molecule exhibits activity and the orientation in the active site belonging to the receptors in contact with the molecule can change. For this reason, depending on the receptor with which it interacts, the conformation of the molecule and its orientation in the receptor must be determined. Thus, the behavior of the anthraquinone molecule in the binding site of the target receptor can be described. The most common method, which simulates the relationship between two molecular structures for this process and has been in use since the 1980s, is Molecular Docking. Experimental difficulties and economic costs in determining the structures of complexes are among the most important advantages of using molecular docking to find the default binding conformation. The first molecular docking experiment was the structural analysis of protein–protein interactions performed by Levinthal *et al.* in 1975 (Levinthal et. al., 1975) and the keystone of this method is the key–lock theory proposed by Emil Fischer in 1894 (Fischer, 1894).

Interaction Mechanism

The molecular docking method can be applied on various interactions that play an important role in many biological processes, such as protein–protein(Ehrlich et. al., 2001), protein–ligand(Rarey, 2001), protein–DNA(Sternberg et. al., 2002) signal transduction, cell regulation, and preservation of genomic DNA structure and integrity, and it can be also applied depending on the rigidity or flexibility of these structures. The protein–protein docking calculation can be described as the study of stable structures resulting from the interaction between two protein structures. In the following years, protein–ligand interactions have been added to these interactions and today they have become one of the most active areas of model-based drug discovery. These protein–ligand interactions are essential for structure-based drug design. All processes in organisms depend on protein–ligand interactions, which are based on biological identities at the molecular level. Understanding the protein–ligand interactions by determining the active site, where the protein–ligand interaction takes place, plays a crucial role in the definition of cellular mechanisms and are involved in the preliminary response to drugs. However, in this interaction, it is difficult to perform the docking process between the ligand and protein considering the flexibility. This is because it is necessary to make calculations involving all conformations of this chemical structure. Thus, most of the programs used assume that the ligand structure is flexible while the protein is considered to be rigid.

This calculation is based on the identification of the conformation of the ligand in the active site of the protein and the identification of the most likely conformation and orientation by ranking these conformations with the specified scores. There are various programs that perform docking depending on the difference of the scoring function and an algorithm, including DOCK, AutoDock, AutoDock Vina, UCSF Dock, GOLD, and ICM-Dock.

The following docking calculation methods are used:

1. **Rigid Docking:** The geometry of the ligand and receptor is kept rigid during the docking procedure.
2. **Flexible Docking:** The ligand and the sidechain of the protein remain flexible during the docking procedure. The energy is calculated for the different conformations of the ligand. Although this analysis is time consuming, conformation or conformations can be obtained very close to those of the experimental results.

Molecular Docking Applications of Anthraquinone Derivatives

The number of studies on this molecule are increasing on a daily basis, and its growing importance is attributable to the biologically-active nature of anthraquinone and its derivatives, which has been mentioned above. Docking analysis is significant, since this molecule is also a guide for determining the activity and interaction of receptors within a cell.

Depending on the interaction between anthraquinones and DNA, the orientation of the molecules was determined by Panigrahi *et al.* in 2018, using the CDOCKER module in *Discovery Studio* (Figure 7) (Panigrahi et. al., 2018). It is thought that the results obtained are consistent with the biophysical data and that emodin has a stronger binding affinity to DNA

Figure 7. Calf Thymus DNA (ctDNA) – Orientation of Ligands as a Result of Anthraquinone Interaction (a) DNA – Emodin, (b) DNA – Aloe-emodin, (c) DNA – Rhein, (d) DNA – Chrysophanol, (e) DNA – Physcion
(*Panigrahi et. al., 2018*)

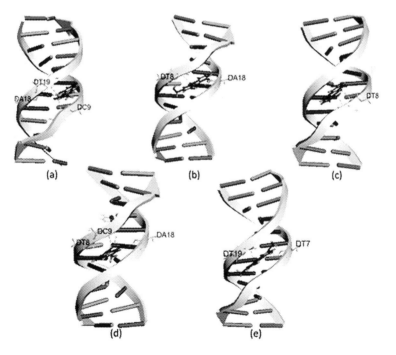

For a more accurate representation see the electronic version.

among the five anthraquinones. Another important assumption is that the affinity for anthraquinone to bind with DNA is related to its cytotoxic potential.

Using docking analysis, the interaction between Alizarin Red S, Acid Blue 129, and Uniblue anthraquinone dyes and lysozyme was determined in 2010 by Paramaguru *et al.*, as shown in Figure 8 (Paramaguru et. al., 2010). This method shows that the receptor Trp62 is in close proximity to the three anthraquinones during this process.

A potential binding mode was determined by Wang *et al.* in 2018 (Figure 9), as a result of the interaction of the 2-(dimethoxymethyl)-1-hydroxyanthracene-9,10-dione molecule with an anthraquinone derivative exhibiting antimicrobial activity with topoisomerase IV and AmpC beta-lactamase (β-lactamase) enzymes (Wang et. al., 2018).

Figure 8. Interaction of Lysozyme with (a) Alizarin Red S, (b) Acid Blue 129, and (c) Uniblue Anthraquinone Dyes
(Paramaguru et. al., 2010)

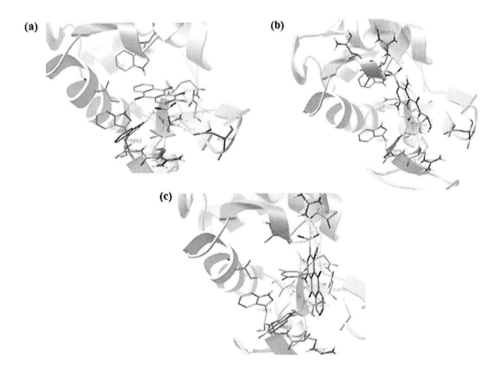

*For a more accurate representation see the electronic version.

Molecular docking studies carried out with these enzymes show that 2-(dimethoxymethyl)-1-hydroxyanthracene-9,10-dione has the least binding energy to support antimicrobial activity.

In 2016, Balachandran *et al.* examined the interaction of the 2-hydroxy-9,10-anthraquinone molecule, which exhibits good antimicrobial activity against bacteria and fungi, with the DNA topoisomerase IV receptor. Thus, the orientation of the ligand with the active site of the receptor was determined (Figure 10) (Balachandran et. al., 2016). Molecular docking studies have shown that the 2-hydroxy-9,10-anthraquinone compound, isolated with topoisomerase, TtgR, and β-lactamase enzymes, has low binding energy.

Figure 9. DNA Topoisomerase IV and AmpC β-lactamase Molecular Docking Analysis with 2-(Dimethoxymethyl)-1-hydroxyanthracene-9,10-dione
(*Wang et. al., 2018*)

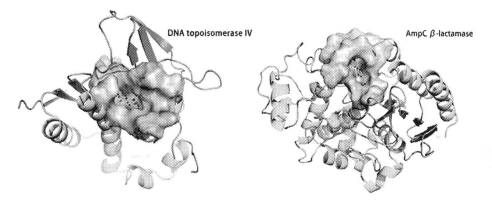

For a more accurate representation see the electronic version.

Figure 10. The Binding Pose of 2-Hydroxy-9,10-anthraquinone with Topoisomerase
(*Balachandran et. al., 2016*)

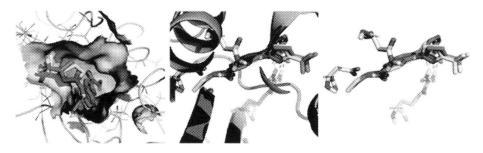

For a more accurate representation see the electronic version.

Docking analysis of the 1,5,7-trihydroxy-3-hydroxy methyl anthraquinone molecule, which has important antimicrobial activity, with DNA topoisomerase IV was performed by Duraipandiyan *et al.* (Duraipandiyan et. al., 2014). As a result of the molecular docking studies, the pose of this compound, isolated using TtgR, topoisomerase IV and AmpC β-lactamase enzymes, has been shown to have the least binding energy (Figure 11).

Li *et al.* simulated the interaction between anthraquinone derivatives with estrogenic activities and the estrogen receptor alpha (α) with the aid of the CDOCKER implementation, thereby determining possible regions of interaction (Figure 12) (Li et. al., 2010). This study found that hydrogen bonding, hydrophobic, and pi to pi (π-π) interactions between anthraquinone derivatives and the estrogen receptor α moderate the estrogenic activities of anthraquinone derivatives.

In 2008, Gan *et al.* investigated 3-alkylaminopropoxy-9,10-anthraquinone derivatives and their interaction with the cyclooxygenase (COX) enzyme. During this study, dock scores and interaction energies were also obtained by molecular simulations. Docking results for the three compounds given in Figure 13 show that they can be used as pharmacophores for the production and optimization of new antithrombotic and anti-inflammatory agents (Gan et. al., 2008).

Figure 11. The Binding Pose Obtained by Docking Analysis of Topoisomerase IV and the 1,5,7-Trihydroxy-3-hydroxy Methyl Anthraquinone Molecule (Duraipandiyan et. al., 2014)

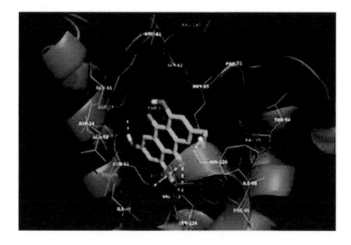

*For a more accurate representation see the electronic version.

Figure 12. Hydrogen Bond and Hydrophobic Interactions between 1,5-diaminoanthraquinone and the Estrogen Receptor α in the Binding Region (Li et. al., 2010)

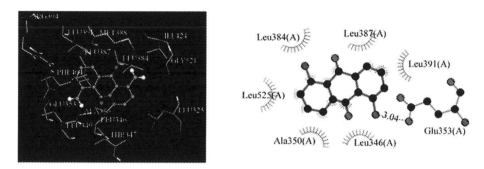

Figure 13. Binding of the 3-Alkylaminopropoxy-9,10-anthraquinone Derivative to the Active Region of the COX-1 Enzyme (Gan et. al., 2008)

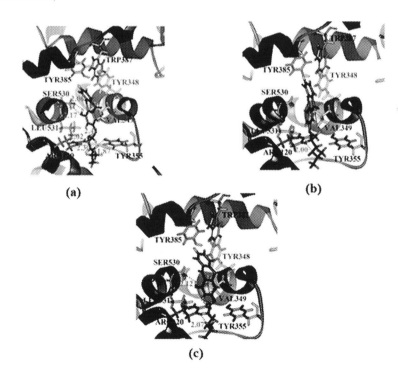

In an experimental study, Jordheim et. al investigated the interaction of human cytosolic 5'-nucleotidase II in complex with anthraquinone-2,6-disulfonic acid by x-ray diffraction. The ligand–receptor interaction, obtained from x-ray diffraction analysis, is shown in Figure 14 (Jordheim et. al., 2013).

In 2014, Ryan et. al. investigated the crystal structure of paAzoR1 which is bound to antrakinon-2-sulfonate. The ligand-receptor interaction, obtained from the X-ray diffraction analysis is shown in Figure 15. (Ryan et. al., 2014)

De Luchi et.al. investigated the crystal structure of telomeric sequence d(UBrAGG) interacting with anthraquinone derivative by x-ray diffraction analysis in 2010. This ligand- receptor interaction is shown in Figure 16 (De Luchi et. al., 2010).

CONCLUSION

Anthraquinones constitute an important class of natural and synthetic compounds with a wide range of applications. This chapter summarizes the

Figure 14. The interaction of human cytosolic 5'-nucleotidase II in complex with anthraquionone-2,6- disulfonic acid
(Jordheim et. al., 2013)

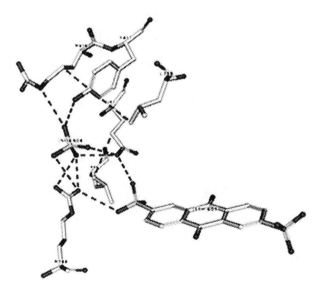

*For a more accurate representation see the electronic version.

Figure 15. Ligand- receptor interaction of paAzoR1 which is bound to antrakinon-2-sulfonate
(Ryan et. al., 2014)

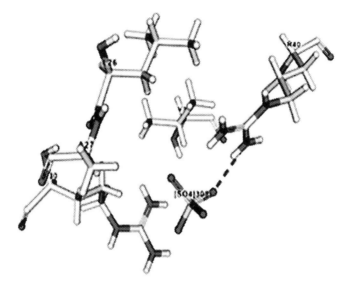

For a more accurate representation see the electronic version.

Figure 16. Ligand- receptor interaction which is obtained from the telomeric sequence d(UBrAGG) interacting with anthraquionone derivate
(De Luchi et. al., 2010)

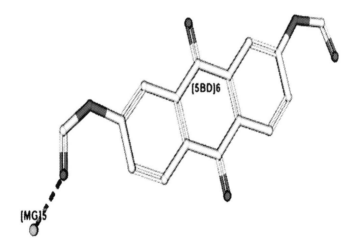

For a more accurate representation see the electronic version.

broad application areas of anthraquinones and the effects of anthraquinone analogues in tumor cells, due to their interaction with DNA. The discovery of new compounds with antitumor activity has become one of the most important objectives in pharmacy. In recent years, an interesting group of chemotherapeutic agents used in the treatment of cancer include molecules which interact with DNA. Molecular docking calculations can determine the level of interaction of anthraquinone analogues with enzymes and DNA.

REFERENCES

Abu, N., Akhtar, M. N., Ho, W. Y., Yeap, S. K., & Alitheen, N. B. (2013). 3-Bromo-1-hydroxy-9, 10-anthraquinone (BHAQ) inhibits growth and migration of the human breast cancer cell lines MCF-7 and MDA-MB231. *Molecules (Basel, Switzerland)*, *18*(9), 10367–10377. doi:10.3390/molecules180910367 PMID:23985955

Agarwal, S. K., Singh, S. S., Verma, S., & Kumar, S. (2000). Antifungal activity of anthraquinone derivatives from Rheum emodi. *Journal of Ethnopharmacology*, *72*(1), 43–46. doi:10.1016/S0378-8741(00)00195-1 PMID:10967452

Ali, A. M., Ismail, N. H., Mackeen, M. M., Yazan, L. S., Mohamed, S. M., Ho, A. S. H., & Lajis, N. H. (2000). Antiviral, cyototoxic and antimicrobial activities of anthraquinones isolated from the roots of Morinda elliptica. *Pharmaceutical Biology*, *38*(4), 298–301. doi:10.1076/1388-0209(200009)38:4;1-A;FT298 PMID:21214480

Almutairi, M. S., Hegazy, G. H., Haiba, M. E., Ali, H. I., Khalifa, N. M., & Soliman, A. E. M. M. (2014). Synthesis, Docking and Biological Activities of Novel Hybrids Celecoxib and Anthraquinone Analogs as Potent Cytotoxic Agents. *International Journal of Molecular Sciences*, *15*(12), 22580–22603. doi:10.3390/ijms151222580 PMID:25490139

Balachandran, C., Duraipandiyan, V., Arun, Y., Sangeetha, B., Emi, N., Al-Dhabi, N. A., ... Perumal, P. T. (2016). Isolation and characterization of 2-hydroxy-9, 10-anthraquinone from Streptomyces olivochromogenes (ERINLG-261) with antimicrobial and antiproliferative properties. *Revista Brasileira de Farmacognosia*, *26*(3), 285–295. doi:10.1016/j.bjp.2015.12.003

Barnard, D. L., Huffman, J. H., Morris, J. L., Wood, S. G., Hughes, B. G., & Sidwell, R. W. (1992). Evaluation of the antiviral activity of anthraquinones, anthrones and anthraquinone derivatives against human cytomegalovirus. *Antiviral Research*, *17*(1), 63–77. doi:10.1016/0166-3542(92)90091-I PMID:1310583

Benjamin, T. V., & Lamikanra, A. (1981). Investigation of Cassia alata, a plant used in Nigeria in the treatment of skin diseases. *Quarterly Journal of Crude Drug Research*, *19*(2-3), 93–96. doi:10.3109/13880208109070583

Brück, T. B., & Brück, D. W. (2011). Oxidative metabolism of the anti-cancer agent mitoxantrone by horseradish, lacto-and lignin peroxidase. *Biochimie*, *93*(2), 217–226. doi:10.1016/j.biochi.2010.09.015 PMID:20887767

Chang, C. H., Lin, C. C., Yang, J. J., Namba, T., & Hattori, M. (1996). Anti-inflammatory effects of emodin from ventilago leiocarpa. *The American Journal of Chinese Medicine*, *24*(02), 139–142. doi:10.1142/S0192415X96000189 PMID:8874670

Chen, R. F., Shen, Y. C., Huang, H. S., Liao, J. F., Ho, L. K., Chou, Y. C., ... Chen, C. F. (2004). Evaluation of the anti-inflammatory and cytotoxic effects of anthraquinones and anthracenes derivatives in human leucocytes. *The Journal of Pharmacy and Pharmacology*, *56*(7), 915–919. doi:10.1211/0022357023781 PMID:15233871

Chen, Y. W., Huang, H. S., Shieh, Y. S., Ma, K. H., Huang, S. H., Hueng, D. Y., ... Lin, G. J. (2014). A novel compound NSC745885 exerts an anti-tumor effect on tongue cancer SAS cells in vitro and in vivo. *PLoS One*, *9*(8), e104703. doi:10.1371/journal.pone.0104703 PMID:25127132

Choi, R. J., Ngoc, T. M., Bae, K., Cho, H. J., Kim, D. D., Chun, J., ... Kim, Y. S. (2013). Anti-inflammatory properties of anthraquinones and their relationship with the regulation of P-glycoprotein function and expression. *European Journal of Pharmaceutical Sciences*, *48*(1), 272–281. doi:10.1016/j.ejps.2012.10.027 PMID:23174748

Chukwujekwu, J. C., Coombes, P. H., Mulholland, D. A., & Van Staden, J. (2006). Emodin, an antibacterial anthraquinone from the roots of Cassia occidentalis. *South African Journal of Botany*, *72*(2), 295–297. doi:10.1016/j.sajb.2005.08.003

Clement, Y. N., Morton-Gittens, J., Basdeo, L., Blades, A., Francis, M. J., Gomes, N., ... Singh, A. (2007). Perceived efficacy of herbal remedies by users accessing primary healthcare in Trinidad. *BMC Complementary and Alternative Medicine*, *7*(1), 4. doi:10.1186/1472-6882-7-4 PMID:17286858

Cohen, P. A., Hudson, J. B., & Towers, G. H. N. (1996). Antiviral activities of anthraquinones, bianthrones and hypericin derivatives from lichens. *Cellular and Molecular Life Sciences*, *52*(2), 180–183. doi:10.1007/BF01923366 PMID:8608821

Comini, L. R., Montoya, S. N., Páez, P. L., Argüello, G. A., Albesa, I., & Cabrera, J. L. (2011). Antibacterial activity of anthraquinone derivatives from Heterophyllaea pustulata (Rubiaceae). *Journal of Photochemistry and Photobiology. B, Biology*, *102*(2), 108–114. doi:10.1016/j.jphotobiol.2010.09.009 PMID:20965744

Cota, B. B., de Oliveira, A. B., Guimarães, K. G., Mendonça, M. P., de Souza Filho, J. D., & Braga, F. C. (2004). Chemistry and antifungal activity of Xyris species (Xyridaceae): A new anthraquinone from Xyris pilosa. *Biochemical Systematics and Ecology*, *32*(4), 391–397. doi:10.1016/j.bse.2003.11.006

Dave, H., & Ledwani, L. (2012). *A review on anthraquinones isolated from Cassia species and their applications*. Academic Press.

De Luchi, D., Usón, I., Wright, G., Gouyette, C., & Subirana, J. A. (2010). Structure of a stacked anthraquinone–DNA complex. *Acta Crystallographica. Section F, Structural Biology and Crystallization Communications*, *66*(9), 1019–1022. doi:10.1107/S1744309110030034 PMID:20823516

Demirezer, L. Ö., Kuruüzüm-Uz, A., Bergere, I., Schiewe, H. J., & Zeeck, A. (2001). The structures of antioxidant and cytotoxic agents from natural source: Anthraquinones and tannins from roots of Rumex patientia. *Phytochemistry*, *58*(8), 1213–1217. doi:10.1016/S0031-9422(01)00337-5 PMID:11738410

Duraipandiyan, V., Al-Dhabi, N. A., Balachandran, C., Raj, M. K., Arasu, M. V., & Ignacimuthu, S. (2014). Novel 1, 5, 7-trihydroxy-3-hydroxy methyl anthraquinone isolated from terrestrial Streptomyces sp.(ERI-26) with antimicrobial and molecular docking studies. *Applied Biochemistry and Biotechnology*, *174*(5), 1784–1794. doi:10.100712010-014-1157-y PMID:25149455

Ehrlich, L. P., & Wade, R. C. (2001). Protein-protein docking. *Reviews in Computational Chemistry*, *17*, 61–98.

Ekpo, B. A., Bala, D. N., Essien, E. E., & Adesanya, S. A. (2008). Ethnobotanical survey of Akwa Ibom state of Nigeria. *Journal of Ethnopharmacology*, *115*(3), 387–408. doi:10.1016/j.jep.2007.10.021 PMID:18053664

El-Gogary, T. M. (2003). Molecular complexes of some anthraquinone anti-cancer drugs: Experimental and computational study. *Spectrochimica Acta. Part A: Molecular and Biomolecular Spectroscopy*, *59*(5), 1009–1015. doi:10.1016/S1386-1425(02)00283-4 PMID:12633717

Fischer, E. (1894). Einfluss der Configuration auf die Wirkung der Enzyme. *European Journal of Inorganic Chemistry*, *27*(3), 2985–2993.

Fisher, G. R., Brown, J. R., & Patterson, L. H. (1990). Involvement of hydroxyl radical formation and DNA strand breakage in the cytotoxicity of anthraquinone antitumour agents. *Free Radical Research Communications*, *11*(1-3), 117–125. doi:10.3109/10715769009109674 PMID:1963615

Gan, K. H., Teng, C. H., Lin, H. C., Chen, K. T., Chen, Y. C., Hsu, M. F., ... Lin, C. N. (2008). Antiplatelet effect and selective binding to cyclooxygenase by molecular docking analysis of 3-alkylaminopropoxy-9, 10-anthraquinone derivatives. *Biological & Pharmaceutical Bulletin*, *31*(8), 1547–1551. doi:10.1248/bpb.31.1547 PMID:18670087

Ganapathy, S., Thomas, P. S., Fotso, S., & Laatsch, H. (2004). Article. *Phytochemistry*, (65): 1265–1271. doi:10.1016/j.phytochem.2004.03.011

Ge, P., & Russell, R. A. (1997). The synthesis of anthraquinone derivatives as potential anticancer agents. *Tetrahedron*, *53*(51), 17469–17476. doi:10.1016/S0040-4020(97)10195-8

Goel, R. K., Das, G. G., Ram, S. N., & Pandey, V. B. (1991). Antiulcerogenic and anti-inflammatory effects of emodin, isolated from Rhamnus triquerta wall. *Indian Journal of Experimental Biology*, *29*(3), 230–232. PMID:1874536

Gupta, N., & Linschitz, H. (1997). Hydrogen-Bonding and Protonation Effects in Electrochemistry of Quinones in Aprotic Solvents. *Journal of the American Chemical Society*, *119*(27), 6384–6391. doi:10.1021/ja970028j

Hahn, E., Patsch, M., & Kilburg, H. (1995). *U.S. Patent No. 5,424,461*. Washington, DC: U.S. Patent and Trademark Office.

Han, W. T., Trehan, A. K., Wright, J. K., Federici, M. E., Seiler, S. M., & Meanwell, N. A. (1995). Azetidin-2-one derivatives as inhibitors of thrombin. *Bioorganic & Medicinal Chemistry*, *3*(8), 1123–1143. doi:10.1016/0968-0896(95)00101-L PMID:7582985

Hsu, S. C., & Chung, J. G. (2012). Anticancer potential of emodin. *BioMedicine*, *2*(3), 108–116. doi:10.1016/j.biomed.2012.03.003

Huang, H. S., Chiou, J. F., Chiu, H. F., Hwang, J. M., Lin, P. Y., Tao, C. W., ... Jeng, W. R. (2002). Synthesis of symmetrical 1, 5-bis-thio-substituted anthraquinones for cytotoxicity in cultured tumor cells and lipid peroxidation. *Chemical & Pharmaceutical Bulletin*, *50*(11), 1491–1494. doi:10.1248/cpb.50.1491 PMID:12419916

Huang, L., Zhang, T., Li, S., Duan, J., Ye, F., Li, H., ... Yang, X. (2014). Anthraquinone G503 induces apoptosis in gastric cancer cells through the mitochondrial pathway. *PLoS One*, *9*(9), e108286. doi:10.1371/journal.pone.0108286 PMID:25268882

Huang, P. H., & Lin, H. (2010). *Abstract B46: Proliferative suppression of anthraquinone derives emodin and aloe-emodin through selective targeting in prostate and breast cancer cells*. Academic Press.

Huang, Q., Lu, G., Shen, H. M., Chung, M., & Ong, C. N. (2007). Anti-cancer properties of anthraquinones from rhubarb. *Medicinal Research Reviews*, *27*(5), 609–630. doi:10.1002/med.20094 PMID:17022020

Jarrahpour, A., Ebrahimi, E., De Clercq, E., Sinou, V., Latour, C., Bouktab, L. D., & Brunel, J. M. (2011). Synthesis of mono-, bis-spiro-and dispiro-β-lactams and evaluation of their antimalarial activities. *Tetrahedron*, *67*(45), 8699–8704. doi:10.1016/j.tet.2011.09.041

Jarrahpour, A., Ebrahimi, E., Khalifeh, R., Sharghi, H., Sahraei, M., Sinou, V., ... Brunel, J. M. (2012). Synthesis of novel β-lactams bearing an anthraquinone moiety, and evaluation of their antimalarial activities. *Tetrahedron*, *68*(24), 4740–4744. doi:10.1016/j.tet.2012.04.011

Johnson, M. G., Kiyokawa, H., Tani, S., Koyama, J., Morris-Natschke, S. L., Mauger, A., ... Lee, K. H. (1997). Antitumor agents—CLXVII. Synthesis and structure-activity correlations of the cytotoxic anthraquinone 1, 4-bis-(2, 3-epoxypropylamino)-9, 10-anthracenedione, and of related compounds. *Bioorganic & Medicinal Chemistry*, *5*(8), 1469–1479. doi:10.1016/S0968-0896(97)00097-7 PMID:9313853

Jordheim, L. P., Marton, Z., Rhimi, M., Cros-Perrial, E., Lionne, C., Peyrottes, S., ... Chaloin, L. (2013). Identification and characterization of inhibitors of cytoplasmic 5'-nucleotidase cN-II issued from virtual screening. *Biochemical Pharmacology*, 85(4), 497–506. doi:10.1016/j.bcp.2012.11.024 PMID:23220537

Lee, S. U., Shin, H. K., Min, Y. K., & Kim, S. H. (2008). Emodin accelerates osteoblast differentiation through phosphatidylinositol 3-kinase activation and bone morphogenetic protein-2 gene expression. *International Immunopharmacology*, 8(5), 741–747. doi:10.1016/j.intimp.2008.01.027 PMID:18387517

Levinthal, C., Wodak, S. J., Kahn, P., & Dadivanian, A. K. (1975). Hemoglobin interaction in sickle cell fibers. I: Theoretical approaches to the molecular contacts. *Proceedings of the National Academy of Sciences of the United States of America*, 72(4), 1330–1334. doi:10.1073/pnas.72.4.1330 PMID:1055409

Li, B., Zhang, D. M., Luo, Y. M., & Chen, X. G. (2006). Three new and antitumor anthraquinone glycosides from Lasianthus acuminatissimus MERR. *Chemical & Pharmaceutical Bulletin*, 54(3), 297–300. doi:10.1248/cpb.54.297 PMID:16508180

Li, F., Li, X., Shao, J., Chi, P., Chen, J., & Wang, Z. (2010). Estrogenic activity of anthraquinone derivatives: In vitro and in silico studies. *Chemical Research in Toxicology*, 23(8), 1349–1355. doi:10.1021/tx100118g PMID:20707409

Li, Y. L., Zhang, J., Min, D., Hongyan, Z., Lin, N., & Li, Q. S. (2016). Anticancer effects of 1, 3-dihydroxy-2-methylanthraquinone and the ethyl acetate fraction of hedyotis diffusa willd against HepG2 carcinoma cells mediated via apoptosis. *PLoS One*, 11(4), e0151502. doi:10.1371/journal.pone.0151502 PMID:27064569

Lown, J. W. (1993). Anthracycline and anthraquinone anticancer agents: Current status and recent developments. *Pharmacology & Therapeutics*, 60(2), 185–214. doi:10.1016/0163-7258(93)90006-Y PMID:8022857

Magassouba, F. B., Diallo, A., Kouyaté, M., Mara, F., Mara, O., Bangoura, O., ... Lamah, K. (2007). Ethnobotanical survey and antibacterial activity of some plants used in Guinean traditional medicine. *Journal of Ethnopharmacology*, 114(1), 44–53. doi:10.1016/j.jep.2007.07.009 PMID:17825510

Manojlovic, N. T., Solujic, S., Sukdolak, S., & Milosev, M. (2005). Antifungal activity of Rubia tinctorum, Rhamnus frangula and Caloplaca cerina. *Fitoterapia*, *76*(2), 244–246. doi:10.1016/j.fitote.2004.12.002 PMID:15752641

Matsui, M., Taniguchi, S., Suzuki, M., Wang, M., Funabiki, K., & Shiozaki, H. (2005). Dyes produced by the reaction of 1, 2, 3, 4-tetrafluoro-9, 10-anthraquinones with bifunctional nucleophiles. *Dyes and Pigments*, *65*(3), 211–220. doi:10.1016/j.dyepig.2004.07.006

McKenzie, N., McNulty, J., McLeod, D., McFadden, M., & Balachandran, N. (2012). Synthesizing novel anthraquinone natural product-like compounds to investigate protein–ligand interactions in both an in vitro and in vivo assay: An integrated research-based third-year chemical biology laboratory course. *Journal of Chemical Education*, *89*(6), 743–749. doi:10.1021/ed200417d

Ozkok, F., & Sahin, Y. M. (2016). *Development of Original Method for Synthesis of Bioactive Anthraquine Anologues*. Patent No: 2016/19610 (Turkish Patent Institute).

Panigrahi, G. K., Verma, N., Singh, N., Asthana, S., Gupta, S. K., Tripathi, A., & Das, M. (2018). Interaction of anthraquinones of Cassia occidentalis seeds with DNA and Glutathione. *Toxicology Reports*, *5*, 164–172. doi:10.1016/j.toxrep.2017.12.024 PMID:29326881

Pankiewicz, F., Zöllmer, A., Gräser, Y., & Hilker, M. (2007). Article. *Archives of Insect Biochemistry and Physiology*, (66), 98–108.

Paramaguru, G., Kathiravan, A., Selvaraj, S., Venuvanalingam, P., & Renganathan, R. (2010). Interaction of anthraquinone dyes with lysozyme: Evidences from spectroscopic and docking studies. *Journal of Hazardous Materials*, *175*(1-3), 985–991. doi:10.1016/j.jhazmat.2009.10.107 PMID:19939563

Patai, S. (1988). *The Chemistry of Quinones Compounds*. New York: Wiley.

Perchellet, E. M., Magill, M. J., Huang, X., Dalke, D. M., Hua, D. H., & Perchellet, J. P. (2000). 1, 4-Anthraquinone: An anticancer drug that blocks nucleoside transport, inhibits macromolecule synthesis, induces DNA fragmentation, and decreases the growth and viability of L1210 leukemic cells in the same nanomolar range as daunorubicin in vitro. *Anti-Cancer Drugs*, *11*(5), 339–352. doi:10.1097/00001813-200006000-00004 PMID:10912950

Pesewu, G. A., Cutler, R. R., & Humber, D. P. (2008). Antibacterial activity of plants used in traditional medicines of Ghana with particular reference to MRSA. *Journal of Ethnopharmacology, 116*(1), 102–111. doi:10.1016/j.jep.2007.11.005 PMID:18096337

Pieme, C. A., Penlap, V. N., Ngogang, J., Kuete, V., Catros, V., & Moulinoux, J. P. (2009). In vitro effects of extract of Senna alata (Ceasalpiniaceae) on the polyamines produced by Leukaemia cells (L1210). *Pharmacognosy Magazine, 5*(17), 8.

Rarey, M. (2001). Protein–ligand docking in drug design. *Bioinformatics-from genomes to drugs*, 315-360.

Rath, G., Ndonzao, M., & Hostettmann, K. (1995). Antifungal anthraquinones from Morinda lucida. *International Journal of Pharmacognosy, 33*(2), 107-114.

Ryan, A., Kaplan, E., Nebel, J. C., Polycarpou, E., Crescente, V., Lowe, E., ... Sim, E. (2014). Identification of NAD (P) H quinone oxidoreductase activity in azoreductases from P. aeruginosa: Azoreductases and NAD (P) H quinone oxidoreductases belong to the same FMN-dependent superfamily of enzymes. *PLoS One, 9*(6), e98551. doi:10.1371/journal.pone.0098551 PMID:24915188

Saturnino, C., Fusco, B., Saturnino, P., De Martino, G., Rocco, F., & Lancelot, J. C. (2000). Evaluation of analgesic and anti-inflammatory activity of novel β-lactam monocyclic compounds. *Biological & Pharmaceutical Bulletin, 23*(5), 654–656. doi:10.1248/bpb.23.654 PMID:10823683

Schinazi, R. F., Chu, C. K., Babu, J. R., Oswald, B. J., Saalmann, V., Cannon, D. L., ... Nasr, M. (1990). Anthraquinones as a new class of antiviral agents against human immunodeficiency virus. *Antiviral Research, 13*(5), 265–272. doi:10.1016/0166-3542(90)90071-E PMID:1697740

Singh, D. N., Verma, N., Raghuwanshi, S., Shukla, P. K., & Kulshreshtha, D. K. (2006). Antifungal anthraquinones from Saprosma fragrans. *Bioorganic & Medicinal Chemistry Letters, 16*(17), 4512–4514. doi:10.1016/j.bmcl.2006.06.027 PMID:16824761

Sperka, T., Pitlik, J., Bagossi, P., & Tözsér, J. (2005). Beta-lactam compounds as apparently uncompetitive inhibitors of HIV-1 protease. *Bioorganic & Medicinal Chemistry Letters, 15*(12), 3086–3090. doi:10.1016/j.bmcl.2005.04.020 PMID:15893929

Sternberg, M. J., & Moont, G. (2002). Modelling protein–protein and protein–DNA docking. *Bioinformatics-From Genomes to Drugs*, 361-404.

Tsang, S. W., Zhang, H., Lin, C., Xiao, H., Wong, M., Shang, H., ... Bian, Z. (2013). Rhein, a natural anthraquinone derivative, attenuates the activation of pancreatic stellate cells and ameliorates pancreatic fibrosis in mice with experimental chronic pancreatitis. *PLoS One*, *8*(12), e82201. doi:10.1371/journal.pone.0082201 PMID:24312641

Wang, W., Chen, R., Luo, Z., Wang, W., & Chen, J. (2018). Antimicrobial activity and molecular docking studies of a novel anthraquinone from a marine-derived fungus Aspergillus versicolor. *Natural Product Research*, *32*(5), 558–563. doi:10.1080/14786419.2017.1329732 PMID:28511613

Wuthi-udomlert, M., Kupittayanant, P., & Gritsanapan, W. (2010). In vitro evaluation of antifungal activity of anthraquinone derivatives of Senna alata. *J Health Res*, *24*(3), 117–122.

Wuthi-Udomlert, M., Prathanturarug, S., & Soonthornchareonnon, N. (2001, July). Antifungal activities of Senna alata extracts using different methods of extraction. In *International Conference on Medicinal and Aromatic Plants (Part II) 597* (pp. 205-208). Academic Press.

Yang, K. L., Wei, M. Y., Shao, C. L., Fu, X. M., Guo, Z. Y., Xu, R. F., ... Wang, C. Y. (2012). Antibacterial anthraquinone derivatives from a sea anemone-derived fungus Nigrospora sp. *Journal of Natural Products*, *75*(5), 935–941. doi:10.1021/np300103w PMID:22545792

Yen, G. C., Duh, P. D., & Chuang, D. Y. (2000). Antioxidant activity of anthraquinones and anthrone. *Food Chemistry*, *70*(4), 437–441. doi:10.1016/S0308-8146(00)00108-4

Zarzeczanska, D., Niedzialkowski, P., Wcislo, A., Chomicz, L., Rak, J., & Ossowski, T. (2014). Synthesis, redox properties, and basicity of substituted 1-aminoanthraquinones: Spectroscopic, electrochemical, and computational studies in acetonitrile solutions. *Structural Chemistry*, *25*(2), 625–634. doi:10.100711224-013-0332-z

Zhang, J., Redman, N., Litke, A. P., Zeng, J., Zhan, J., Chan, K. Y., & Chang, C. W. T. (2011). Synthesis and antibacterial activity study of a novel class of cationic anthraquinone analogs. *Bioorganic & Medicinal Chemistry*, *19*(1), 498–503. doi:10.1016/j.bmc.2010.11.001 PMID:21111625

Zhang, X., Thuong, P. T., Jin, W., Su, N. D., Bae, K., & Kang, S. S. (2005). Antioxidant Activity of Anthraquinones and Flavonoids from Flower ofReynoutria sachalinensis. *Archives of Pharmacal Research*, *28*(1), 22–27. doi:10.1007/BF02975130 PMID:15742803

Zheng, Y., Zhu, L., Fan, L., Zhao, W., Wang, J., Hao, X., ... Wang, W. (2017). Synthesis, SAR and pharmacological characterization of novel anthraquinone cation compounds as potential anticancer agents. *European Journal of Medicinal Chemistry*, *125*, 902–913. doi:10.1016/j.ejmech.2016.10.012 PMID:27769031

Chapter 8
The Importance of Ionic Liquids and Applications on Their Molecular Modeling

Sefa Celik
Istanbul University – Cerrahpasa, Turkey

Ali Tugrul Albayrak
Istanbul University – Cerrahpasa, Turkey

Sevim Akyuz
Istanbul Kultur University, Turkey

Aysen E. Ozel
Istanbul University, Turkey

ABSTRACT

Ionic liquids are salts with melting points generally below 100 °C made of entirely ions by the combination of a large cation and a group of anions. Some ionic liquids are found to have therapeutic properties due to their toxic effects (e.g., anticancer, antibacterial, and antifungal properties). The determination of the most stable molecular structures, that is, the lowest energy conformer of these ionic liquids with versatile biological activities, is of particular importance. Density function theory (DFT) based on quantum mechanical calculation method, one of the molecular modeling methods, is widely used in physics and chemistry to determine the electronic structures of these stable geometries and molecules. With the theory, the energy of the molecule is determined by using the electron density instead of the wave function. It is observed that the theoretical models developed on the ionic liquids in the literature are in agreement with the experimental results because of electron correlations included in the calculation.

DOI: 10.4018/978-1-5225-7467-5.ch008

INTRODUCTION

The first ionic liquid was synthesized by Paul Walden 104 years ago. Ionic liquids are eutectic salt mixtures that consist completely of ions and their melting point is normally below 100 °C. Ionic liquids have been of interest by reason of their many unique features such as superior capacity to dissolve organic and inorganic substances, enormously low volatility, adjustable nature, high thermal stability, high chemical inertness, adjustable viscosity, high conductivity, high heat capacity, wide electrochemical range. Ionic liquids have outstanding handling advantages like nearly zero probability of explosion in high-temperature chemical reactions on account of their low volatilities and non-flammability, their use over a broad range of reaction temperatures owing to their high thermal stabilities (ie thermal decay generally above 350 °C) and high boiling points, dissolution of several organic and inorganic materials in this liquids and usage of polar aprotic ionic liquids to replace harmful and flammable polar aprotic solvents such as dimethylsulfoxide, acetonitrile and dimethylformamide. As long as the synthesis routes and purification methods are more complicated, the costs of ionic liquids become even higher (Ozokwelu et al., 2017; Dupont et al., 2015).

General Synthesis Methods of Ionic Liquids

Lately, more ionic liquids have been synthesized by different methods. The reactions of the processes are commonly neutralization, quaternization and ion exchange reactions.

1. Acid-Base Neutralization

The exothermic neutralization reaction between equimolar Brönsted acid and Brönsted base that is performed either in a vessel equipped with a cooling jacket or in a flask immersed into a water bath, or an ice bath brings about the formation of ionic liquids through proton transfer, which is among the easiest synthesis routes. Following the reaction, remaining unreacted starting materials in ionic liquid can be readily removed from the formed product by washing with water, and the final product is dried in a vacuum oven (Wasserscheid and Welton, 2002). When carboxylic acids are treated with some amines at high temperatures, amides can form in place of ionic liquid.

Consequently, the process must be performed at low temperatures to prevent amide formation and also to achieve high ionic liquid yield (Kirchner, 2009).

2. Quaternization

This type of reactions is very simple: by protonation reaction in which amine reacts with an acid to form an amine salt or by reaction of an amine or a phosphine with a haloalkane under mixing and heating. An example is complete reaction of 1-methyl imidazole with chloroalkanes at about 80 °C for 2-3 days. This process is economically pretty favorable as it is carried out with cheap starting materials (e.g. haloalkanes) at mild temperatures (Wasserscheid and Welton, 2002).

3. Anion-Exchange

These reactions of ionic liquids are usually classified as the direct reaction of halide salts with Lewis acids and the formation of ionic liquids via anion metathesis (Wasserscheid and Welton, 2002).

a. Halometallate Ionic Liquids

They are obtained simply by mixing a quaternary halide salt Q^+X^- with a Lewis acid MX_n (usually $AlCl_3$) and this reaction, which is quite exothermic, can generate multiple anion species based on different molar ratios of MX_n to Q^+X^-. The synthesis must be carried out either in an externally cooled vessel or by adding one component to the other in small portions to hinder the occurrence of extreme heat from which the thermal degradation of the final product may result.

Due to the water-sensitive character of the ionic liquid formed and many starting materials, the reactions must be accomplished in an inert medium both not to affect the physical properties of the resultant product and to reach high purity (Wasserscheid and Welton, 2002).

b. Anion Metathesis

Alkylated methylimidazolium cation-based ionic liquids, which are unaffected by air and water, were first synthesized in 1992 by Wilkes and Zaworotko through a metathesis reaction between silver salts such as $AgNO_3$, $AgBF_4$ and [EMIM] I in methanol. Since the by-product silver iodide precipitates in methanol solution and the reaction solvent is volatile, AgI and methanol can be facilely separated from the ionic liquid by filtration and distillation, respectively, thereby providing ionic liquids with high yield and purity. However, this synthesis is not cost-effective since the silver salts are expensive.

Hydrophobic ionic liquids obtained by the cation-anion metathesis between the halide salt in water and free acid or metal salt are composed of the cation of the halide salt and the anion of free acid or metal salt. When free acid is used, the remaining trace amounts of acid can degrade the ionic liquid in time if water-wash procedure to remove the resulting by-product hydrogen halide and also the unreacted acid is not completely carry out. Therefore, to solve this problem, metal salt can be used instead of free acid. Due to the exothermic nature of most metathesis reactions, indirect cooling should be provided throughout the reaction (Wasserscheid and Welton, 2002).

Removal of Impurities From Ionic Liquids

The properties of ionic liquids formed are substantially influenced by various contaminants such as organic starting materials, organic solvents used through the reaction, halide impurities stemmed from metathesis reactions and water (Ozokwelu et al., 2017).

The following points must be borne in mind to prevent the above-mentioned impurities: The impure starting chemicals reduce the purity and yield of the ionic liquid formed. If not pure, they should be purified before the synthesis. Throughout the synthesis reaction, it is necessary to keep the reaction temperature as low as possible since, as a result of the elevated temperatures, possible side reactions can cause the discoloration of the final product and a decrease in yield. Since the ionic liquid formed in the synthesis time can be affected by oxygen and moisture in the atmosphere depending on its structure, the quaternization reactions must be done within an inert atmosphere (nitrogen and helium). It is favorable to use starting materials in low quantities (<0.3 mole) since quaternization reactions release high heat (Ozokwelu et al., 2017; Endres et al., 2008).

Some Physical and Chemical Properties of Ionic Liquids

The solubility of an ionic liquid in water can be modulated by altering the alkyl side chain of the cation. Furthermore, depending on anion species on the ionic liquid, ILs can differ considerably in physical and chemical properties (Mohammad and Inamuddin, 2012).

- **Melting Point:** The melting point of several ionic liquids can be indefinite as ionic liquids undergo a greatly varying phase transition temperature depending on considerable over-cooling by heating or cooling the sample. They generally melt below 100 °C and are mostly liquid at 20-25 °C. The reduction of the melting point of ionic liquids is attributed to both cations and anions. As the size of the anion increases, the melting point of ionic liquid decreases (Mohammad and Inamuddin, 2012).

- **Volatility:** Ionic liquids are used in the field of green chemistry by virtue of their negligible vapor pressure even at high temperatures, meaning they are considered non-flammable due to their non-volatility in the environment with higher temperatures. Thermogravimetric analyses show a large number of ionic liquids undergo thermal decomposition at temperatures greater than 350 °C depending the anion and cation type (Mohammad and Inamuddin, 2012).

- **Viscosity:** Ionic liquids generally have a much lower fluidity than organic solvents at 20-25 °C. The viscosity of ionic liquids has an important effect on mixing, blending, pumping operations and friction as it can influence the mass transfer properties and machinery lubrication (Mohammad and Inamuddin, 2012).

- **Density:** Densities of ionic liquids, whose densities are found to decrease with an increase in alkyl chain length of the cation, are generally between 1 and 1.6 g cm^{-3}. For similar ionic liquids, the density of ionic liquid decreases as the size of the organic cation increases (Mohammad and Inamuddin, 2012).

- **Toxicity:** Ionic liquids are used in sustainable chemistry as a substitute for conventional organic solvents. Though it is assumed that ionic liquids are not toxic, this is not the case. Some anions and cations of ionic liquids can show toxicity and accordingly, they can be harmful to the environment. Alternatively, introducing different functional groups into ionic liquids can cause a change in the toxicity of ionic liquids (Mohammad and Inamuddin, 2012).

- **Water and Air-Stability:** Many ionic liquids are not affected by air and moisture, whereas many hydrophilic imidazolium and ammonium salts can be exposed to hydration in a humid ambient. The hydrophobicity of ionic liquids has been reported to decrease with decreasing alkyl chain length (Mohammad and Inamuddin, 2012).

- **Production Cost and Biodegradation:** Owing to the high cost and biodegradability issues of ionic liquids, novel green solvents have been synthesized from low-cost starting materials or renewable raw materials. Especially in the recent times, cheap choline chlorine-based deep eutectic liquids have been produced. Ionic liquids with choline cations have been reported to demonstrate biodegradable properties. The inclusion of an ester group into long alkyl chains can diminish not only the degree that the ionic liquid can harm living organisms but also its ecological toxicity (Mohammad and Inamuddin, 2012).

Toxicological Issues

As ionic liquids are used in vast amounts, toxicity and environmental problems are becoming increasingly crucial. 1-butyl-3-methylimidazolium-based ionic liquids were usually found to be slightly biodegradable. Ionic liquids with short alkyl group are usually not active against microbes and fungi but become activated by an alkyl chain length of 8 or more carbon atoms. The criterion for becoming active (i.e. showing toxicity) is that the ionic liquid can enter microbial or fungal cells. As long as they are virtually eliminated from other organic chemicals and that biodegradation products are not toxic and that ionic liquids are not volatile, humans are barely exposed to them (Dyson and Geldbach, 2005).

Biological Properties

Both cations and anions of ionic liquids affect their biological properties. Ionic liquids with long alkyl substituents generally inhibit the growth of pathogenic microorganisms and exhibit poor capacity to induce mutation on the plants. They are not significantly toxic for most animals (Dupont et al., 2015).

Anticancer Activities

The primary organic cations found in ionic liquids are imidazolium, pyridinium, ammonium, phosphonium and guanidium (Kokorin, 2011; Florindo et al., 2013; Dias et al., 2017). In the synthesis of ILs, inorganic or organic anions such as halides, tetrafluoroborate, hexafluorophosphate, bis (trifluoromethylsulfonyl) amide (TF_2N), acetate, dicyanamide, cyanoborate, sulfate, $[ClO_4]^-$, $[NO_3]^-$ etc.) can be used (Kokorin, 2011; Ferraz et al., 2011; Bubalo et al., 2014; Plechkova and Seddon,2014; Handy,2011).

Recently, the biggest challenges in the pharmaceutical sector are bioavailability, solubility, stability and polymorphism (Hilfiker, 2006). When solid drugs are used, their solubility changes by undergoing polymorphic transformation, thus affecting bioavailability (Bauer, 2008). When incorporated into drugs, ionic liquids can exhibit biological activity and also can result in increased bioavailability by solving the above-mentioned problems (especially by inhibiting polymorphism) (Ferraz et al., 2011; Marrucho et al., 2014; Kaushik et al., 2012; Malhotra, 2010). However, the ionic liquid may not be biologically active alone. For this purpose, it is necessary to introduce active pharmaceutical additives (biologically active ingredients (Beken, 2007)) into the ionic liquid (Dias et al., 2017). In addition, pharmaceutical products with higher yield can be synthesized using ionic liquids instead of toxic organic solvents as reaction media at shorter reaction times (Moniruzzaman and Goto, 2011; Ahfad-Hosseini et al., 2017; Modugu and Pittala, 2017).

Cancer is one of the fatal diseases such as AIDS, Ebola, yellow fever and malaria in the World (The World Health Report, 1996) and most people are ever-increasingly getting cancer due to poor diet, smoking, obesity and air pollution (Schottenfeld and Fraumeni, 2018). Conventional cancer treatments such as chemotherapy and radiotherapy kill the fast-growing cancer cells, whereas those therapies can damage healthy cells, which causes some adverse side effects (Senapati et al., 2018). Therefore, there is a need to use new compounds which are not harmful to normal human cells and which show high toxicity towards cancer cells. To achieve this goal, ionic liquids can be used as anticancer agent for new cancer treatments (Kaushik et al., 2012). By changing the constituent cations and anions, not only the physical and the pharmacological properties of ionic liquids but also their toxicity to destroy cancer cells can easily be tailored (Marrucho et al., 2014; Kumar and Malhotra, 2009).

Effect of Cation Side Chain Length of Ionic Liquid on Human Cancer Cells

In studies carried out with different parent groups such as imidazolium, ammonium, phosphonium and pyridinium with different halides, it was demonstrated an increase in the alkyl side chain length from C_1 to C_{18} leads to increased toxicity and thus a decline in cell viability (Florindo et al., 2013; Arning and Matzke, 2011). In another study investigating anticancer activity and cytotoxicity of phosphonium and ammonium-based ionic liquids, it has been revealed that the capability to destroy tumor increased with the alkyl chain length and also phosphonium-based ionic liquids were even more bioactive and less cytotoxic than ammonium-based ionic liquids (Kumar and Malhotra, 2009).

Effect of a Functional Group in Ionic Liquid

In addition to the effects of toxicity of cation side chain length on human cancer cell lines, the effect of functional groups on the main cation side chain of ionic liquids on tumor cell lines has been examined. The polar groups in the cation of the methylimidazolium-based ionic liquids have been shown to enhance HT-29 cell viability in the presence of PF_6 and BF_4 anions (Frade et al., 2007). In other comparable studies, it has been reported that incorporation of ether functionality, an oxygen, terminal hydroxyl group and nitrile function into the side chains of ionic liquid cations cause a lower toxicity (Stolte et al., 2007; Frade et al., 2009; Samori et al., 2010).

The Effects of Ionic Liquids on Bacteria, Fungi and Enzymes

In a study concerning the effect of a series of imidazolium-based ionic liquids on antibacterial activity, it was found that the antibacterial activity decreased in the following order: Vibrio Cholera > Micro coccus luteus > Klebsiella aerogenes > Staphylo coccus aureus and BBMIMBr is the most toxic ionic liquid towards the bacteria (Rajathi and Rajendran, 2013). Ionic liquids based on imidazolium, pyridinium, pyrrolidinium, piperidinium, ammonium and other cations have been reported to have antibacterial and antifungal activity (Egorova and Ananikov, 2014; Docherty and Kulpa, 2005; Pernak et al., 2007; Dipeolu et al., 2009; Hough-Troutman et al., 2009; Papaiconomou et al., 2010; Cornellas et al., 2011; Iwai et al., 2011; Pretti et al., 2011; Wang et al., 2011; Ventura et al., 2012[a]; Ventura et al., 2012[b]; Ventura et al., 2014; Anvari et al., 2016; Yu et al., 2016; Egorova et al., 2017).

It has been observed that ionic liquids with BF_4^-, PF_6^- ve Tf_2N^- anions which have lower hydrogen bond basicity and nucleophilicity improves the stability and activity of the enzymes as compared to ionic liquids with $CF_3CO_2^-, CF_3SO_3^-, NO_3^-, Cl^-, Br^-, CH_3CO_2^-$ anions which have high hydrogen bond basicity and nucleophilicity (Patel et al., 2014; Zhao, 2010; Anderson et al., 2002; Armstrong et al., 1999; Park and Kazlauskas, 2003; Sheldon et al., 2002; Lozano et al., 2001; Zhao et al., 2006; Lue et al., 2010; Kaar et al., 2003; Noritomi et al., 2011; Lee et al., 2006; Dabirmanesh et al., 2011; Constatinescu et al., 2010). It was established that enzymes in hydrophobic ionic liquids such as [omim][PF_6], [bmim][PF_6], [hmim][PF_6] and [hmim] [Tf_2N] have generally a higher activity than in hydrophilic ones such as [bmim] [CF_3COO], [bmim][BF_4], [bmim][Cl] and [bmim][NO_3], thus more stable (Kaar et al., 2003; Laszlo and Compton,2001; Yang and Pan, 2005 ; Nara et al., 2002; de Gonzalo et al., 2007; Shen et al., 2008; Hernandez-Fernandez et al., 2009). In some studies, it is reported that ionic liquids based on cations with short alkyl chains have a higher stabilizing effect than ionic liquids based on cations with long alkyl chain on the enzymes (Dabirmanesh et al., 2011; Lange et al., 2005; Yamamoto et al., 2011; Yan et al., 2012). Besides, it is found that some ionic liquids improve the thermal stability of proteins (Fujita et al., 2005; Micaelo and Soares, 2008; Byrne et al., 2007).

Molecular Modeling

Molecular modelling offers applications to drug design and chemistry, to investigate wide range of molecular systems, from small molecules to large molecular systems. In this way, the process of discovering new drug molecules has gained speed. The molecules having a flexible structure are in motion at room temperature and the spatial positions of the atoms forming the molecule are constantly changing. Thus, molecules may have different conformers having different energy. However, there are more low-energy conformations among these conformers. The fact that the activity of the drugs depends on the low-energy conformation shows the importance of investigating these conformations. Molecular modeling simulations make it possible to find all possible low-energy conformations. One of the widely used quantum mechanical calculations in molecular modeling is the Density Functional Theory (DFT). This method is increasingly used due to the high-accuracy predictions of the molecular properties and the reduction of the calculation time.

DFT Method

By using the DFT method based on the electron density of a many-body system, the physical and chemical properties can be found and the structures can be clarified in detail. DFT can be applied to atoms, molecules, liquids and solids. The basis of this approach was put by Llewellyn Thomas-Enrico Fermi. It was developed by the theorems introduced by Pierre Hohenber and Walter Kohn in 1964 and by Walter Kohn-Lu Jeu Sham in 1965, with the inclusion of Coulomb interactions between the electrons, e.g., the exchange and correlation interactions. After the approximations used in the theory were greatly refined to better model the exchange and correlation interactions, both the reliability and the usage of DFT have increased exponentially. DFT is a widely used electronic structure method, because of its short calculation time and its compatibility with experimental results.

DFT Applications of Ionic Liquids

In 2009, Katsyuba and colleagues, modeled the structure of imidazolium ionic liquid in dichloromethane (Katsyuba et al., 2009) at B3LYP level with 6-31G* basis set. They calculated the energies of the molecular structures obtained by considering possible hydrogen bonds between molecules (Figure 1). Among these structures, the most stable (viz. the lowest-energy) structure of the ionic liquid has been determined. Furthermore, C-H stretching frequencies and IR intensities of seven possible molecular structures have been calculated using the same method with the same basis set.

Lassegues and his collaborates first optimized the geometry of cis, trans, planar and non-planar conformation of 1-ethyl-3-methyl-imidazolium bis (trifluoromethanesulfonyl) imide ionic liquid by HF/6-311+ G* method. Geometry and vibration spectrum calculations (HF + DFT) were performed at the B3LYP level with 6-311+ G * basis set (Lassegues et al., 2007).

In 2010, Zhang and his collaborates investigated the structure of 1-Ethyl-3-Methylimidazolium Ethyl Sulfate ionic liquid and calculated the hydrogen bond interaction between the ionic liquid and the water molecule. The optimized geometries (Figure 2), bonding energy, harmonic vibrational frequencies and IR intensities were calculated by the 6-31++G(d,p) basis set (Zhang et al., 2010).

Figure 1. The energies obtained by taking into account possible hydrogen bonds of the ionic liquid: 1-Ethyl-3-methylimidazolium tetrafluoroborate
(Katsyuba et al., 2009)

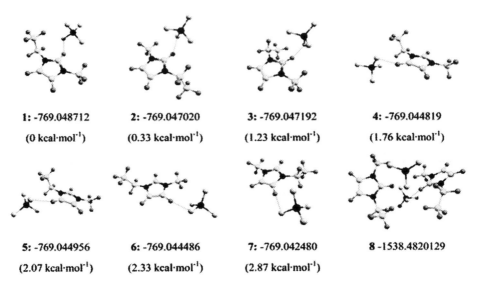

1: -769.048712   **2: -769.047020**   **3: -769.047192**   **4: -769.044819**

(0 kcal·mol⁻¹)   (0.33 kcal·mol⁻¹)   (1.23 kcal·mol⁻¹)   (1.76 kcal·mol⁻¹)

5: -769.044956   **6: -769.044486**   **7: -769.042480**   **8 -1538.4820129**

(2.07 kcal·mol⁻¹)   (2.33 kcal·mol⁻¹)   (2.87 kcal·mol⁻¹)

Figure 2. Molecular modeling of 1-Ethyl-3-Methylimidazolium Ethyl Sulfate ionic liquid and its components with water
(Zhang et al., 2010)

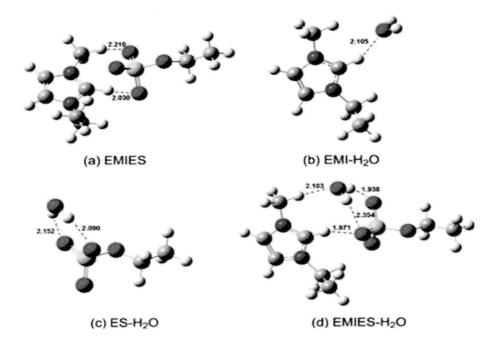

(a) EMIES   (b) EMI-H₂O

(c) ES-H₂O   (d) EMIES-H₂O

In a study carried out by Katsyuba et al. on 1-Ethyl-3-methyl-1H-imidazolium tetrafluoroborate ionic liquid, the stable molecular geometry was found as in Figure 3 using the DFT method at the B3LYP level with the 6-31G* and 6-31 +G* basis sets. They compared the experimental IR and Raman spectra with the theoretical ones obtained by calculating the vibrational frequency and IR Raman intensities using the DFT/B3LYP method with the 6-31G* basis set (Katsyuba et al., 2004).

In another study reported in 2004 on the modeling of a series of alkyl imidazolium-based ionic liquids, their optimized molecular structures (Figure 4), their theoretical vibration frequencies and their IR intensities have been calculated at the 6-311+G(2d,p) basis sets (Talaty et al., 2004).

In 2006, Heimer et al. fulfilled a study on the three ionic liquids containing tetrafluoroborate anions using DFT/B3LYP/6-311+G(2d,p) basis set and the theoretical vibration frequencies of these ionic liquids have been determined via their molecular geometries with the lowest energy (Figure 5) (Heimer et al., 2006).

Figure 3. Molecular structure (optimized at the B3LYP/6-31+ G* basis set) of 1-Ethyl-3-methyl-1H-imidazolium Tetrafluoroborate ionic liquid (Katsyuba et al., 2004)

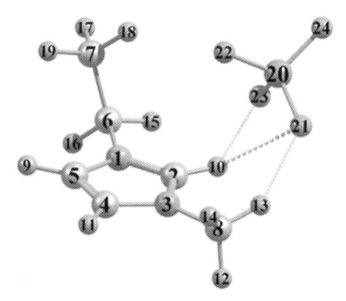

Figure 4. The molecular structures of the ionic liquids: 1-ethyl-3-methyl imidazolium hexafluorophosphate (a), 1-propyl-3-methyl imidazolium hexafluorophosphate (b) and 1-butyl-3-methylimidazolium hexafluorophosphate (c) at the 6-311+G(2d,p) basis set
(Talaty et al., 2004)

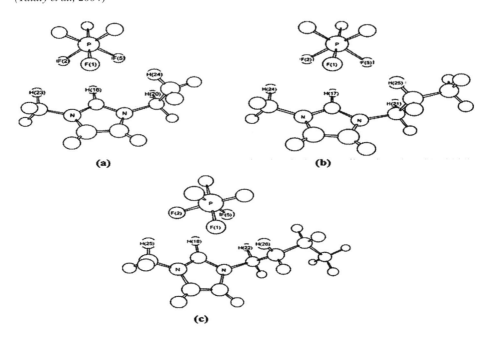

(a)　　　　　　　(b)

(c)

In 2013, in an other study, the optimized molecular structure of the complex obtained as a result of the interaction of 1-ethyl-3-methylimidazolium ethylsulphate ionic liquid with carbazole molecule using Hartree-Fock method and 6-31G* basis set was determined (Figure 6) (Ramalingam et al., 2013).

In 2012, Roth and his collaborates determined the stable molecular geometry of imidazolium-based ionic liquids [C_nMIM] [NTf_2] and their hydrogen bond lengths with DFT / B3LYP function and 6-31+ G(d) basis set (Figure 7)(Roth et al., 2012).

Zorn et al. have found the optimized geometries of tetrazolium-based ionic liquids with the DFT/ B3LYP function employing 6-311G(d, p) basis set (Zorn et al., 2006).

Figure 5. The optimized molecular structures of 1-ethyl-3-methylimidazolium tetrafluoroborate (a,b), 1-propyl-3-methylimidazolium tetrafluoroborate (c,d), 1-butyl-3-methylimidazolium tetrafluoroborate (e-g) and their conformers determined at the 6-311+G(2d, p) basis set
(Heimer et al., 2006)

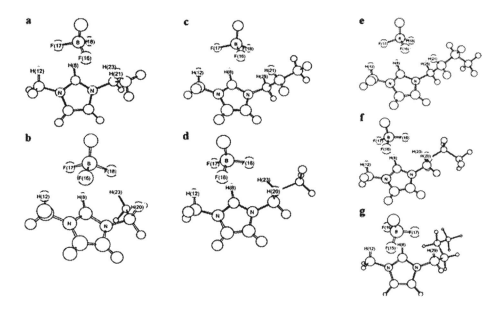

Figure 6. The optimized molecular structures of 1-ethyl-3-methylimidazolium ethylsulphate ionic liquid and its carbazole complex
(Ramalingam et al., 2013)

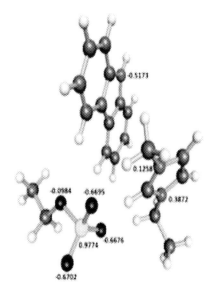

Figure 7. The stable geometry obtained at B3LYP/6-31+G(d) level of theory for [C₂MIM][NTf₂] ionic liquid
(Roth et al., 2012)

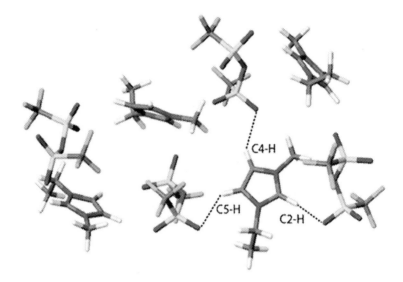

Figure 8. The stable conformers of 1-ethyl-3-methyl imidazolium tetracyanoborate ([Emim]⁺[TCB]⁻) ionic liquid
(Mao et al., 2013)

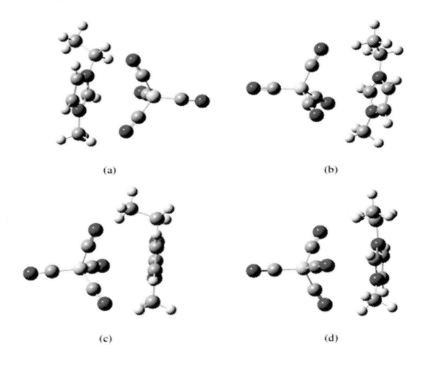

The stable optimized geometries of 1-ethyl-3-methyl imidazolium tetracyanoborate ([Emim]$^+$[TCB]$^-$) ionic liquid have been determined by Mao et al. using the DFT method [B3LYP/6-31+G(d,p) basis set]. The theoretical vibration frequencies belonging to the conformers are also calculated (Figure 8)(Mao et al., 2013).

REFERENCES

Ahfad-Hosseini, H. R., Bagheri, H., & Amidi, S. (2017). Ionic liquid-assisted synthesis of celexocib using tris-(2-hydroxyethyl) ammonium acetate as an efficient and reusable catalyst. *Iranian Journal of Pharmaceutical Research*, *16*(1), 158–164. PMID:28496471

Anderson, J. L., Ding, J., Welton, T., & Armstrong, D. W. (2002). Characterizing ionic liquids on the basis of multiple solvation interactions. *Journal of the American Chemical Society*, *124*(47), 14247–14254. doi:10.1021/ja028156h PMID:12440924

Anvari, S., Hajfarajollah, H., Mokhtarani, B., Enayati, M., Sharifi, A., & Mirzaei, M. (2016). Antibacterial and anti-adhesive properties of ionic liquids with various cationic and anionic heads toward pathogenic bacteria. *Journal of Molecular Liquids*, *221*, 685–690. doi:10.1016/j.molliq.2016.05.093

Armstrong, D. W., He, L., & Liu, Y. S. (1999). Examination of ionic liquids and their interaction with molecules, when used as stationary phases in gas chromatography. *Analytical Chemistry*, *71*(17), 3873–3876. doi:10.1021/ac990443p PMID:10489532

Arning, J., & Matzke, M. (2011). Toxicity of ionic liquids towards mammalian cell lines. *Current Organic Chemistry*, *15*(12), 1905–1917. doi:10.2174/138527211795703694

Bauer, J. F. (2008). Polymorphism--a critical consideration in pharmaceutical development, manufacturing, and stability. *Journal of Validation Technology*, *14*(5), 15-24.

Beken, T. V. (2007). *The European Pharmaceutical Sector and Crime Vulnerabilities*. Antwerb, Belgium: Maklu Publishers.

Bubalo, M. C., Radošević, K., Redovniković, I. R., Halambek, J., & Srček, V. G. (2014). A brief overview of the potential environmental hazards of ionic liquids. *Ecotoxicology and Environmental Safety*, *99*, 1–12. doi:10.1016/j. ecoenv.2013.10.019 PMID:24210364

Byrne, N., Wang, L. M., Belieres, J. P., & Angell, C. A. (2007). Reversible folding–unfolding, aggregation protection, and multi-year stabilization, in high concentration protein solutions, using ionic liquids. *Chemical Communications*, (26): 2714–2716. doi:10.1039/B618943A PMID:17594030

Constatinescu, D., Herrmann, C., & Weingärtner, H. (2010). Patterns of protein unfolding and protein aggregation in ionic liquids. *Physical Chemistry Chemical Physics*, *12*(8), 1756–1763. doi:10.1039/b921037g PMID:20145840

Cornellas, A., Perez, L., Comelles, F., Ribosa, I., Manresa, A., & Garcia, M. T. (2011). Self-aggregation and antimicrobial activity of imidazolium and pyridinium based ionic liquids in aqueous solution. *Journal of Colloid and Interface Science*, *355*(1), 164–171. doi:10.1016/j.jcis.2010.11.063 PMID:21186035

Dabirmanesh, B., Daneshjou, S., Sepahi, A. A., Ranjbar, B., Khavari-Nejad, R. A., Gill, P., ... Khajeh, K. (2011). Effect of ionic liquids on the structure, stability and activity of two related α-amylases. *International Journal of Biological Macromolecules*, *48*(1), 93–97. doi:10.1016/j. ijbiomac.2010.10.001 PMID:20946913

de Gonzalo, G., Lavandera, I., Durchschein, K., Wurm, D., Faber, K., & Kroutil, W. (2007). Asymmetric biocatalytic reduction of ketones using hydroxy-functionalised water-miscible ionic liquids as solvents. *Tetrahedron, Asymmetry*, *18*(21), 2541–2546. doi:10.1016/j.tetasy.2007.10.010

Dias, A. R., Costa-Rodrigues, J., Fernandes, M. H., Ferraz, R., & Prudencio, C. (2017). The anticancer potential of ionic liquids. *ChemMedChem*, *12*(1), 11–18. doi:10.1002/cmdc.201600480 PMID:27911045

Dipeolu, O., Green, E., & Stephens, G. (2009). Effects of water-miscible ionic liquids on cell growth and nitro reduction using Clostridium sporogenes. *Green Chemistry*, *11*(3), 397–401. doi:10.1039/b812600c

Docherty, K. M., & Kulpa, C. F. Jr. (2005). Toxicity and antimicrobial activity of imidazolium and pyridinium ionic liquids. *Green Chemistry*, *7*(4), 185–189. doi:10.1039/b419172b

Dupont, J., Itoh, T., Lozano, P., & Malhotra, S. V. (2015). *Environmentally Friendly Syntheses Using Ionic Liquids.* CRC Press.

Dyson, P. J., & Geldbach, T. J. (2005). *Metal Catalysed Reactions in Ionic Liquids* (Vol. 29). Dordrecht, Netherlands: Springer. doi:10.1007/1-4020-3915-8

Egorova, K. S., & Ananikov, V. P. (2014). Toxicity of ionic liquids: Eco (cyto) activity as complicated, but unavoidable parameter for task-specific optimization. *ChemSusChem, 7*(2), 336–360. doi:10.1002/cssc.201300459 PMID:24399804

Egorova, K. S., Gordeev, E. G., & Ananikov, V. P. (2017). Biological activity of ionic liquids and their application in pharmaceutics and medicine. *Chemical Reviews, 117*(10), 7132–7189. doi:10.1021/acs.chemrev.6b00562 PMID:28125212

Endres, F., MacFarlane, D., & Abbott, A. (2008). *Electrodeposition from Ionic Liquids.* Weinheim, Germany: Wiley-VCH Verlag GmbH&Co. KgaA. doi:10.1002/9783527622917

Ferraz, R., Branco, L. C., Prudencio, C., Noronha, J. P., & Petrovski, Z. (2011). Ionic liquids as active pharmaceutical ingredients. *ChemMedChem, 6*(6), 975–985. doi:10.1002/cmdc.201100082 PMID:21557480

Florindo, C., Araujo, J. M., Alves, F., Matos, C., Ferraz, R., Prudencio, C., ... Marrucho, I. M. (2013). Evaluation of solubility and partition properties of ampicillin-based ionic liquids. *International Journal of Pharmaceutics, 456*(2), 553–559. doi:10.1016/j.ijpharm.2013.08.010 PMID:23978632

Frade, R. F., Matias, A., Branco, L. C., Afonso, C. A., & Duarte, C. M. (2007). Effect of ionic liquids on human colon carcinoma HT-29 and CaCo-2 cell lines. *Green Chemistry, 9*(8), 873–877. doi:10.1039/b617526k

Frade, R. F., Rosatella, A. A., Marques, C. S., Branco, L. C., Kulkarni, P. S., Mateus, N. M., ... Duarte, C. M. (2009). Toxicological evaluation on human colon carcinoma cell line (CaCo-2) of ionic liquids based on imidazolium, guanidinium, ammonium, phosphonium, pyridinium and pyrrolidinium cations. *Green Chemistry, 11*(10), 1660–1665. doi:10.1039/b914284n

Fujita, K., MacFarlane, D. R., & Forsyth, M. (2005). Protein solubilising and stabilising ionic liquids. *Chemical Communications*, (38): 4804–4806. doi:10.1039/b508238b PMID:16193120

Handy, S. T. (2011). *Applications of Ionic Liquids in Science and Technology.* Croatia: InTech Publisher. doi:10.5772/1769

Heimer, N. E., Del Sesto, R. E., Meng, Z., Wilkes, J. S., & Carper, W. R. (2006). Vibrational spectra of imidazolium tetrafluoroborate ionic liquids. *Journal of Molecular Liquids, 124*(1-3), 84–95. doi:10.1016/j.molliq.2005.08.004

Hernandez-Fernandez, F. J., De los Rios, A. P., Tomás-Alonso, F., Gomez, D., & Víllora, G. (2009). Stability of hydrolase enzymes in ionic liquids. *Canadian Journal of Chemical Engineering, 87*(6), 910–914. doi:10.1002/cjce.20227

Hilfiker, R. (2006). *Polymorphism: in the Pharmaceutical Industry.* Weinheim, Germany: WILEY-VCH Verlag GmbH&Co. doi:10.1002/3527607889

Hough-Troutman, W. L., Smiglak, M., Griffin, S., Reichert, W. M., Mirska, I., Jodynis-Liebert, J., ... Pernak, J. (2009). Ionic liquids with dual biological function: Sweet and anti-microbial, hydrophobic quaternary ammonium-based salts. *New Journal of Chemistry, 33*(1), 26–33. doi:10.1039/B813213P

Inamuddin. (2012). Green Solvents II-Properties and Applications of Ionic Liquids. Springer Science+Business Media.

Iwai, N., Nakayama, K., & Kitazume, T. (2011). Antibacterial activities of imidazolium, pyrrolidinium and piperidinium salts. *Bioorganic & Medicinal Chemistry Letters, 21*(6), 1728–1730. doi:10.1016/j.bmcl.2011.01.081 PMID:21324694

Kaar, J. L., Jesionowski, A. M., Berberich, J. A., Moulton, R., & Russell, A. J. (2003). Impact of ionic liquid physical properties on lipase activity and stability. *Journal of the American Chemical Society, 125*(14), 4125–4131. doi:10.1021/ja028557x PMID:12670234

Katsyuba, S. A., Dyson, P. J., Vandyukova, E. E., Chernova, A. V., & Vidiš, A. (2004). Molecular Structure, Vibrational Spectra, and Hydrogen Bonding of the Ionic Liquid 1-Ethyl-3-methyl-1H-imidazolium Tetrafluoroborate. *Helvetica Chimica Acta, 87*(10), 2556–2565. doi:10.1002/hlca.200490228

Katsyuba, S. A., Griaznova, T. P., Vidis, A., & Dyson, P. J. (2009). Structural studies of the ionic liquid 1-ethyl-3-methylimidazolium tetrafluoroborate in dichloromethane using a combined DFT-NMR spectroscopic approach. *The Journal of Physical Chemistry B, 113*(15), 5046–5051. doi:10.1021/jp8083327 PMID:19309104

Kaushik, N., Attri, P., Kaushik, N., & Choi, E. (2012). Synthesis and antiproliferative activity of ammonium and imidazolium ionic liquids against T98G brain cancer cells. *Molecules (Basel, Switzerland), 17*(12), 13727–13739. doi:10.3390/molecules171213727 PMID:23174892

Kirchner, B. (2009). Ionic Liquids. *Topics in Current Chemistry, 290*. PMID:21107799

Kokorin, A. (2011). *Ionic Liquids: Applications and Perspectives*. Rijeka: InTech Publishing. doi:10.5772/1782

Kumar, V., & Malhotra, S. V. (2009). Study on the potential anti-cancer activity of phosphonium and ammonium-based ionic liquids. *Bioorganic & Medicinal Chemistry Letters, 19*(16), 4643–4646. doi:10.1016/j.bmcl.2009.06.086 PMID:19615902

Lange, C., Patil, G., & Rudolph, R. (2005). Ionic liquids as refolding additives: N′-alkyl and N′-(ω-hydroxyalkyl) N-methylimidazolium chlorides. *Protein Science, 14*(10), 2693–2701. doi:10.1110/ps.051596605 PMID:16195554

Lassegues, J. C., Grondin, J., Holomb, R., & Johansson, P. (2007). Raman and ab initio study of the conformational isomerism in the 1-ethyl-3-methyl-imidazolium bis (trifluoromethanesulfonyl) imide ionic liquid. *Journal of Raman Spectroscopy: JRS, 38*(5), 551–558. doi:10.1002/jrs.1680

Laszlo, J. A., & Compton, D. L. (2001). α-Chymotrypsin catalysis in imidazolium-based ionic liquids. *Biotechnology and Bioengineering, 75*(2), 181–186. doi:10.1002/bit.1177 PMID:11536140

Lee, S. H., Ha, S. H., Lee, S. B., & Koo, Y. M. (2006). Adverse effect of chloride impurities on lipase-catalyzed transesterifications in ionic liquids. *Biotechnology Letters, 28*(17), 1335–1339. doi:10.100710529-006-9095-6 PMID:16820978

Lozano, P., de Diego, T., Guegan, J. P., Vaultier, M., & Iborra, J. L. (2001). Stabilization of α-chymotrypsin by ionic liquids in transesterification reactions. *Biotechnology and Bioengineering, 75*(5), 563–569. doi:10.1002/bit.10089 PMID:11745132

Lue, B. M., Guo, Z., & Xu, X. (2010). Effect of room temperature ionic liquid structure on the enzymatic acylation of flavonoids. *Process Biochemistry, 45*(8), 1375–1382. doi:10.1016/j.procbio.2010.05.024

Malhotra, S. V. (2010). *Ionic Liquid Applications: Pharmaceuticals, Therapeutics, and Biotechnology.* Washington, DC: ACS. doi:10.1021/bk-2010-1038

Mao, J. X., Lee, A. S., Kitchin, J. R., Nulwala, H. B., Luebke, D. R., & Damodaran, K. (2013). Interactions in 1-ethyl-3-methyl imidazolium tetracyanoborate ion pair: Spectroscopic and density functional study. *Journal of Molecular Structure, 1038,* 12–18. doi:10.1016/j.molstruc.2013.01.046

Marrucho, I. M., Branco, L. C., & Rebelo, L. P. N. (2014). Ionic liquids in pharmaceutical applications. *Annual Review of Chemical and Biomolecular Engineering, 5*(1), 527–546. doi:10.1146/annurev-chembioeng-060713-040024 PMID:24910920

Micaelo, N. M., & Soares, C. M. (2008). Protein structure and dynamics in ionic liquids. Insights from molecular dynamics simulation studies. *The Journal of Physical Chemistry B, 112*(9), 2566–2572. doi:10.1021/jp0766050 PMID:18266354

Modugu, N. R., & Pittala, P. K. (2017). Ionic liquid mediated and promoted one-pot green synthesis of new isoxazolyl dihydro-1 H-indol-4 (5 H)-one derivatives at ambient temperature. *Cogent Chemistry, 3*(1), 1318693. doi:10.1080/23312009.2017.1318693

Moniruzzaman, M., & Goto, M. (2011). Ionic Liquids: Future Solvents and Reagents for Pharmaceuticals. *Journal of Chemical Engineering of Japan, 44*(6), 370–381. doi:10.1252/jcej.11we015

Nara, S. J., Harjani, J. R., & Salunkhe, M. M. (2002). Lipase-catalysed transesterification in ionic liquids and organic solvents: A comparative study. *Tetrahedron Letters, 43*(16), 2979–2982. doi:10.1016/S0040-4039(02)00420-3

Noritomi, H., Minamisawa, K., Kamiya, R., & Kato, S. (2011). Thermal stability of proteins in the presence of aprotic ionic liquids. *Journal of Biomedical Science and Engineering, 4*(2), 94–99. doi:10.4236/jbise.2011.42013

Ozokwelu, D., Zhang, S., Okafor, O. C., Cheng, W., & Litombe, N. (2017). *Novel Catalytic and Separation Processes Based On Ionic Liquids.* Elsevier Inc.

Papaiconomou, N., Estager, J., Traore, Y., Bauduin, P., Bas, C., Legeai, S., ... Draye, M. (2010). Synthesis, physicochemical properties, and toxicity data of new hydrophobic ionic liquids containing dimethylpyridinium and trimethylpyridinium cations. *Journal of Chemical & Engineering Data*, *55*(5), 1971–1979. doi:10.1021/je9009283

Park, S., & Kazlauskas, R. J. (2003). Biocatalysis in ionic liquids–advantages beyond green technology. *Current Opinion in Biotechnology*, *14*(4), 432–437. doi:10.1016/S0958-1669(03)00100-9 PMID:12943854

Patel, R., Kumari, M., & Khan, A. B. (2014). Recent advances in the applications of ionic liquids in protein stability and activity: A review. *Applied Biochemistry and Biotechnology*, *172*(8), 3701–3720. doi:10.100712010-014-0813-6 PMID:24599667

Pernak, J., Syguda, A., Mirska, I., Pernak, A., Nawrot, J., Prądzyńska, A., ... Rogers, R. D. (2007). Choline-derivative-based ionic liquids. *Chemistry (Weinheim an der Bergstrasse, Germany)*, *13*(24), 6817–6827. doi:10.1002/chem.200700285 PMID:17534999

Plechkova, N. V., & Seddon, K. R. (2014). *Ionic Liquids Further UnCOILed: Critical Expert Overviews.* John Wiley & Sons, Inc. doi:10.1002/9781118839706

Pretti, C., Renzi, M., Focardi, S. E., Giovani, A., Monni, G., Melai, B., ... Chiappe, C. (2011). Acute toxicity and biodegradability of N-alkyl-N-methylmorpholinium and N-alkyl-DABCO based ionic liquids. *Ecotoxicology and Environmental Safety*, *74*(4), 748–753. doi:10.1016/j.ecoenv.2010.10.032 PMID:21093055

Rajathi, K., & Rajendran, A. (2013). Synthesis, Characterization and Biological Evaluation of Imidazolium Based Ionic Liquids. *RRJC*, *2*(1), 36–41.

Ramalingam, A., Hizaddin, H. F., Jayakumar, N. S., & Hashim, M. A. B. (2013). A quantum chemical study on interaction energy between halogen free ionic liquid and aromatic nitrogen compounds. *Journal of Innovative Engineering*, *1*(1), 3.

Roth, C., Chatzipapadopoulos, S., Kerle, D., Friedriszik, F., Lütgens, M., Lochbrunner, S., ... Ludwig, R. (2012). Hydrogen bonding in ionic liquids probed by linear and nonlinear vibrational spectroscopy. *New Journal of Physics*, *14*(10), 105026. doi:10.1088/1367-2630/14/10/105026

Samorì, C., Malferrari, D., Valbonesi, P., Montecavalli, A., Moretti, F., Galletti, P., ... Pasteris, A. (2010). Introduction of oxygenated side chain into imidazolium ionic liquids: Evaluation of the effects at different biological organization levels. *Ecotoxicology and Environmental Safety*, *73*(6), 1456–1464. doi:10.1016/j.ecoenv.2010.07.020 PMID:20674022

Schottenfeld, D., & Fraumeni, J. F. (2018). *Cancer Epidemiology and Prevention* (4th ed.). Oxford University Press.

Senapati, S., Mahanta, A. K., Kumar, S., & Maiti, P. (2018). Controlled drug delivery vehicles for cancer treatment and their performance. *Signal Transduction and Targeted Therapy, 3*(1), 7.

Sheldon, R. A., Lau, R. M., Sorgedrager, M. J., van Rantwijk, F., & Seddon, K. R. (2002). Biocatalysis in ionic liquids. *Green Chemistry*, *4*(2), 147–151. doi:10.1039/b110008b

Shen, Z. L., Zhou, W. J., Liu, Y. T., Ji, S. J., & Loh, T. P. (2008). One-pot chemoenzymatic syntheses of enantiomerically-enriched O-acetyl cyanohydrins from aldehydes in ionic liquid. *Green Chemistry*, *10*(3), 283–286. doi:10.1039/b717235d

Stolte, S., Arning, J., Bottin-Weber, U., Müller, A., Pitner, W. R., Welz-Biermann, U., ... Ranke, J. (2007). Effects of different head groups and functionalised side chains on the cytotoxicity of ionic liquids. *Green Chemistry*, *9*(7), 760–767. doi:10.1039/B615326G

Talaty, E. R., Raja, S., Storhaug, V. J., Dölle, A., & Carper, W. R. (2004). Raman and infrared spectra and ab initio calculations of C2-4MIM imidazolium hexafluorophosphate ionic liquids. *The Journal of Physical Chemistry B*, *108*(35), 13177–13184. doi:10.1021/jp040199s

The World Health Report. (1996). *Fighting disase, Fostering development*. WHO.

Ventura, S. P., de Barros, R. L., Sintra, T., Soares, C. M., Lima, Á. S., & Coutinho, J. A. (2012). Simple screening method to identify toxic/non-toxic ionic liquids: Agar diffusion test adaptation. *Ecotoxicology and Environmental Safety*, *83*, 55–62. doi:10.1016/j.ecoenv.2012.06.002 PMID:22742861

Ventura, S. P., Marques, C. S., Rosatella, A. A., Afonso, C. A., Gonçalves, F., & Coutinho, J. A. (2012). Toxicity assessment of various ionic liquid families towards Vibrio fischeri marine bacteria. *Ecotoxicology and Environmental Safety*, *76*, 162–168. doi:10.1016/j.ecoenv.2011.10.006 PMID:22019310

Ventura, S. P., Silva, F. A., Gonçalves, A. M., Pereira, J. L., Gonçalves, F., & Coutinho, J. A. (2014). Ecotoxicity analysis of cholinium-based ionic liquids to Vibrio fischeri marine bacteria. *Ecotoxicology and Environmental Safety*, *102*, 48–54. doi:10.1016/j.ecoenv.2014.01.003 PMID:24580821

Wang, H., Malhotra, S. V., & Francis, A. J. (2011). Toxicity of various anions associated with methoxyethyl methyl imidazolium-based ionic liquids on Clostridium sp. *Chemosphere*, *82*(11), 1597–1603. doi:10.1016/j. chemosphere.2010.11.049 PMID:21159360

Wasserscheid, P., & Welton, T. (2002). *Ionic Liquids in Synthesis*. Weinheim, Germany: Wiley-VCH Verlag GmbH&Co. KgaA. doi:10.1002/3527600701

Yamamoto, E., Yamaguchi, S., & Nagamune, T. (2011). Protein refolding by N-alkylpyridinium and N-alkyl-N-methylpyrrolidinium ionic liquids. *Applied Biochemistry and Biotechnology*, *164*(6), 957–967. doi:10.100712010-011-9187-1 PMID:21302144

Yan, H., Wu, J., Dai, G., Zhong, A., Chen, H., Yang, J., & Han, D. (2012). Interaction mechanisms of ionic liquids [Cnmim] Br (n= 4, 6, 8, 10) with bovine serum albumin. *Journal of Luminescence*, *132*(3), 622–628. doi:10.1016/j. jlumin.2011.10.026

Yang, Z., & Pan, W. (2005). Ionic liquids: Green solvents for nonaqueous biocatalysis. *Enzyme and Microbial Technology*, *37*(1), 19–28. doi:10.1016/j. enzmictec.2005.02.014

Yu, J., Zhang, S., Dai, Y., Lu, X., Lei, Q., & Fang, W. (2016). Antimicrobial activity and cytotoxicity of piperazinium-and guanidinium-based ionic liquids. *Journal of Hazardous Materials*, *307*, 73–81. doi:10.1016/j. jhazmat.2015.12.028 PMID:26775108

Zhang, Q. G., Wang, N. N., & Yu, Z. W. (2010). The hydrogen bonding interactions between the ionic liquid 1-ethyl-3-methylimidazolium ethyl sulfate and water. *The Journal of Physical Chemistry B*, *114*(14), 4747–4754. doi:10.1021/jp1009498 PMID:20337406

Zhao, H. (2010). Methods for stabilizing and activating enzymes in ionic liquids—A review. *Journal of Chemical Technology and Biotechnology (Oxford, Oxfordshire), 85*(7), 891–907. doi:10.1002/jctb.2375

Zhao, H., Olubajo, O., Song, Z., Sims, A. L., Person, T. E., Lawal, R. A., & Holley, L. A. (2006). Effect of kosmotropicity of ionic liquids on the enzyme stability in aqueous solutions. *Bioorganic Chemistry, 34*(1), 15–25. doi:10.1016/j.bioorg.2005.10.004 PMID:16325223

Zorn, D. D., Boatz, J. A., & Gordon, M. S. (2006). Electronic structure studies of tetrazolium-based ionic liquids. *The Journal of Physical Chemistry B, 110*(23), 11110–11119. doi:10.1021/jp060854r PMID:16771373

Chapter 9
Sequential Importance Sampling for Logistic Regression Model

Ruriko Yoshida
Naval Postgraduate School, USA

Hisayuki Hara
Doshisha University, Japan

Patrick M. Saluke
Naval Postgraduate School, USA

ABSTRACT

Logistic regression is one of the most popular models to classify in data science, and in general, it is easy to use. However, in order to conduct a goodness-of-fit test, we cannot apply asymptotic methods if we have sparse datasets. In the case, we have to conduct an exact conditional inference via a sampler, such as Markov Chain Monte Carlo (MCMC) or Sequential Importance Sampling (SIS). In this chapter, the authors investigate the rejection rate of the SIS procedure on a multiple logistic regression models with categorical covariates. Using tools from algebra, they show that in general SIS can have a very high rejection rate even though we apply Linear Integer Programming (IP) to compute the support of the marginal distribution for each variable. More specifically, the semigroup generated by the columns of the design matrix for a multiple logistic regression has infinitely many "holes." They end with application of a hybrid scheme of MCMC and SIS to NUN study data on Alzheimer disease study.

DOI: 10.4018/978-1-5225-7467-5.ch009

INTRODUCTION

Sampling from two-way and multiway contingency tables has a wide range of applications such as computing exact p-values of goodness-of-fit, estimating the number of contingency tables satisfying given marginal sums and more (Besag and Clifford 1989; Y. Chen et al. 2005; Diaconis and Efron 1985; Guo and Thompson 1992). For some problems, such as sparse tables, the data of interest does not permit the use of asymptotic methods. In such cases, one can apply Monte Carlo Markov Chain (MCMC) procedures using *Markov bases* (Diaconis and Sturmfels 1998). In order to run MCMC over the state space, all states must be connected via a Markov chain. A Markov basis is a set of moves on all contingency tables (the state space) guaranteed to be connected via a Markov chain (Diaconis and Sturmfels 1998). One important quality of a Markov basis is that the moves will work for any marginal sums under a fixed model. The two major advantages to using a MCMC approach, if a Markov basis is already known, is that it is easy to program, and it is not memory intensive. However MCMC methods are not without drawbacks where one bottleneck is the computation of a Markov basis. In fact, for 3-way contingency tables with fixed 2-margins, De Loera and Onn (2005) showed that the number of Markov basis elements can be arbitrary. To try to circumvent the difficulty of computing a Markov basis which may be large, Yuguo Chen et al. (2005; Bunea and Besag 2000) studied computing a smaller set of moves by allowing entries of the contingency table to be negative. The trade off to this approach is longer running time of the Markov chains. Even using a standard MCMC approach, to sample a table independently from the distribution, the Markov chains can take a long time to converge to a stationary distribution in order to satisfy the independent assumption. Lastly, it is not clear in general how long the chain must be run to converge.

A sequential importance sampling (SIS) procedure is easy to implement and was first applied to sampling two-way contingency tables under the independence model in (Y. Chen et al. 2005). It proceeds by simply sampling cell entries of the contingency table sequentially such that the final distribution approximates the target distribution. This method will terminate at the last cell and sample independently and identically distributed (iid) tables from the proposal distribution. Thus the SIS procedure does not require expensive or prohibitive pre-computations, as is the case of computing a Markov basis for a MCMC approach. Second, when attempting to sample a single table, the

SIS procedure is guaranteed to sample a table from the distribution, where in an MCMC approach the chain may require a long time to run in order to satisfy the independent condition. In these regards, the SIS overcomes the disadvantages of MCMC but presents a new set of problems. One major difficulty is computing the marginal distribution of each cell. Typically an interval from which the support of the marginal distribution lies is computed using Integer Programming (IP), Linear Programming (LP), or the Shuttle Algorithm (Dobra and Fienberg 2010). When the support of the marginal distribution does not equal the interval, the SIS procedure may reject the partially sampled table. The SIS has been successful on two-way contingency tables due to the fact that the computed interval often equals the support of the marginal distribution. For example, under the independence model, the SIS procedure will always produce tables satisfying the marginal sums, i.e. there are no rejections (Chen, Dinwoodie, and Sullivant 2006). Moreover, for zero-one two-way contingency tables (Y. Chen et al. 2005) provided an algorithm to sample using the SIS with Conditional Poisson distributions which also avoids rejections and relies on the Gale-Ryser Theorem. (Chen, Dinwoodie, and Sullivant 2006) extended the SIS to multiway contingency tables, and gave excellent algebraic interpretations of precisely when an interval will equal the support of the marginal distribution. Regardless, one of the major disadvantages of the SIS is the fact that rejections lead to increased computational time.

In this paper we focus on the rejection rate of the SIS procedure on a multiple logistic regression model with categorical covariates. In order to study we use the notion of the *semigroup* (defined in Subsection 2.4), of the columns of the *design matrix* (defined in Subsection 2.1). In general, we show that the rejection rate of the SIS procedure for the multiple logistic regression with categorical covariates can be arbitrary high.

We end this paper with simulation studies and application of a hybrid scheme of MCMC with a set of moves which was proposed in (Hara, Takemura, and Yoshida 2010) and SIS procedures to a multidimensional study data set of nuns with Alzheimer's Disease from (Mortimer 2012). We attempt to ascertain the performance of our method for predicting the propensity among Alzheimer's patients to transition to a state of senility or death. We hope to use this research to validate our methodology and develop a general approach that analysts and researchers could replicate on a variety of similar problems.

PRELIMINARIES

Basic Notation

Let $\mathbf{n}$ be a contingency table with k cells. In order to simplify the notation, we denote by $\mathcal{X} = \{1, \ldots, k\}$ the sample space of contingency tables.

Let $\mathbb{Z}_+$ be the set of nonnegative integers, i.e., $\mathbb{Z}_+ = \{0, 1, 2, \ldots\}$ and let $\mathbb{Z}$ be the set of all integers, i.e., $\mathbb{Z} = \{\ldots, -2, -1, 0, 1, 2, \ldots\}$. Without loss of generality, in this paper, we represent a table by a vector of counts $\mathbf{n} = (n_1, \ldots, n_k)$. With this point of view, a contingency table $\mathbf{n}$ can be regarded as a function $\mathbf{n} : \mathcal{X} \rightarrow \mathbb{Z}_+$, and it can also be viewed as a vector $\mathbf{n} \in \mathbb{Z}_+^k$.

The fiber of an observed table $\mathbf{n}_{\text{obs}}$ with respect to a function $T : \mathbb{Z}_+^k \rightarrow \mathbb{Z}_+^d$ is the set

$$\mathcal{F}_T\left(\mathbf{n}_{\text{obs}}\right) = \left\{\mathbf{n} \mid \mathbf{n} \in \mathbb{Z}_+^k, T\left(\mathbf{n}\right) = T\left(\mathbf{n}_{\text{obs}}\right)\right\}. \tag{1}$$

When the dependence on the specific observed table is irrelevant, we will write simply $\mathcal{F}_T$ instead of $\mathcal{F}_T\left(\mathbf{n}_{\text{obs}}\right)$.

In a mathematical statistics framework, the function T is usually the minimal sufficient statistic of some statistical model and the usefulness of enumeration of the fiber $\mathcal{F}_T\left(\mathbf{n}_{\text{obs}}\right)$ follows from classical theorems such as the Rao-Blackwell theorem, see e.g. (Shao 1998).

When the function T is linear, it can be extended in a natural way to a homomorphism from $\mathbb{R}^k$ to $\mathbb{R}^d$. The function T is represented by an $d \times k$-matrix A_T, and its element $A_T\left(\ell, h\right)$ is

$$A_T\left(\ell, h\right) = T_\ell\left(h\right), \tag{2}$$

where T_ℓ is the ℓ-th component of the function T. The matrix A_T is called the *design matrix* of the model T. In terms of the matrix A_T, the fiber $\mathcal{F}_T$ can be easily rewritten in the form:

$$\mathcal{F}_T = \left\{ \mathbf{n} \mid \mathbf{n} \in \mathbb{Z}_+^k, A_T \mathbf{n} = A_T \mathbf{n}_{\text{obs}} \right\}. \tag{3}$$

When the context is clear, we will simply write A instead of A_T.

Since the cell counts of a contingency table are nonnegative integers and usually the sufficient statistics are a set of marginals of cell counts, the design matrix A of a model T is a nonnegative $d \times k$ matrix.

Logistic Regression

We assume the sufficient statistic is fixed under the binomial logistic regression model with several covariates. In this section we remind readers of the sufficient statistic for the observed contingency table ($\mathbf{n}_0$) under a logistic regression with multiple covariates.

Let $\mathbf{X}$ be the $2 \times I_1 \times I_2 \times \ldots \times I_s$ table under the logistic regression with s many covariates. Let $X_{0i_1 i_2 \ldots i_s}$ be the $\left(0, i_1, i_2, \ldots, i_s \right)$th cell count for the response equal to 0 and $X_{1i_1 i_2 \ldots i_s}$ be the $\left(1, i_1, i_2, \ldots, i_s \right)$th cell count for the response equal to 1 of the table $\mathbf{X}$. Then the sufficient statistic for estimating regression $s+1$ coefficients consists of the following sums:

$$\sum_{i_1=1}^{I_1} \sum_{i_2=1}^{I_2} \cdots \sum_{i_s=1}^{I_s} X_{0i_1 i_2 \ldots i_s},$$

$$\sum_{i_1=1}^{I_1} \sum_{i_2=1}^{I_2} \cdots \sum_{i_s=1}^{I_s} i_1 \cdot X_{0i_1 i_2 \ldots i_s},$$

$$\sum_{i_1=1}^{I_1} \sum_{i_2=1}^{I_2} \cdots \sum_{i_s=1}^{I_s} i_2 \cdot X_{0i_1 i_2 \ldots i_s},$$

$$\vdots$$

$$\sum_{i_1=1}^{I_1} \sum_{i_2=1}^{I_2} \cdots \sum_{i_s=1}^{I_s} i_s \cdot X_{0i_1 i_2 \ldots i_s}.$$

In the binomial logistic regression models, the column sums

$$X_{0i_1i_2\cdots i_s} + X_{1i_1i_2\cdots i_s}, \text{ for } i_1 = 1,\ldots,I_1,\ldots,i_s = 1,\ldots,I_s$$

are also fixed.

In order to compute the design matrix (Hara, Takemura, and Yoshida 2010) used Segre Product of matrices and Lawrence lifting of a matrix. Following (Hara, Takemura, and Yoshida 2010), we consider two configurations $B = \left(\mathbf{b}_1,\cdots,\mathbf{b}_I\right)$ and $C = \left(\mathbf{c}_1,\cdots,\mathbf{c}_J\right)$, where $\mathbf{b}_i$ and $\mathbf{c}_j$ are column vectors. The Segre product of B and C is defined as

$$B \otimes C = \left(\mathbf{b}_i \oplus \mathbf{c}_j, i = 1,\cdots,I, j = 1,\cdots,J\right), \mathbf{b}_i \oplus \mathbf{c}_j = \begin{pmatrix} \mathbf{b}_i \\ \mathbf{c}_j \end{pmatrix}. \tag{4}$$

First, for each ith factor, we make a matrix:

$$A_i = \begin{bmatrix} 1 & 1 & \cdots & 1 \\ 1 & 2 & \cdots & I_i \end{bmatrix}.$$

Then we apply Segre Product on matrices $A_1,\ldots,A_s$.

For example, suppose we have a $2 \times 2 \times 3 \times 4$ table $\mathbf{X}$. To calculate the sufficient statistic from the observed table, we first flatten $\mathbf{n}_0$ from dimension $2 \times 2 \times 3 \times 4$ to a vector of 48×1. This simple transformation preserves the data exactly and allows for easier conceptualization of the sufficient statistic calculations through common 2-dimensional linear algebra.

For a factor with I levels, a configuration matrix is generated as

$$\mathrm{B} = \begin{bmatrix} 1 & 1 & \cdots & 1 \\ 1 & 2 & \cdots & I \end{bmatrix}. \tag{5}$$

Suppose we have three factors with levels $= 2, 3$, and 4 respectively. Using Equation (5), the Segre product of B, C, and D is:

$$\begin{bmatrix} 1 & 1 & 1 & 1 & 1 & 1 & 1 & 1 & 1 & 1 & 1 & 1 & 1 & 1 & 1 & 1 & 1 & 1 & 1 & 1 & 1 & 1 & 1 & 1 \\ 1 & 1 & 1 & 1 & 1 & 1 & 1 & 1 & 1 & 1 & 1 & 1 & 2 & 2 & 2 & 2 & 2 & 2 & 2 & 2 & 2 & 2 & 2 & 2 \\ 1 & 1 & 1 & 1 & 1 & 1 & 1 & 1 & 1 & 1 & 1 & 1 & 1 & 1 & 1 & 1 & 1 & 1 & 1 & 1 & 1 & 1 & 1 & 1 \\ 1 & 1 & 1 & 1 & 2 & 2 & 2 & 2 & 3 & 3 & 3 & 3 & 1 & 1 & 1 & 1 & 2 & 2 & 2 & 2 & 3 & 3 & 3 & 3 \\ 1 & 1 & 1 & 1 & 1 & 1 & 1 & 1 & 1 & 1 & 1 & 1 & 1 & 1 & 1 & 1 & 1 & 1 & 1 & 1 & 1 & 1 & 1 & 1 \\ 1 & 2 & 3 & 4 & 1 & 2 & 3 & 4 & 1 & 2 & 3 & 4 & 1 & 2 & 3 & 4 & 1 & 2 & 3 & 4 & 1 & 2 & 3 & 4 \end{bmatrix}.$$

The modified Segre product (Z) is obtained by removing the redundant rows (rows 3 and 5).

$$Z^{3 \times 24} = \begin{bmatrix} 1 & 1 & 1 & 1 & 1 & 1 & 1 & 1 & 1 & 1 & 1 & 1 & 1 & 1 & 1 & 1 & 1 & 1 & 1 & 1 & 1 & 1 & 1 & 1 \\ 1 & 1 & 1 & 1 & 1 & 1 & 1 & 1 & 1 & 1 & 1 & 1 & 2 & 2 & 2 & 2 & 2 & 2 & 2 & 2 & 2 & 2 & 2 & 2 \\ 1 & 1 & 1 & 1 & 2 & 2 & 2 & 2 & 3 & 3 & 3 & 3 & 1 & 1 & 1 & 1 & 2 & 2 & 2 & 2 & 3 & 3 & 3 & 3 \end{bmatrix}.$$

The row corresponding to Y_3, which has levels $= \{1, 2, 3, 4\}$, has been removed.

A Lawrence lifting of the modified Segre product (Z) yields the appropriate matrix for calculating the sufficient statistic (b). From (Xie 2016), the Lawrence lifting matrix (A) of the modified Segre product (Z) with C columns ($C = 24$ cells in this example with $L = 1$) is defined as:

$$A = \Lambda(Z) = \begin{bmatrix} Z & 0 \\ I_C & I_C \end{bmatrix} \tag{6}$$

where I_C is the identity matrix of dimension C.

Applying the Lawrence lifting matrix (A; Equation (6)) to our example facilitates the calculation of all 27 elements of $\mathbf{b}$ that satisfy the equation $A\mathbf{n}_0 = \mathbf{b}$ where $\mathbf{b}$ is the sufficient statistic vector.

Sequential Importance Sampling

Let $\mathcal{F}_T$ be the set of all tables satisfying marginal conditions (for example, under the independence model, all tables satisfying given row and column sums). Let $p(\mathbf{n})$, for any $\mathbf{n} \in \mathcal{F}_T$, be the uniform distribution over $\mathcal{F}_T$, so $p(\mathbf{n}) = 1 / |\mathcal{F}_T|$. Let $q(\cdot)$ be a trial distribution such that $q(\mathbf{n}) > 0$ for all $\mathbf{n} \in \mathcal{F}_T$. Then we have

$$\mathbb{E}\left[\frac{1}{q(\mathbf{n})}\right] = \sum_{\mathbf{n} \in \mathcal{F}_T} \frac{1}{q(\mathbf{n})} q(\mathbf{n}) = |\mathcal{F}_T|.$$

Thus we can estimate $|\mathcal{F}_T|$ by

$$|\hat{\mathcal{F}}_T| = \frac{1}{N} \sum_{i=1}^{N} \frac{1}{q(\mathbf{n}_i)},$$

where $\mathbf{n}_1, \ldots, \mathbf{n}_N$ are tables drawn iid from $q(\mathbf{n})$. Here, this proposed distribution $q(\mathbf{n})$ is the distribution (approximate) of tables sampled via the SIS.

If we vectorize the table $\mathbf{n} = (n_1, \cdots, n_k)$ then by the multiplication rule we have

$$q\left(\mathbf{n} = (n_1, \cdots, n_k)\right) = q(n_1) q(n_2 \mid n_1) q(n_3 \mid n_2, n_1) \cdots q(n_k \mid n_{k-1}, \ldots, n_1).$$

Since we sample each cell count of a table from a interval we can easily compute $q(n_i \mid n_{i-1}, \ldots, n_1)$ for $i = 2, 3, \ldots, k$.

When an interval of integers between the lower bound l_i and the upper bound u_i is the support of the marginal distribution $n_i \mid (n_{i-1}, \ldots, n_1)$ for n_i, Chen, Dinwoodie, and Sullivant (2006) noticed that one can sample a value from the interval at each step for n_i from the interval $[l_i, u_i]$ and this procedure always produces a table which satisfies the marginal constraints. Therefore if we can obtain l_i and u_i for each n_i sequentially we can apply the SIS.

Usually we obtain l_i and u_i for each n_i by Integer Programming (IP) to obtain tight bounds, namely we solve the linear integer programming problem for the lower bound:

$$\min\ x_i$$
$$\text{s.t.}\quad \mathbf{a}_i x_i + \cdots + \mathbf{a}_k x_k = \mathbf{b} - \left(\mathbf{a}_1 x_1^* + \cdots + \mathbf{a}_{i-1} x_{i-1}^*\right), \tag{7}$$
$$x_i, \ldots x_k \in \mathbb{Z}_+,$$

where $x_1^*, \ldots x_{i-1}^*$ are integers already sampled by the SIS, $\mathbf{b} = A\mathbf{n}_{\text{obs}}$, and $\mathbf{a}_j$ is the jth column of A. To compute the upper bound via IP we set $\max$ instead of $\min$ in Equation (7). One can approximate these bounds by linear programming (LP) or the Shuttle Algorithm (Buzzigoli and Giusti 1998), however they might not give tight bounds.

Based on this observation Chen, Dinwoodie, and Sullivant (2006) developed a sequential importance sampling (SIS) method to sample a table from $\mathcal{F}_T$. The outline of the SIS procedure is the following:

Algorithm 2.2 [Sequential Importance Sampling Procedure]

1. For $i = 1, \ldots, k$ do:
    a. Compute l_i and u_i by solving an integer programming problem (7).
    b. Sample an integer x_i^* from the interval $\left[l_i, u_i\right]$ according to the distribution q.
2. Return the table $\mathbf{x}^* = \left(x_1^*, \ldots, x_k^*\right)$.

Remark 2.3: If we want to estimate $\left|\mathcal{F}_T\right|$ then q is the uniform distribution over $\left[l_i, u_i\right] \cap \mathbb{Z}$. Thus we sample x_i^* from $\left[l_i, u_i\right] \cap \mathbb{Z}$ with a probability $1 / \left(u_i - l_i + 1\right)$.

When we have rejections, this means that we are sampling tables from a bigger set $\mathcal{F}_T^*$ such that $\mathcal{F}_T \subset \mathcal{F}_T^*$. In this case, as long as the conditional probability $q(n_i \mid n_{i-1}, \ldots, n_1)$ for $i = 2, 3, \ldots$ and $q(n_1)$ are normalized, $q(\mathbf{n})$ is normalized over $\mathcal{F}_T^*$ since

$$\sum_{\mathbf{n}\in\mathcal{F}_T^*} q(\mathbf{n}) = \sum_{n_1,\dots n_k} q(n_1)q(n_2\mid n_1)q(n_3\mid n_2,n_1)\cdots q(n_k\mid n_{k-1},\dots,n_1)$$

$$= \sum_{n_1} q(n_1)\left[\sum_{n_2} q(n_1\mid n_2)\left[\cdots\left[\sum_{n_k} q(n_k\mid n_{k-1},\dots,n_1)\right]\right]\right]$$

$$= 1.$$

Thus we have

$$\mathbb{E}\left[\frac{\mathbb{I}_{\mathbf{n}\in\mathcal{F}_T}}{q(\mathbf{n})}\right] = \sum_{\mathbf{n}\in\mathcal{F}_T^*}\frac{\mathbb{I}_{\mathbf{n}\in\mathcal{F}_T}}{q(\mathbf{n})}q(\mathbf{n}) = \left|\mathcal{F}_T\right|,$$

where $\mathbb{I}_{\mathbf{n}\in\mathcal{F}_T}$ is an indicator function for the set $\mathcal{F}_T$. . By the law of large numbers this estimator is unbiased.

Semigroup

Consider the following system of linear equations and inequalities:

$$A\mathbf{x} = \mathbf{b}, \mathbf{x} \geq 0, \tag{8}$$

where $A \in \mathbb{Z}^{d\times k}$ and $\mathbf{b} \in \mathbb{Z}^d$. Suppose the solution set

$$\left\{x \in \mathbb{R}^k : Ax = b, x \geq 0\right\} \neq \varnothing.$$

Note that there exists an integral solution for the system in (8) if and only if $\mathbf{b}$ is in the *semigroup* generated by the column vectors $\mathbf{a}_1,\dots,\mathbf{a}_k$ of A, that is, the set of all nonnegative integer combinations of the columns of A, namely

$$Q = Q(A) = \left\{\mathbf{a}_1 x_1 + \cdots + \mathbf{a}_k x_k \middle| x_1,\dots,x_k \in \mathbb{Z}_+\right\}.$$

Let $K = K(A)$ be the cone generated by the columns $\mathbf{a}_1,\dots,\mathbf{a}_k$ of A, that is:

$$K = K(A) = \left\{ \mathbf{a}_1 x_1 + \cdots + \mathbf{a}_k x_k \,\middle|\, x_1, \ldots, x_k \in \mathbb{R}_+ \right\}.$$

The lattice $L = L(A)$ generated by the columns $\mathbf{a}_1, \ldots, \mathbf{a}_k$ of A is:

$$L = L(A) = \left\{ \mathbf{a}_1 x_1 + \cdots + \mathbf{a}_n x_n \,\middle|\, x_1, \ldots, x_k \in \mathbb{Z} \right\}.$$

The semigroup $Q_{sat}(A) = K(A) \cap L(A)$ is called the *saturation* of the semigroup Q. It follows that $Q \subset Q_{sat}$ and we call Q *saturated* if $Q = Q_{sat}$ (this also is called *normal*). We define $H = H(A) = Q_{sat}(A) \setminus Q(A)$ the set of *holes* of the semigroup $Q(A)$.

If $b \in H \subset Q_{sat}$, then the system

$$A\mathbf{x} = \mathbf{b}, \mathbf{x} \geq 0, \mathbf{x} \in \mathbb{R}^k$$

has a feasible solution. However, the system

$$A\mathbf{x} = \mathbf{b}, \mathbf{x} \geq 0, \mathbf{x} \in \mathbb{Z}^k$$

does not have a feasible solution.

REJECTION RATE OF SIS PROCEDURE

Suppose we have a given set of marginals for contingency tables. Here in order to make sure the SIS can sample a table from the conditional state space, we want to decide whether there exists a table satisfying the given marginals.

This is called the *multi-dimensional integer planar transportation problem*. In terms of Optimization, we can rewrite this problem as an *integral feasibility problem*, that is: Decide whether there exists an integral solution in the system

$$A\mathbf{x} = \mathbf{b}, \mathbf{x} \geq 0,$$

where $A \in \mathbb{Z}^{d_1 \times d_2}$ and $b \in \mathbb{Z}^{d_1}$.

Remark 3.1: Assume the lattice L generated by the columns of A is $\mathbb{Z}^{d_1 \times d_2}$. Let $\operatorname{cone}(A)$ be the cone generated by the columns of A and $P_b = \{\mathbf{x} \in \mathbb{R}^{d_2} : A\mathbf{x} = \mathbf{b}, \mathbf{x} \geq 0\}$.

$$P_b \neq \varnothing \Leftrightarrow \mathbf{b} \in \operatorname{cone}(A).$$

Let $Q(A)$ be the semigroup generated by the columns A_i of A, i.e.

$$Q(A) = \{\sum_{i=1}^{d_2} \alpha_i A_i, | \, \alpha_i \in \mathbb{Z}_+ \} \subset \operatorname{cone}(A) \cap \mathbb{Z}^{d_1}.$$

$$P_b \neq \varnothing \Leftrightarrow \mathbf{b} \in \operatorname{cone}(A),$$

$$(P_b \neq \varnothing) \wedge (P_b \cap \mathbb{Z}^{d_2} \neq \varnothing) \Leftrightarrow b \in (\operatorname{cone}(A) \cap \mathbb{Z}^{d_1} - Q).$$

We study on the set of *holes* of $Q(A)$, $H(A) := \operatorname{cone}(A) \cap L(A) - Q(A)$, where $L(A)$ is the lattice generated by the columns of A.

Geometrically, we can see the picture as follows: The first quadrant is mapped to the semigroup generated by the columns of A (Figure 1).

In terms of SIS, we can view as shown in Figure 2.

Figure 1.

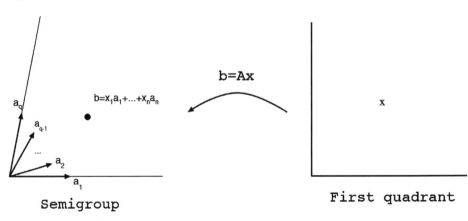

Semigroup   First quadrant

Figure 2.

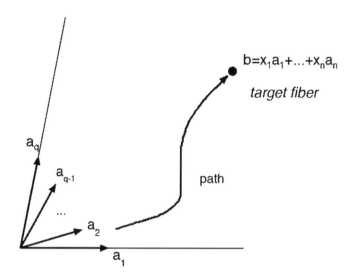

Here is a better example.

Example 3.2: Let

$$A = \begin{pmatrix} 1 & 1 & 1 & 1 \\ 2 & 0 & 3 & 4 \end{pmatrix},$$

and $b = (7,7)^T$ where x^T is the transpose of x. Then we have the lower and upper bounds for x_1 as $L_1 = 0$ and $U_1 = 2$ via Integer Programming. Then suppose we pick $x_1 = 1$. Then we have a new system of equalities:

$$A' = \begin{pmatrix} 1 & 1 & 1 \\ 0 & 3 & 4 \end{pmatrix},$$

and $b' = (7,7)^T - (1,2)^T = (6,5)$. Since the holes of the semigroup generated by the columns of A' is

$$H' = \left\{ \left(k, s \right) : s = 1, 2, 5, \ \text{and} \ k = 1, 2, 3, \ldots \right\}$$

and since $b' \in H'$, we cannot have a solution for the system

$$A'x = b' \ x \geq \mathbb{Z}_+^3.$$

In this example, the polytope has only two integer points, namely: $\left(2, 4, 1, 0 \right)$ and $\left(0, 5, 1, 1 \right)$.

Here we have the following theorem for the holes of the semigroup generated by the columns of the design matrix for the binary logistic regression model with more than one covariates.

Theorem 3.3: We consider the semigroup $Q\left(A \right)$ generated by the columns of the design matrix A for the univariate logistic regression model for $I = 2, J \geq 3$. Then $H(A) \neq \varnothing$.

Proof. Consider the design matrix for the univariate logistic regression with the level equal to three, i.e., $J = 3$, so that we have 2×3 contingency tables. The design matrix forms as follows:

```
1 1 1 0 0 0
1 2 3 0 0 0
1 0 0 1 0 0
0 1 0 0 1 0
0 0 1 0 0 1
```

Using the software normaliz (Bruns et al. 2017), the semigroup generated by the columns of this matrix is not normal. Therefore, the semigroup generated by the columns of the design matrix for 2×3 contingency tables under the univariate logistic regression model has holes. For $I \times J$ tables under the univariate logistic regression model, where $I = 2$ and $J \geq 3$, this 2×3 contingency table can be seen as a special case where cell count X_{ijk} with the indeces $i = 1, 2$ and $J \geq j \geq 3$ equals to zero. Therefore, the semigoup generated by the columns of the design matrix for the univariate logistic regression model has holes.

Theorem 3.4: We consider the semigroup $Q(A)$ generated by the columns of the design matrix A for the univariate logistic regression model for $I = 2, J \geq 3$. Then $Q(A)$ has infinitely many holes.

Proof. We use Theorem 3.7 from (Takemura and Yoshida 2008) to the semigroup $Q(A)$ generated by the columns of the design matrix of the logistic regression model with $J = 2$ and $K = 3$ shown in the proof for Theorem [thm:holes]. Let $\mathbf{b}_s$ be the sth column of the matrix A for $s = 1, \ldots, 6$. After using the software normaliz, the Hilbert basis consists of the 6 columns of the matrix A and one additional vector:

$$\mathbf{b}_7 = \left(1, 2, 1, 0, 1\right).$$

Therefore $\mathbf{b}_7 \notin Q(A)$. Then we set the following system of linear equations such that:

$$\mathbf{b}_1 x_1 + \mathbf{b}_2 x_2 + \ldots + \mathbf{b}_6 x_6 = \mathbf{b}_7$$
$$x_1 \in \mathbb{Z}_-, \; x_i \in \mathbb{Z}_+, \; \text{for } i = 2, 3, \ldots, 6.$$

We used R package lpSolve (Buttrey 2015) to solve the system of equations using the linear programming with the cost function $\min x_1$, then it shows that there is no real solution in the system of linear equations and inequalities. Thus, $\mathbf{b}_7 \notin \left(-\mathbb{N}A_1\right) + Q(A)_1$, where $Q(A)_1$ is the semigroup generated by $\mathbf{b}_2, \ldots, \mathbf{b}_{12}$. Therefore, by Theorem 3.7 from (Takemura and Yoshida 2008), the number of elements in $H(A)$ is infinite. We can generalize this to $I \times J$ tables for $I = 2, J \geq 3$ since a 2×3 table is a sub-table of $I \times J$ tables for $I = 2, J \geq 3$ as shown in the proof of Theorem 3.3.

Theorem 3.5: We consider the semigroup $Q(A)$ generated by the columns of the design matrix A for the bivariate logistic regression model for $I = 2, J \geq 2, K \geq 3$. Then $H(A) \neq \varnothing$.

Proof. Consider the design matrix for the bivariate logistic regression with the level equal to two and the level equal to three, i.e., $J = 2$ and $K = 3$, so that we have $2 \times 2 \times 3$ contingency tables. The design matrix forms as follows:

```
1 1 1 1 1 1 0 0 0 0 0 0
1 1 1 2 2 2 0 0 0 0 0 0
1 2 3 1 2 3 0 0 0 0 0 0
1 0 0 0 0 0 1 0 0 0 0 0
0 1 0 0 0 0 0 1 0 0 0 0
0 0 1 0 0 0 0 0 1 0 0 0
0 0 0 1 0 0 0 0 0 1 0 0
0 0 0 0 1 0 0 0 0 0 1 0
0 0 0 0 0 1 0 0 0 0 0 1
```

Using the software normaliz (Bruns et al. 2017), the semigroup generated by the columns of this matrix is not normal. Therefore, the semigroup generated by the columns of the design matrix for $2 \times 2 \times 3$ contingency tables under the bivariate logistic regression model has holes. For $I \times J \times K$ tables under the multivariate logistic regression model, where $I = 2, J \geq 2, K \geq 3$, this $2 \times 2 \times 3$ contingency table can be seen as a special case where cell count X_{ijk} with the indeces $I \geq i \geq 2$, $J \geq j \geq 2$, and $K \geq k \geq 3$ equals to zero. Therefore, the semigoup generated by the columns of the design matrix for the multivariate logistic regression model has holes.

Theorem 3.6: We consider the semigroup $Q(A)$ generated by the columns of the design matrix A for the bivariate logistic regression model for $I = 2, J \geq 2, K \geq 3$. Then $Q(A)$ has infinitely many holes.

Proof. We use Theorem 3.7 from (Takemura and Yoshida 2008) to the semigroup $Q(A)$ generated by the columns of the design matrix of the logistic regression model with $J = 2$ and $K = 3$ shown in the proof for Theorem 3.5. Let $\mathbf{b}_s$ be the sth column of the matrix A for $s = 1,...,12$. After using the software normaliz, the Hilbert basis consists of the 12 columns of the matrix A and two additional vectors:

$$\mathbf{b}_{13} = (1, 2, 2, 0, 1, 0, 0, 0, 1)$$
$$\mathbf{b}_{14} = (2, 1, 1, 0, 0, 0, 1, 0).$$

Therefore $\mathbf{b}_{13}, \mathbf{b}_{14} \notin Q(A)$. Then we set the following system of linear equations such that:

$$\mathbf{b}_1 x_1 + \mathbf{b}_2 x_2 + \ldots + \mathbf{b}_{12} x_{12} = \mathbf{b}_{13}$$
$$x_1 \in \mathbb{Z}_-, \, x_i \in \mathbb{Z}_+, \text{ for } i = 2, 3, \ldots, 12.$$

We used R package lpSolve (Buttrey 2015) to solve the system of equations using the linear programming with the cost function $\min x_1$, then it shows that there is no real solution in the system of linear equations and inequalities. Thus, $\mathbf{b}_{13} \notin (-\mathbb{N}A_1) + Q(A)_1$, where $Q(A)_1$ is the semigroup generated by $\mathbf{b}_2, \ldots, \mathbf{b}_{12}$. Therefore, by Theorem 3.7 from (Takemura and Yoshida 2008), the number of elements in $H(A)$ is infinite. We can generalize this to $I \times J \times K$ tables for $I = 2, J \geq 2, K \geq 3$ since a $2 \times 2 \times 3$ table is a sub-table of $I \times J \times K$ tables for $I = 2, J \geq 2, K \geq 3$ as shown in the proof of Theorem 3.5.

Using Theorem 3.6 we have immediately the following corollary.

Corollary 3.7: We consider the semigroup $Q(A)$ generated by the columns of the design matrix A for the multivariate logistic regression model for $I = 2, J \geq 2, K \geq 3$. Then $Q(A)$ is not very ample.

Theorem 3.8: We consider the semigroup $Q(A)$ generated by the columns of the design matrix A for the multivariate logistic regression model for $2 \times I_1 \times I_2 \times \ldots \times I_s$ contingency tables for $I_i \geq 2$ and $I_s \geq 3$. Then $Q(A)$ has infinitely many holes.

Proof. One can think that the univariate 2×3 contingency table is a special case of $2 \times I_1 \times I_2 \times \ldots \times I_s$ contingency tables for $I_i \geq 2$ and $I_s \geq 3$ since this is a hierarchical model. Using Theorem 3.4 we are done.

NUN STUDY DATA SET

The NUN study data set is from (Mortimer 2012). This study was conducted on 672 participants from 1031 eligible Catholic sisters born before 1917 from the School Sisters of Notre Dame religious order. After removal of data with missing values, the final data set had 461 participants with 2480 total observations (Wei and Kryscio 2016). They were asked to participate in the study from 1991 to 1993 and were all aged 75 years and older at the time of the study (Mortimer 2012). Each participant agreed on the release of the information collected for future analysis. This study has been used extensively in academic papers for application of sampling techniques and insights into factors affecting Alzheimer's disease.

The data has five factors: prior cognitive status, current cognitive status, presence of APOE-4 allele, education, and age.

- The prior/current cognitive status has five levels: intact cognition (noted as level 1), mild cognitive impairments (MCI) (2), global impairment (GI) (3), dementia (4), and death (5).
- The presence of APOE-4 allele (noted as APOE4) has two levels, not present (1) and present (2).
- Education has three levels: no college (noted as 1), college degree (2), and post graduate degree (3).
- In the data set, age is a continuous variable. In our analysis, we categorize age into four quantiles. For the age factor, we set level 1 as age from 77 to 83.61, level 2 as age from 83.61 to 87.12, level 3 as age from 87.12 to 90.54, and level 4 as age from 90.54 to 104.34.

(Tyas et al. 2007) applied a Markov chain model and (Wei and Kryscio 2016) used a Semi-Markov model to fit the data set. In both models, the researchers used the following set up: they modeled the transitions between cognitive status as a DTMC with a finite state space with five states (1,2,3,4,5) and a transition probability matrix:

$$\begin{pmatrix} P_{11} & P_{12} & P_{13} & P_{14} & P_{15} \\ P_{21} & P_{22} & P_{23} & P_{24} & P_{25} \\ P_{31} & P_{32} & P_{33} & P_{34} & P_{35} \\ 0 & 0 & 0 & 1 & 0 \\ 0 & 0 & 0 & 0 & 1 \end{pmatrix}.$$

Here dementia (4) and death (5) status are considered absorbing states, and other status are considered transient states. Figure 1 depicts the state transitions graphically. We are interested in which factors contribute to increased relative transition probabilities.

Figure 3 shows the five states which comprise the Markov state space. Numbers displayed on the edges represent the number of observed transitions from state i to state j, including transitions to the same state. Source (Wei and Kryscio 2016).

We would like to compare the fit of the observed data to two log-linear models (H_0 and H_1) using a goodness-of-fit test. More specifically, we are interested in the associations between transition ratios and three factors of interest: the presence of APOE-4 allele, education, and age. Following the basic modeling of Salazar et. al. (Salazar et al. 2007), Wei and Kryscio (Wei and Kryscio 2016), and Xie (Xie 2016), we model the relationships as a multivariate logistic regression model such that:

$$\log\left(\frac{P_{s4}}{P_{sv}}\right) = \alpha_{sv} + \beta_{1sv}Y_1 + \beta_{2sv}Y_2 + \beta_{3sv}Y_3,$$

for $s = 1, 2, 3$ and $v = 1, 2, 3$. Here $\left(\frac{P_{s4}}{P_{sv}}\right)$ mimics the odds ratio. The numerator is the number of transitions from state s to dementia (state 4). The denominator is the number of transitions from state s to state v.

Figure 3. DTMC for NUN data

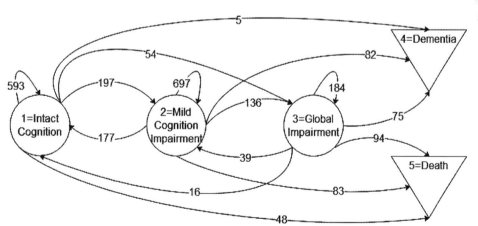

COMPUTATIONAL RESULT

MCMC and SIS Combination for Goodness-of-Fit Tests

In this computational experiment, we employ the hybrid scheme proposed by (Kahle, Yoshida, and Garcia-Puente 2017) of the MCMC with a set of moves computed in (Hara, Takemura, and Yoshida 2010) in order to improve mixing.

In this experiment, we conduct a statistical test with the following hypotheses: bivariate logistic regression as the null hypothesis and trivariate logistic regression.

Algorithm 5.1: MCMC and SIS Hybrid for Goodness-of-Fit Tests

Input: The observed contingency table $\mathbf{n}_0$ and sufficient statistic $\mathbf{b}$. The number of SIS samples K and the sample size N for each MCMC chain. The number of burn-in samples B. The thinning interval Q. Model for H_0 (F_0) and model for H_1 (F_1).

Output: A list of log likelihood ratios ($\mathbf{T}$) from tables sampled according to the hypergeometric distribution.

Algorithm:

1. Sample K many starting tables using SIS. The sample is denoted as $\left\{\mathbf{X}_{11}, ..., \mathbf{X}_{1K}\right\}$.

2. [step2:hybrid] For $k = 1, \cdots, K$:

    a. Sample N many tables with MCMC using starting table $\mathbf{X}_{1k}$. Markov chain $\mathbf{R}_k = \left\{\mathbf{X}_{1k}, ..., \mathbf{X}_{Nk}\right\}$.

    b. Initialize the vector of test statistics $\mathbf{T}_k = \varnothing$.

    c. Burn-In: Eliminate the first B tables from $\mathbf{R}_k$ to minimize dependence of MCMC on SIS starting point $\mathbf{X}_{1k}$. $m = B + 1$.

    d. While $m \leq N$:

        i. Take table $\mathbf{X}_{mk}$ from $\mathbf{R}_k$.

        ii. Compute the maximum log likelihood (residual deviance) under H_0.

       iii. Compute maximum log likelihood (residual deviance) under H_1.

       iv. Compute the log likelihood ratio test statistic (G^2) as the difference in the residual deviance.

       v. Add G^2 to $\mathbf{T}_k$.

       vi. [stepe6] Thinning: Advance m by Q, the thinning interval to minimize dependence between successive test statistics.

   e. Return $\mathbf{T}_k$.

3. The test statistic distribution is approximated by combining samples from each Markov chain ($\mathbf{R}_k$). $\mathbf{T} = \left\{\mathbf{T}_1, ..., \mathbf{T}_K\right\}$.

Results

We set the following simulation settings for Algorithm 5.1. $K = 100$ independent SIS samples. $N = 2201$ contingency tables in each MCMC chain, beginning with an SIS sample. Burn-in $B = 100$ and thinning iterval $Q = 20$. We run our hybrid SIS and MCMC approach to ascertain a test statistic distribution ($T(\mathbf{X})$) for all $s \in \{1, 2, 3\}$, $v \in \{1, 2, 3\}$, and $i \in \{1, 2, 3\}$. After burn-in and thinning, each test statistic distribution sample for a given (s, v, i) will have 10100 samples from the distribution.

    Recall the null and alternative hypotheses being tested through a goodness-of-fit hypothesis test given s, v, i.

$$\log\left(\frac{P_{s4}}{P_{sv}}\right) = \alpha_{sv} + \beta_{1sv}Y_1 + \beta_{2sv}Y_2 + \beta_{3sv}Y_3.$$

$$H_0^{isv} : \beta_{isv} = 0,$$

$$H_1^{isv} : \beta_{isv} \neq 0.$$

    The results of the 27 different goodness-of-fit tests are summarized in Table 1.

    The hybrid sampling methodology proposed in this paper produces estimated p-values similar to the asymptotic approximation p-values. In conducting the 27 hypothesis tests on the NUN dataset, the asymptotic and

Table 1. p-values and rejections for (s,v,i) goodness-of-fit tests. For each (s,v,i) combination, the approximate p-value from SIS and MCMC sampling is reported. The p-value using a χ^2_1 approximation is also stated. Finally, the number of rejections from the sampling of 1000 tables via SIS is shown.

s	v	i	χ^2 p-value	Sampling p-value	SIS rejections
1	1	1	0.005	0.005	10
1	1	2	0.0001	0.008	3
1	1	3	0.36	0.33	0
1	2	1	0.053	0.12	16
1	2	2	0.007	0.009	3
1	2	3	0.51	0.66	0
1	3	1	0.039	0.12	24
1	3	2	0.0008	0.0007	26
1	3	3	0.77	0.98	0
2	1	1	0.003	0.007	74
2	1	2	0.10	0.11	39
2	1	3	<.0001	0.000	35
2	2	1	0.73	0.75	77
2	2	2	0.43	0.49	33
2	2	3	0.002	0.007	11
2	3	1	0.13	0.13	104
2	3	2	0.17	0.21	89
2	3	3	0.34	0.39	52
3	1	1	0.08	0.14	56
3	1	2	0.040	0.064	26
3	1	3	0.09	0.12	4
3	2	1	0.007	0.012	60
3	2	2	0.71	0.77	79
3	2	3	0.10	0.11	67
3	3	1	0.14	0.16	81
3	3	2	0.39	0.41	42
3	3	3	0.54	0.56	30

hybrid methodologies agree in each case on the reject/fail to reject decision regarding H_0.

This result occurs despite the contingency tables being sparse and, in the case of s=1, producing test statistic distributions with only a handful of possible values.

We infer this as evidence of the applicability of the χ^2 asymptotic approximation even to relatively sparse contingency tables. Contrary to our initial conjectures, the asymptotic approximation works well for this dataset of sparse, multidimensional contingency tables.

Rejections for 1000 SIS samples ranged from 0 to 104.

ACKNOWLEDGMENT

R.Y. is supported by NSF Division of Mathematical Sciences: CDS&E-MSS program. Proposal number:1622369.

REFERENCES

Besag, J., & Clifford, P. (1989). Generalized Monte Carlo Significance Tests. *Biometrika*, *76*(4), 633–642. doi:10.1093/biomet/76.4.633

Bruns, W., Ichim, B., Römer, T., Sieg, R., & Söger, C. (2017). *Normaliz. Algorithms for Rational Cones and Affine Monoids*. Available at https://www.normaliz.uni-osnabrueck.de

Bunea, F., & Besag, J. (2000). MCMC in I x J x K Contingency Tables. In Monte Carlo Methods (vol. 26, pp. 25–36). Fields Institute Communications.

Buttrey, S. E. (2015). *LpSolve, Version 5.6.13*. Available at https://cran.r-project.org/web/packages/lpSolve/index.html

Buzzigoli & Giusti. (1998). An Algorithm to Calculate the Lower and Upper Bounds of the Elements of an Array Given Its Marginals. *Statistical Data Protection (SDP'98) Proceedings*, 131–47.

Chen, Y., Diaconis, P., Holmes, S. P., & Liu, J. S. (2005). Sequential Monte Carlo Methods for Statistical Analysis of Tables. *American Statistical Association*, *100*(469), 109–120. doi:10.1198/016214504000001303

Chen, Y., Dinwoodie, I., Dobra, A., & Huber, M. (2005). Lattice Points, Contingency Tables, and Sampling. In *Integer Points in Polyhedra—Geometry, Number Theory, Algebra Optimization*, *374*, 65–78.

Chen, Y., Dinwoodie, I. H., & Sullivant, S. (2006). Sequential Importance Sampling for Multiway Tables. *Annals of Statistics*, *34*(1), 523–545. doi:10.1214/009053605000000822

De Loera, J., & Onn, S. (2005). Markov Bases of Three-Way Tables Are Arbitrarily Complicated. *Journal of Symbolic Computation*, *41*(2), 173–181. doi:10.1016/j.jsc.2005.04.010

Diaconis, P., & Efron, B. (1985). Testing for Independence in a Two-Way Table: New Interpretations of the Chi-Square Statistic (with Discussion). *Annals of Statistics*, *13*(3), 845–913. doi:10.1214/aos/1176349634

Diaconis, P., & Sturmfels, B. (1998). Algebraic Algorithms for Sampling from Conditional Distributions. *Annals of Statistics*, *26*(1), 363–397. doi:10.1214/aos/1030563990

Dobra, A., & Fienberg, S. E. (2010). The Generalized Shuttle Algorithm. In P. Gibilisco, E. Riccomagno, M. P. Rogantin, & H. P. Wynn (Eds.), *Algebraic and Geometric Methods in Statistics* (pp. 135–156). Cambridge University Press.

Guo, S. W., & Thompson, E. A. (1992). Performing the Exact Test of Hardy–Weinberg Proportion for Multiple Alleles. *Biometrics*, *48*(2), 361–372. doi:10.2307/2532296 PMID:1637966

Hara, H., Takemura, A., & Yoshida, R. (2010). On Connectivity of Fibers with Positive Marginals in Multiple Logistic Regression. *Journal of Multivariate Analysis*, *101*(4), 909–925. doi:10.1016/j.jmva.2009.12.014

Kahle, D., Yoshida, R., & Garcia-Puente, L. (2017, September). Hybrid Schemes for Exact Conditional Inference in Discrete Exponential Families. *Annals of the Institute of Statistical Mathematics*, 1–29.

Mortimer, J. A. (2012). The Nun Study: Risk Factors for Pathology and Clinical-Pathologic Correlations. *Current Alzheimer Research*, *9*(6), 621–627. doi:10.2174/156720512801322546 PMID:22471869

Salazar, J. C., Schmitt, F. A., Yu, L., Mendiondo, M., & Kryscio, R. J. (2007). Shared Random Effects Analysis of Multi-State Markov Models: Application to a Longitudinal Study of Transitions to Dementia. *Statistics in Medicine*, *26*(3), 568–580. doi:10.1002im.2437 PMID:16345024

Shao, J. (1998). *Mathematical Statistics*. New York: Springer Verlag.

Takemura, A., & Yoshida, R. (2008). A Generalization of the Integer Linear Infeasibility Problem. *Discrete Optimization*, 5(1), 36–52. doi:10.1016/j. disopt.2007.10.004

Tyas, S. L., Salazar, J., Snowdon, D., Desrosiers, M., Riley, K., Mendiondo, M., & Kryscio, R. (2007). Transitions to Mild Cognitive Impairments, Dementia, and Death: Findings from the Nun Study. *American Journal of Epidemiology*, 165(11), 1231–1238. doi:10.1093/aje/kwm085 PMID:17431012

Wei, S., & Kryscio, R. J. (2016). Semi-Markov Models for Interval Censored Transient Cognitive States with Back Transitions and a Competing Risk. *Statistical Methods in Medical Research*, 25(6), 2909–2924. doi:10.1177/0962280214534412 PMID:24821001

Xie, Z. (2016). *Topics in Logistic Regression Analysis* (PhD thesis). Lexington, KY: Dept. Statistics, Univ. Kentucky.

Compilation of References

Abdulhay, E., Alafeef, M., Hadoush, H., & Alomari, N. (2017). Frequency 3d mapping and inter-channel stability of EEG intrinsic function pulsation: Indicators towards autism spectrum diagnosis. In *Electrical and Electronics Engineering Conference (JIEEEC), 2017 10th Jordanian International*. IEEE. 10.1109/JIEEEC.2017.8051416

Abibullaev, B., & An, J. (2012). Decision support algorithm for diagnosis of adhd using electroencephalograms. *Journal of Medical Systems*, *36*(4), 2675–2688. doi:10.100710916-011-9742-x PMID:21671069

Abu, N., Akhtar, M. N., Ho, W. Y., Yeap, S. K., & Alitheen, N. B. (2013). 3-Bromo-1-hydroxy-9, 10-anthraquinone (BHAQ) inhibits growth and migration of the human breast cancer cell lines MCF-7 and MDA-MB231. *Molecules (Basel, Switzerland)*, *18*(9), 10367–10377. doi:10.3390/molecules180910367 PMID:23985955

Adolphs, R. (2009). The social brain: Neural basis of social knowledge. *Annual Review of Psychology*, *60*(1), 693–716. doi:10.1146/annurev.psych.60.110707.163514 PMID:18771388

Agarwal, S. K., Singh, S. S., Verma, S., & Kumar, S. (2000). Antifungal activity of anthraquinone derivatives from Rheum emodi. *Journal of Ethnopharmacology*, *72*(1), 43–46. doi:10.1016/S0378-8741(00)00195-1 PMID:10967452

Ahfad-Hosseini, H. R., Bagheri, H., & Amidi, S. (2017). Ionic liquid-assisted synthesis of celexocib using tris-(2-hydroxyethyl) ammonium acetate as an efficient and reusable catalyst. *Iranian Journal of Pharmaceutical Research*, *16*(1), 158–164. PMID:28496471

Alderson, R. M., Kasper, L. J., Hudec, K. L., & Patros, C. H. (2013). Attention-deficit/hyperactivity disorder (ADHD) and working memory in adults: a meta-analytic review. *Neuropsychology, 27*(3), 287.

Al-Fahoum, A. S., & Al-Fraihat, A. A. (2014). Methods of EEG signal features extraction using linear analysis in frequency and time-frequency domains. *ISRN Neuroscience, 2014*, 1–7. doi:10.1155/2014/730218

Ali, A. M., Ismail, N. H., Mackeen, M. M., Yazan, L. S., Mohamed, S. M., Ho, A. S. H., & Lajis, N. H. (2000). Antiviral, cyototoxic and antimicrobial activities of anthraquinones isolated from the roots of Morinda elliptica. *Pharmaceutical Biology, 38*(4), 298–301. doi:10.1076/1388-0209(200009)38:4;1-A;FT298 PMID:21214480

Alie, D., Mahoor, M. H., Mattson, W. I., Anderson, D. R., & Messinger, D. S. (2011). Analysis of eye gaze pattern of infants at risk of autism spectrum disorder using Markov models. In *Applications of Computer Vision (WACV), 2011 IEEE Workshop on.* IEEE. 10.1109/WACV.2011.5711515

Almutairi, M. S., Hegazy, G. H., Haiba, M. E., Ali, H. I., Khalifa, N. M., & Soliman, A. E. M. M. (2014). Synthesis, Docking and Biological Activities of Novel Hybrids Celecoxib and Anthraquinone Analogs as Potent Cytotoxic Agents. *International Journal of Molecular Sciences, 15*(12), 22580–22603. doi:10.3390/ijms151222580 PMID:25490139

American Psychiatric Association. (2000). *Diagnostic and Statistical Manual of Mental Disorders: DSM-IV-TR* (4th ed.). Washington, DC: American Psychiatric Association.

Anderson, J. L., Ding, J., Welton, T., & Armstrong, D. W. (2002). Characterizing ionic liquids on the basis of multiple solvation interactions. *Journal of the American Chemical Society, 124*(47), 14247–14254. doi:10.1021/ja028156h PMID:12440924

Anvari, S., Hajfarajollah, H., Mokhtarani, B., Enayati, M., Sharifi, A., & Mirzaei, M. (2016). Antibacterial and anti-adhesive properties of ionic liquids with various cationic and anionic heads toward pathogenic bacteria. *Journal of Molecular Liquids, 221*, 685–690. doi:10.1016/j.molliq.2016.05.093

Argyle, M., & Cook, M. (1976). *Gaze and Mutual Gaze*. Cambridge, MA: Cambridge University Press.

Armstrong, D. W., He, L., & Liu, Y. S. (1999). Examination of ionic liquids and their interaction with molecules, when used as stationary phases in gas chromatography. *Analytical Chemistry*, *71*(17), 3873–3876. doi:10.1021/ac990443p PMID:10489532

Arning, J., & Matzke, M. (2011). Toxicity of ionic liquids towards mammalian cell lines. *Current Organic Chemistry*, *15*(12), 1905–1917. doi:10.2174/138527211795703694

Asha, K., Ajay, K., Naznin, V., George, T., & Peter, D. (2005). *Gesture-based affective computing on motion capture data*. Paper presented at the International Conference on Affective Computing and Intelligent Interaction.

Azuma, M., Minamoto, T., Yaoi, K., Osaka, M., & Osaka, N. (2014). Effect of memory load in eye movement control: A study using the reading span test. *Journal of Eye Movement Research*, *7*(5), 1–9.

Bal, E., Harden, E., Lamb, D., Van Hecke, A. V., Denver, J. W., And Porges, S. W. 2010. Emotion Recognition in Children with Autism Spectrum Disorders: Relations to Eye Gaze and Autonomic State. *Journal of Autism and Developmental Disorders, 40*(3), 358–370.

Balachandran, C., Duraipandiyan, V., Arun, Y., Sangeetha, B., Emi, N., Al-Dhabi, N. A., ... Perumal, P. T. (2016). Isolation and characterization of 2-hydroxy-9, 10-anthraquinone from Streptomyces olivochromogenes (ERINLG-261) with antimicrobial and antiproliferative properties. *Revista Brasileira de Farmacognosia, 26*(3), 285–295. doi:10.1016/j.bjp.2015.12.003

Barkley, R. A. (1997). Behavioral inhibition, sustained attention, and executive functions: constructing a unifying theory of adhd. *Psychological Bulletin, 121*(1), 65.

Barkley, R. A. (1998). *Attention Deficit Hyperactivity Disorder: A Handbook for Diagnosis and Treatment* (2nd ed.). New York: Guilford Press.

Barnard, D. L., Huffman, J. H., Morris, J. L., Wood, S. G., Hughes, B. G., & Sidwell, R. W. (1992). Evaluation of the antiviral activity of anthraquinones, anthrones and anthraquinone derivatives against human cytomegalovirus. *Antiviral Research*, *17*(1), 63–77. doi:10.1016/0166-3542(92)90091-I PMID:1310583

Baron-Cohen, S., Leslie, A. M., & And Frith, U. (1985). Does the autistic child have a "theory of mind"? *Cognition*, *21*(1), 37–46. doi:10.1016/0010-0277(85)90022-8 PMID:2934210

Barresi, J., & And Moore, C. (1996). Intentional relations and social understanding. *Behavioral and Brain Sciences*, *19*(1), 107–122. doi:10.1017/S0140525X00041790

Bartlett, M. S., Littlewort, G., Fasel, I., & Movellan, J. R. (2003). *Real Time Face Detection and Facial Expression Recognition: Development and Applications to Human Computer Interaction*. Paper presented at the Conference on Computer Vision and Pattern Recognition Workshop. 10.1109/CVPRW.2003.10057

Bauer, J. F. (2008). Polymorphism--a critical consideration in pharmaceutical development, manufacturing, and stability. *Journal of Validation Technology*, *14*(5), 15-24.

Bedford, R., Elsabbagh, M., Gliga, T., Pickles, A., Senju, A., Charman, T., & Johnson, M. H. (2012). Precursors to Social and Communication Difficulties in Infants At-Risk for Autism: Gaze Following and Attentional Engagement. *Journal of Autism and Developmental Disorders*, *42*(10), 2208–2218.

Beken, T. V. (2007). *The European Pharmaceutical Sector and Crime Vulnerabilities*. Antwerb, Belgium: Maklu Publishers.

Ben Shalom, D., Mostofsky, S. H., Hazlett, R. L., Goldberg, M. C., Landa, R. J., Faran, Y., ... Hoehn-Saric, R. (2006). Normal physiological emotions but differences in expression of conscious feelings in children with high-functioning autism. *Journal of Autism and Developmental Disorders*, *36*(3), 395–400. doi:10.100710803-006-0077-2 PMID:16565884

Bengio, Y. (2012, June). Deep learning of representations for unsupervised and transfer learning. In *Proceedings of ICML Workshop on Unsupervised and Transfer Learning* (pp. 17-36). Academic Press.

Benjamin, T. V., & Lamikanra, A. (1981). Investigation of Cassia alata, a plant used in Nigeria in the treatment of skin diseases. *Quarterly Journal of Crude Drug Research, 19*(2-3), 93–96. doi:10.3109/13880208109070583

Bernard-Opitz, V., Sriram, N., & Nakhoda-Sapuan, S. (2001). Enhancing social problem solving in children with autism and normal children through computer-assisted instruction. *Journal of Autism and Developmental Disorders, 31*(4), 377–384. doi:10.1023/A:1010660502130 PMID:11569584

Besag, J., & Clifford, P. (1989). Generalized Monte Carlo Significance Tests. *Biometrika, 76*(4), 633–642. doi:10.1093/biomet/76.4.633

Bethel, C., Salomon, K., Murphy, R., & Burke, J. (2007). *Survey of psychophysiology measurements applied to human-robot interaction.* Paper presented at the IEEE International Symposium on Robot and Human Interactive Communication, Jeju, South Korea. 10.1109/ROMAN.2007.4415182

Biederman, J., Hammerness, P., Sadeh, B., Peremen, Z., Amit, A., Or-Ly, H., ... Faraone, S. (2017). Diagnostic utility of brain activity flow patterns analysis in attention deficit hyperactivity disorder. *Psychological Medicine, 47*(7), 1259–1270. doi:10.1017/S0033291716003329 PMID:28065167

Billeci, L., Narzisi, A., Campatelli, G., Crifaci, G., Calderoni, S., Gagliano, A., ... Muratori, F. (2016). Disentangling the initiation from the response in joint attention: An eye-tracking study in toddlers with autism spectrum disorders. *Translational Psychiatry, 6*(5), e808. doi:10.1038/tp.2016.75 PMID:27187230

Bishop, C. M. (2006). *Pattern recognition and machine learning.* Springer.

Black, M. H., Chen, N. T. M., Iyer, K. K., Lipp, O. V., Bölte, S., Falkmer, M., ... Girdler, S. (2017). Mechanisms of facial emotion recognition in autism spectrum disorders: Insights from eye tracking and electroencephalography. *Neuroscience and Biobehavioral Reviews, 80*, 488–515. doi:10.1016/j.neubiorev.2017.06.016 PMID:28698082

Blake, M. (2015). An Internet of Things for Healthcare. *IEEE Internet Computing, 19*(4), 4–6. doi:10.1109/MIC.2015.89

Blazey, R. N., Patton, D. L., & Parks, P. A. (2003). *ADHD Detection By Eye Saccades.* US Patent 6,652,458.

Bosl, W. J., Tager-Flusberg, H., & Nelson, C. A. (2018). EEG analytics for early detection of autism spectrum disorder: a data-driven approach. *Scientific Reports, 8*(1), 6828.

Bosl, W., Tierney, A., Tager-Flusberg, H., &Nelson, C. (2011). EEG complexity as a biomarker for autism spectrum disorder risk. *BMC Medicine, 9,* 1, 18.

Bradley, M. M. (2000). Emotion and motivation. In J. T. Cacioppo, L. G. Tassinary, & G. Berntson (Eds.), *Handbook of Psychophysiology* (pp. 602–642). New York: Cambridge University Press.

Brain, L., Tshilidzi, M., Taryn, T., & Monica, L. (2006). Prediction of HIV Status from Demographic Data using Neural Networks. IEEE Conference on Systems Man and Cybernetics, Taipei, Taiwan.

Brown, R. M., Hall, L. R., Holtzer, R., Brown, S. L., & Brown, N. L. (1997). Gender and video game performance. *Sex Roles, 36*(11/12), 793–812. doi:10.1023/A:1025631307585

Brück, T. B., & Brück, D. W. (2011). Oxidative metabolism of the anti-cancer agent mitoxantrone by horseradish, lacto-and lignin peroxidase. *Biochimie, 93*(2), 217–226. doi:10.1016/j.biochi.2010.09.015 PMID:20887767

Bruns, W., Ichim, B., Römer, T., Sieg, R., & Söger, C. (2017). *Normaliz. Algorithms for Rational Cones and Affine Monoids*. Available at https://www.normaliz.uni-osnabrueck.de

Bubalo, M. C., Radošević, K., Redovniković, I. R., Halambek, J., & Srček, V. G. (2014). A brief overview of the potential environmental hazards of ionic liquids. *Ecotoxicology and Environmental Safety, 99,* 1–12. doi:10.1016/j.ecoenv.2013.10.019 PMID:24210364

Buescher, A. V., Cidav, Z., Knapp, M., & Mandell, D. S. (2014). Costs of autism spectrum disorders in the United Kingdom and the united states. *JAMA Pediatrics, 168*(8), 721–728. doi:10.1001/jamapediatrics.2014.210 PMID:24911948

Bunea, F., & Besag, J. (2000). MCMC in I x J x K Contingency Tables. In *Monte Carlo Methods* (vol. 26, pp. 25–36). Fields Institute Communications.

Butterworth, G., & Jarrett, N. (1991). What minds have in common is space: Spatial mechanisms serving joint visual attention in infancy. *British Journal of Developmental Psychology, 9*(1), 55–72. doi:10.1111/j.2044-835X.1991.tb00862.x

Buttrey, S. E. (2015). *LpSolve, Version 5.6.13*. Available at https://cran.r-project.org/web/packages/lpSolve/index.html

Buzzigoli & Giusti. (1998). An Algorithm to Calculate the Lower and Upper Bounds of the Elements of an Array Given Its Marginals. *Statistical Data Protection (SDP'98) Proceedings*, 131–47.

Byrne, N., Wang, L. M., Belieres, J. P., & Angell, C. A. (2007). Reversible folding–unfolding, aggregation protection, and multi-year stabilization, in high concentration protein solutions, using ionic liquids. *Chemical Communications*, (26): 2714–2716. doi:10.1039/B618943A PMID:17594030

Cai, S., Zhou, B., Liao, H., & Tan, C. (2017). Imaging Diagnosis of Chronic Encapsulated Intracerebral Hematoma, a Comparison of Computed Tomography (CT) and Magnetic Resonance Imaging (MRI) characteristics. *Polish Journal of Radiology / Polish Medical Society of Radiology*, 82, 578–582. doi:10.12659/PJR.902417 PMID:29662588

Cantwell, D. P., Lewinsohn, P. M., Rohde, P., & Seeley, J. R. (1997). Correspondence between adolescent report and parent report of psychiatric diagnostic data. *Journal of the American Academy of Child and Adolescent Psychiatry*, *36*(5), 610–619. doi:10.1097/00004583-199705000-00011 PMID:9136495

Caruana, N., Brock, J., & Woolgar, A. (2015). A front temporoparietal network common to initiating and responding to joint attention bids. *NeuroImage*, *108*, 34–46. doi:10.1016/j.neuroimage.2014.12.041 PMID:25534111

Castelli, F., Frith, C., Happé, F., & Frith, U. (2002). Autism, Asperger syndrome and brain mechanisms for the attribution of mental states to animated shapes. *Brain*, *125*(8), 1839–1849. doi:10.1093/brain/awf189 PMID:12135974

Centers for Disease Control and Prevention (CDC). (2018). Prevalence of Autism Spectrum Disorder Among Children Aged 8 Years-ADDM Network, United States, 2014. *Morbidity and Mortality Weekly Report (MMWR) Surveillance Summaries, 67*, 1-23.

Chalmers, I., Altman, D., McHaffie, H., Owens, N., & Cooke, R. (2013). Data sharing among data monitoring committees and responsibilities to patients and science. *Trials*, *14*(1), 102. doi:10.1186/1745-6215-14-102 PMID:23782486

Chang, C. H., Lin, C. C., Yang, J. J., Namba, T., & Hattori, M. (1996). Anti-inflammatory effects of emodin from ventilago leiocarpa. *The American Journal of Chinese Medicine*, *24*(02), 139–142. doi:10.1142/S0192415X96000189 PMID:8874670

Chen, R. F., Shen, Y. C., Huang, H. S., Liao, J. F., Ho, L. K., Chou, Y. C., ... Chen, C. F. (2004). Evaluation of the anti-inflammatory and cytotoxic effects of anthraquinones and anthracenes derivatives in human leucocytes. *The Journal of Pharmacy and Pharmacology*, *56*(7), 915–919. doi:10.1211/0022357023781 PMID:15233871

Chen, S. H., & Bernard-Opitz, V. (1993). Comparison of personal and computer-assisted instruction for children with autism. *Mental Retardation*, *31*(6), 368–376. PMID:8152382

Chen, Y. W., Huang, H. S., Shieh, Y. S., Ma, K. H., Huang, S. H., Hueng, D. Y., ... Lin, G. J. (2014). A novel compound NSC745885 exerts an anti-tumor effect on tongue cancer SAS cells in vitro and in vivo. *PLoS One*, *9*(8), e104703. doi:10.1371/journal.pone.0104703 PMID:25127132

Chen, Y., Diaconis, P., Holmes, S. P., & Liu, J. S. (2005). Sequential Monte Carlo Methods for Statistical Analysis of Tables. *American Statistical Association*, *100*(469), 109–120. doi:10.1198/016214504000001303

Chen, Y., Dinwoodie, I. H., & Sullivant, S. (2006). Sequential Importance Sampling for Multiway Tables. *Annals of Statistics*, *34*(1), 523–545. doi:10.1214/009053605000000822

Chen, Y., Dinwoodie, I., Dobra, A., & Huber, M. (2005). Lattice Points, Contingency Tables, and Sampling. In *Integer Points in Polyhedra—Geometry, Number Theory, Algebra Optimization*, *374*, 65–78.

Chita-Tegmark, M. (2016). Social attention in ASD: A review and meta-analysis of eye-tracking studies. *Research in Developmental Disabilities*, *48*, 79–93. doi:10.1016/j.ridd.2015.10.011 PMID:26547134

Choi, R. J., Ngoc, T. M., Bae, K., Cho, H. J., Kim, D. D., Chun, J., ... Kim, Y. S. (2013). Anti-inflammatory properties of anthraquinones and their relationship with the regulation of P-glycoprotein function and expression. *European Journal of Pharmaceutical Sciences*, *48*(1), 272–281. doi:10.1016/j.ejps.2012.10.027 PMID:23174748

Chukwujekwu, J. C., Coombes, P. H., Mulholland, D. A., & Van Staden, J. (2006). Emodin, an antibacterial anthraquinone from the roots of Cassia occidentalis. *South African Journal of Botany, 72*(2), 295–297. doi:10.1016/j.sajb.2005.08.003

Chung, H. (2017). Endoscopic Accessories Used for More Advanced Endoluminal Therapeutic Procedures. *Clinical Endoscopy, 50*(3), 234–241. doi:10.5946/ce.2017.079 PMID:28609821

Clement, Y. N., Morton-Gittens, J., Basdeo, L., Blades, A., Francis, M. J., Gomes, N., ... Singh, A. (2007). Perceived efficacy of herbal remedies by users accessing primary healthcare in Trinidad. *BMC Complementary and Alternative Medicine, 7*(1), 4. doi:10.1186/1472-6882-7-4 PMID:17286858

Coben, R., Clarke, A. R., Hudspeth, W., & Barry, R. J. (2008). EEG power and coherence in autistic spectrum disorder. *Clinical Neurophysiology, 119*(5), 1002–1009. doi:10.1016/j.clinph.2008.01.013 PMID:18331812

Cohen, H., Amerine-Dickens, M., & Smith, T. (2006). Early intensive behavioral treatment: replication of the UCLA model in a community setting. *Journal of Developmental & Behavioral Pediatrics, 27*(2), S145-155.

Cohen, P. A., Hudson, J. B., & Towers, G. H. N. (1996). Antiviral activities of anthraquinones, bianthrones and hypericin derivatives from lichens. *Cellular and Molecular Life Sciences, 52*(2), 180–183. doi:10.1007/BF01923366 PMID:8608821

Colburn, A., Drucker, S., & Cohen, M. (2000). The role of eye-gaze in avatar-mediated conversational interfaces. Paper presented at SIGGRAPH Sketches and Applications, New Orleans, LA.

Colflesh, G. J., & Conway, A. R. (2007). Individual differences in working memory capacity and divided attention in dichotic listening. *Psychonomic Bulletin & Review, 14*(4), 699–703. doi:10.3758/BF03196824 PMID:17972736

Comini, L. R., Montoya, S. N., Páez, P. L., Argüello, G. A., Albesa, I., & Cabrera, J. L. (2011). Antibacterial activity of anthraquinone derivatives from Heterophyllaea pustulata (Rubiaceae). *Journal of Photochemistry and Photobiology. B, Biology, 102*(2), 108–114. doi:10.1016/j.jphotobiol.2010.09.009 PMID:20965744

Conati, C., Chabbal, R., & Maclaren, H. (2003). *A study on using biometric sensors for detecting user emotions in educational games*. Paper presented at the Workshop on Assessing and Adapting to User Attitude and Affects: Why, When and How, Pittsburgh, PA.

Constatinescu, D., Herrmann, C., & Weingärtner, H. (2010). Patterns of protein unfolding and protein aggregation in ionic liquids. *Physical Chemistry Chemical Physics*, *12*(8), 1756–1763. doi:10.1039/b921037g PMID:20145840

Conway, A. R., Kane, M. J., Bunting, M. F., Hambrick, D. Z., Wilhelm, O., & Engle, R. W. (2005). Working memory span tasks: A methodological review and user's guide. *Psychonomic Bulletin & Review*, *12*(5), 769–786. doi:10.3758/BF03196772 PMID:16523997

Conway, A., Jarrold, C., & Kane, M. (2008). *Variation in working memory*. Oxford University Press. doi:10.1093/acprof:oso/9780195168648.001.0001

Cornellas, A., Perez, L., Comelles, F., Ribosa, I., Manresa, A., & Garcia, M. T. (2011). Self-aggregation and antimicrobial activity of imidazolium and pyridinium based ionic liquids in aqueous solution. *Journal of Colloid and Interface Science*, *355*(1), 164–171. doi:10.1016/j.jcis.2010.11.063 PMID:21186035

Cota, B. B., de Oliveira, A. B., Guimarães, K. G., Mendonça, M. P., de Souza Filho, J. D., & Braga, F. C. (2004). Chemistry and antifungal activity of Xyris species (Xyridaceae): A new anthraquinone from Xyris pilosa. *Biochemical Systematics and Ecology*, *32*(4), 391–397. doi:10.1016/j.bse.2003.11.006

Cowie, R., Douglas-Cowie, E., Tsapatsoulis, N., Votsis, G., Kollias, S., Fellenz, W., & Taylor, J. G. (2001). Emotion recognition in human-computer interaction. *IEEE Signal Processing Magazine*, *18*(1), 32–80. doi:10.1109/79.911197

Cresswell, K., & Sheikh, A. (2012). Electronic Health Record Technology. *Journal of the American Medical Association*, *307*(21). doi:10.1001/jama.2012.3520 PMID:22706825

Cromby, J. J., Standen, P. J., & Brown, D. J. (1996). The potentials of virtual environments in the education and training of people with learning disabilities. *Journal of Intellectual Disability Research*, *40*(6), 489–501. doi:10.1111/j.1365-2788.1996.tb00659.x PMID:9004109

Cruz-Cunha, M., Simoes, R., Varajão, J., & Miranda, I. (2014). Information Technology Supporting Healthcare and Social Care Services. *Journal of Information Technology Research, 7*(1), 41–58. doi:10.4018/jitr.2014010104

Cybenko, G. (1989). Approximation by superpositions of a sigmoidal function. *Mathematics of Control, Signals, and Systems, 2*(4), 303–314. doi:10.1007/BF02551274

Dabirmanesh, B., Daneshjou, S., Sepahi, A. A., Ranjbar, B., Khavari-Nejad, R. A., Gill, P., ... Khajeh, K. (2011). Effect of ionic liquids on the structure, stability and activity of two related α-amylases. *International Journal of Biological Macromolecules, 48*(1), 93–97. doi:10.1016/j.ijbiomac.2010.10.001 PMID:20946913

Dalessandro, B., Perlich, C., & Raeder, T. (2014). Bigger is Better, but at What Cost?Estimating the Economic Value of Incremental Data Assets. *Big Data, 2*(2), 87–96. doi:10.1089/big.2014.0010 PMID:27442302

Damarla, S. R., Keller, T. A., Kana, R. K., Cherkassky, V. L., Williams, D. L., Minshew, N. J., & Just, M. A. (2010). Cortical underconnectivity coupled with preserved visuospatial cognition in autism: Evidence from an FMRI study of an embedded figures task. *Autism Research, 3*(5), 273–279. doi:10.1002/aur.153 PMID:20740492

Daneman, M., & Carpenter, P. A. (1983). Individual differences in integrating information between and within sentences. *Journal of Experimental Psychology: Learning, Memory, and Cognition, 9*(4), 561.

Dautenhahn, K., Werry, I., Salter, T., & te Boekhorst, R. (2003). *Towards adaptive autonomous robots in autism therapy: Varieties of interactions.* Paper presented at the IEEE International Symposium on Computational Intelligence in Robotics and Automation, Kobe, Japan. 10.1109/CIRA.2003.1222245

Dautenhahn, K., & Werry, I. (2004). Towards interactive robots in autism therapy: Background, motivation and challenges. *Pragmatics & Cognition, 12*(1), 1–35. doi:10.1075/pc.12.1.03dau

Dave, H., & Ledwani, L. (2012). *A review on anthraquinones isolated from Cassia species and their applications.* Academic Press.

Dawson, G. (2008). Early behavioral intervention, brain plasticity, and the prevention of autism spectrum disorder. *Development and Psychopathology*, *20*(3), 775–803. doi:10.1017/S0954579408000370 PMID:18606031

de Gonzalo, G., Lavandera, I., Durchschein, K., Wurm, D., Faber, K., & Kroutil, W. (2007). Asymmetric biocatalytic reduction of ketones using hydroxy-functionalised water-miscible ionic liquids as solvents. *Tetrahedron, Asymmetry*, *18*(21), 2541–2546. doi:10.1016/j.tetasy.2007.10.010

De Loera, J., & Onn, S. (2005). Markov Bases of Three-Way Tables Are Arbitrarily Complicated. *Journal of Symbolic Computation*, *41*(2), 173–181. doi:10.1016/j.jsc.2005.04.010

De Luchi, D., Usón, I., Wright, G., Gouyette, C., & Subirana, J. A. (2010). Structure of a stacked anthraquinone–DNA complex. *Acta Crystallographica. Section F, Structural Biology and Crystallization Communications*, *66*(9), 1019–1022. doi:10.1107/S1744309110030034 PMID:20823516

Del Valle Rubido, M., Mccracken, J. T., Hollander, E., Shic, F., Noeldeke, J., Boak, L., ... Umbricht, D. (2018). In Search of Biomarkers for Autism Spectrum Disorder. *Autism Research*, *11*(11), 1567–1579. doi:10.1002/aur.2026 PMID:30324656

Delorme, A., & Makeig, S. (2004). EEGLab: An open source toolbox for analysis of single-trial EEG dynamics including independent component analysis. *Journal of Neuroscience Methods*, *134*(1), 1, 9–21. doi:10.1016/j.jneumeth.2003.10.009 PMID:15102499

Demirezer, L. Ö., Kuruüzüm-Uz, A., Bergere, I., Schiewe, H. J., & Zeeck, A. (2001). The structures of antioxidant and cytotoxic agents from natural source: Anthraquinones and tannins from roots of Rumex patientia. *Phytochemistry*, *58*(8), 1213–1217. doi:10.1016/S0031-9422(01)00337-5 PMID:11738410

Deng, J., Dong, W., Socher, R., Li, L. J., Li, K., & Fei-Fei, L. (2009, June). Imagenet: A large-scale hierarchical image database. In *Computer Vision and Pattern Recognition, 2009. CVPR 2009. IEEE Conference on* (pp. 248-255). IEEE. 10.1109/CVPR.2009.5206848

Diaconis, P., & Efron, B. (1985). Testing for Independence in a Two-Way Table: New Interpretations of the Chi-Square Statistic (with Discussion). *Annals of Statistics*, *13*(3), 845–913. doi:10.1214/aos/1176349634

Diaconis, P., & Sturmfels, B. (1998). Algebraic Algorithms for Sampling from Conditional Distributions. *Annals of Statistics*, *26*(1), 363–397. doi:10.1214/aos/1030563990

Dias, A. R., Costa-Rodrigues, J., Fernandes, M. H., Ferraz, R., & Prudencio, C. (2017). The anticancer potential of ionic liquids. *ChemMedChem*, *12*(1), 11–18. doi:10.1002/cmdc.201600480 PMID:27911045

Dipeolu, O., Green, E., & Stephens, G. (2009). Effects of water-miscible ionic liquids on cell growth and nitro reduction using Clostridium sporogenes. *Green Chemistry*, *11*(3), 397–401. doi:10.1039/b812600c

Djemal, R., Alsharabi, K., Ibrahim, S., & Alsuwailem, A. (2017). EEG-based computer aided diagnosis of autism spectrum disorder using wavelet, entropy, and ann. *BioMed Research International*. PMID:28484720

Dobra, A., & Fienberg, S. E. (2010). The Generalized Shuttle Algorithm. In P. Gibilisco, E. Riccomagno, M. P. Rogantin, & H. P. Wynn (Eds.), *Algebraic and Geometric Methods in Statistics* (pp. 135–156). Cambridge University Press.

Docherty, K. M., & Kulpa, C. F. Jr. (2005). Toxicity and antimicrobial activity of imidazolium and pyridinium ionic liquids. *Green Chemistry*, *7*(4), 185–189. doi:10.1039/b419172b

Duchowski, A. T., Krejtz, K., Krejtz, I., Biele, C., Niedzielska, A., Kiefer, P., ... Giannopoulos, I. (2018). The Index of Pupillary Activity: Measuring Cognitive Load Vis-à-vis Task Difficulty with Pupil Oscillation. In *Proceedings of the 2018 CHI Conference on Human Factors in Computing Systems*. ACM. 10.1145/3173574.3173856

Dupont, J., Itoh, T., Lozano, P., & Malhotra, S. V. (2015). *Environmentally Friendly Syntheses Using Ionic Liquids*. CRC Press.

Duraipandiyan, V., Al-Dhabi, N. A., Balachandran, C., Raj, M. K., Arasu, M. V., & Ignacimuthu, S. (2014). Novel 1, 5, 7-trihydroxy-3-hydroxy methyl anthraquinone isolated from terrestrial Streptomyces sp.(ERI-26) with antimicrobial and molecular docking studies. *Applied Biochemistry and Biotechnology*, *174*(5), 1784–1794. doi:10.100712010-014-1157-y PMID:25149455

Dyson, P. J., & Geldbach, T. J. (2005). *Metal Catalysed Reactions in Ionic Liquids* (Vol. 29). Dordrecht, Netherlands: Springer. doi:10.1007/1-4020-3915-8

Egorova, K. S., & Ananikov, V. P. (2014). Toxicity of ionic liquids: Eco (cyto) activity as complicated, but unavoidable parameter for task-specific optimization. *ChemSusChem*, *7*(2), 336–360. doi:10.1002/cssc.201300459 PMID:24399804

Egorova, K. S., Gordeev, E. G., & Ananikov, V. P. (2017). Biological activity of ionic liquids and their application in pharmaceutics and medicine. *Chemical Reviews*, *117*(10), 7132–7189. doi:10.1021/acs.chemrev.6b00562 PMID:28125212

Ehrlich, L. P., & Wade, R. C. (2001). Protein-protein docking. *Reviews in Computational Chemistry*, *17*, 61–98.

Ekpo, B. A., Bala, D. N., Essien, E. E., & Adesanya, S. A. (2008). Ethnobotanical survey of Akwa Ibom state of Nigeria. *Journal of Ethnopharmacology*, *115*(3), 387–408. doi:10.1016/j.jep.2007.10.021 PMID:18053664

El-Gogary, T. M. (2003). Molecular complexes of some anthraquinone anti-cancer drugs: Experimental and computational study. *Spectrochimica Acta. Part A: Molecular and Biomolecular Spectroscopy*, *59*(5), 1009–1015. doi:10.1016/S1386-1425(02)00283-4 PMID:12633717

Endres, F., MacFarlane, D., & Abbott, A. (2008). *Electrodeposition from Ionic Liquids*. Weinheim, Germany: Wiley-VCH Verlag GmbH&Co. KgaA. doi:10.1002/9783527622917

Engle, R. W., Tuholski, S. W., Laughlin, J. E., & Conway, A. R. (1999). Working memory, short-term memory, and general fluid intelligence: a latent-variable approach. *Journal of Experimental Psychology: General, 128*(3), 309.

Engle, R. W. (2002). Working memory capacity as executive attention. *Current Directions in Psychological Science, 11*(1), 19–23. doi:10.1111/1467-8721.00160

Ernsperger, L. (2003). *Keys to Success for Teaching Students with Autism*. Arlington, TX: Future Horizons.

Falck-Ytter, T., Fernell, E., Hedvall, L., Von Hofsten, C., & Gillberg, C. (2012). Gaze Performance in Children with Autism Spectrum Disorder when Observing Communicative Actions. *Journal of Autism and Developmental Disorders, 42*(10), 2236–2245.

Falck-Ytter, T., Thorup, E., & Bölte, S. (2015). Brief Report: Lack of Processing Bias for the Objects Other People Attend to in 3-Year-Olds with Autism. *Journal of Autism and Developmental Disorders, 45*(6), 1897–1904.

Fatt, Q., & Ramadas, A. (2018). The Usefulness and Challenges of Big Data in Healthcare. *Journal of Health Communication, 3*(2). doi:10.4172/2472-1654.100131

Ferraz, R., Branco, L. C., Prudencio, C., Noronha, J. P., & Petrovski, Z. (2011). Ionic liquids as active pharmaceutical ingredients. *ChemMedChem, 6*(6), 975–985. doi:10.1002/cmdc.201100082 PMID:21557480

Fields, S. A., Johnson, W. M., & Hassig, M. B. (2017). Adult adhd: Addressing a unique set of challenges. *The Journal of Family Practice, 66*(2), 68–74. PMID:28222452

Fife, C., & Eckert, K. (2017). Harnessing electronic healthcare data for wound care research: Standards for reporting observational registry data obtained directly from electronic health records. *Wound Repair and Regeneration, 25*(2), 192–209. doi:10.1111/wrr.12523 PMID:28370796

Fischer, E. (1894). Einfluss der Configuration auf die Wirkung der Enzyme. *European Journal of Inorganic Chemistry, 27*(3), 2985–2993.

Fisher, G. R., Brown, J. R., & Patterson, L. H. (1990). Involvement of hydroxyl radical formation and DNA strand breakage in the cytotoxicity of anthraquinone antitumour agents. *Free Radical Research Communications, 11*(1-3), 117–125. doi:10.3109/10715769009109674 PMID:1963615

Fitts, P. M., Jones, R. E., & Milton, J. L. (1950). Eye Movements of Aircraft Pilots During Instrument-Landing Approaches. *Aeronautical Engineering Review, 9*(2), 24–29.

Fletcher-Watson, S., Leekam, S. R., Benson, V., Frank, M., & Findlay, J. (2009). Eye-movements reveal attention to social information in autism spectrum disorder. *Neuropsychologia, 47*(1), 248–257. doi:10.1016/j.neuropsychologia.2008.07.016 PMID:18706434

Florindo, C., Araujo, J. M., Alves, F., Matos, C., Ferraz, R., Prudencio, C., ... Marrucho, I. M. (2013). Evaluation of solubility and partition properties of ampicillin-based ionic liquids. *International Journal of Pharmaceutics*, *456*(2), 553–559. doi:10.1016/j.ijpharm.2013.08.010 PMID:23978632

Fong, T., Nourbakhsh, I., & Dautenhahn, K. (2003). A survey of socially interactive robots. *Robotics and Autonomous Systems*, *42*(3/4), 143–166. doi:10.1016/S0921-8890(02)00372-X

Fostick, L. (2017). The effect of attention-deficit/hyperactivity disorder and methylphenidate treatment on the adult auditory temporal order judgment threshold. *Journal of Speech, Language, and Hearing Research: JSLHR*, *60*(7), 2124–2128. doi:10.1044/2017_JSLHR-H-16-0074 PMID:28672285

Frade, R. F., Matias, A., Branco, L. C., Afonso, C. A., & Duarte, C. M. (2007). Effect of ionic liquids on human colon carcinoma HT-29 and CaCo-2 cell lines. *Green Chemistry*, *9*(8), 873–877. doi:10.1039/b617526k

Frade, R. F., Rosatella, A. A., Marques, C. S., Branco, L. C., Kulkarni, P. S., Mateus, N. M., ... Duarte, C. M. (2009). Toxicological evaluation on human colon carcinoma cell line (CaCo-2) of ionic liquids based on imidazolium, guanidinium, ammonium, phosphonium, pyridinium and pyrrolidinium cations. *Green Chemistry*, *11*(10), 1660–1665. doi:10.1039/b914284n

Frazier, T. W., Klingemier, E. W., Parikh, S., Speer, L., Strauss, M. S., Eng, C., ... Youngstrom, E. A. (2018). Development and Validation of Objective and Quantitative Eye Tracking-Based Measures of Autism Risk and Symptom Levels. *Journal of the American Academy of Child and Adolescent Psychiatry*, *57*(11), 858–866. doi:10.1016/j.jaac.2018.06.023 PMID:30392627

Freivalds, K., & Liepins, R. (2017). *Improving the neural GPU architecture for algorithm learning.* arXiv preprint arXiv:1702.08727

Fromenteze, T., Decroze, C., Abid, S., & Yurduseven, O. (2018). Sparsity-Driven Reconstruction Technique for Microwave/Millimeter-Wave Computational Imaging. *Sensors (Basel)*, *18*(5), 1536. doi:10.339018051536 PMID:29757241

Fujita, K., MacFarlane, D. R., & Forsyth, M. (2005). Protein solubilising and stabilising ionic liquids. *Chemical Communications*, (38): 4804–4806. doi:10.1039/b508238b PMID:16193120

Ganapathy, S., Thomas, P. S., Fotso, S., & Laatsch, H. (2004). Article. *Phytochemistry*, (65): 1265–1271. doi:10.1016/j.phytochem.2004.03.011

Gan, K. H., Teng, C. H., Lin, H. C., Chen, K. T., Chen, Y. C., Hsu, M. F., ... Lin, C. N. (2008). Antiplatelet effect and selective binding to cyclooxygenase by molecular docking analysis of 3-alkylaminopropoxy-9, 10-anthraquinone derivatives. *Biological & Pharmaceutical Bulletin*, *31*(8), 1547–1551. doi:10.1248/bpb.31.1547 PMID:18670087

Gan, M., & Dai, H. (2014). Detecting and monitoring abrupt emergences and submergences of episodes over data streams. *Information Systems*, *39*, 277–289. doi:10.1016/j.is.2012.05.009

Ge, P., & Russell, R. A. (1997). The synthesis of anthraquinone derivatives as potential anticancer agents. *Tetrahedron*, *53*(51), 17469–17476. doi:10.1016/S0040-4020(97)10195-8

Gilleade, K., Dix, A., & Allanson, J. (2005). *Affective videogames and modes of affective gaming: Assist me, challenge me, emote me*. Paper presented at the Digital Games Research Association Conference.

Gillott, A., Furniss, F., & Walter, A. (2001). Anxiety in high-functioning children with autism. *Autism*, *5*(3), 277–286. doi:10.1177/1362361301005003005 PMID:11708587

Gloss, D., Varma, J. K., Pringsheim, T., & Nuwer, M. R. (2016). Practice advisory: The utility of EEG theta/beta power ratio in ADHD diagnosis report of the guideline development, dissemination, and implementation subcommittee of the American academy of neurology. *Neurology*, 10–1212. PMID:27760867

Goel, R. K., Das, G. G., Ram, S. N., & Pandey, V. B. (1991). Antiulcerogenic and anti-inflammatory effects of emodin, isolated from Rhamnus triquerta wall. *Indian Journal of Experimental Biology*, *29*(3), 230–232. PMID:1874536

Gonzalez, R. C. (2016). *Digital image processing*. Pearson.

Goodfellow, I., Bengio, Y., Courville, A., & Bengio, Y. (2016). *Deep learning* (Vol. 1). Cambridge, MA: MIT Press.

Goodwin, M. S. (2008). Enhancing and accelerating the pace of Autism Research and Treatment: The promise of developing Innovative Technology. *Focus on Autism and Other Developmental Disabilities, 23*(2), 125–128. doi:10.1177/1088357608316678

Gordon, I., Eilbott, J. A., Feldman, R., Pelphrey, K. A., & Vander Wyk, B. C. (2013). Social, reward, and attention brain networks are involved when online bids for joint attention are met with congruent versus incongruent responses. *Social Neuroscience, 8*(6), 544–554. doi:10.1080/17470919.201 3.832374 PMID:24044427

Gotham, K., Risi, S., Pickles, A., & Lord, C. (2007). The autism diagnostic observation schedule: revised algorithms for improved diagnostic validity. *Journal of Autism and Developmental Disorders, 37*(4), 613.

Green, D., Baird, G., Barnett, A. L., Henderson, L., Huber, J., & Henderson, S. E. (2002). The severity and nature of motor impairment in Asperger's syndrome: A comparison with specific developmental disorder of motor function. *Journal of Child Psychology and Psychiatry, and Allied Disciplines, 43*(5), 655–668. doi:10.1111/1469-7610.00054 PMID:12120861

Greenhill, L. L. (1998). Diagnosing attention-deficit/hyperactivity disorder in children. *The Journal of Clinical Psychiatry, 59*, 31–41. PMID:9680051

Groden, J., Goodwin, M. S., Baron, M. G., Groden, G., Velicer, W. F., Lipsitt, L. P., ... Plummer, B. (2005). Assessing cardiovascular responses to stressors in individuals with autism spectrum disorders. *Focus on Autism and Other Developmental Disabilities, 20*(4), 244–252. doi:10.1177/1088357605020 0040601

Grossi, E., Olivieri, C., & Buscema, M. (2017). Diagnosis of autism through EEG processed by advanced computational algorithms: A pilot study. *Computer Methods and Programs in Biomedicine, 142*, 73–79. doi:10.1016/j. cmpb.2017.02.002 PMID:28325448

Guillon, Q., Hadjikhani, N., Baduel, S., & Rogé, B. (2014). Visual social attention in autism spectrum disorder: Insights from eye tracking studies. *Neuroscience and Biobehavioral Reviews, 42*, 279–297. doi:10.1016/j. neubiorev.2014.03.013 PMID:24694721

Guo, S. W., & Thompson, E. A. (1992). Performing the Exact Test of Hardy–Weinberg Proportion for Multiple Alleles. *Biometrics*, *48*(2), 361–372. doi:10.2307/2532296 PMID:1637966

Gupta, N., & Linschitz, H. (1997). Hydrogen-Bonding and Protonation Effects in Electrochemistry of Quinones in Aprotic Solvents. *Journal of the American Chemical Society*, *119*(27), 6384–6391. doi:10.1021/ja970028j

Hahn, E., Patsch, M., & Kilburg, H. (1995). *U.S. Patent No. 5,424,461*. Washington, DC: U.S. Patent and Trademark Office.

Handy, S. T. (2011). *Applications of Ionic Liquids in Science and Technology*. Croatia: InTech Publisher. doi:10.5772/1769

Han, W. T., Trehan, A. K., Wright, J. K., Federici, M. E., Seiler, S. M., & Meanwell, N. A. (1995). Azetidin-2-one derivatives as inhibitors of thrombin. *Bioorganic & Medicinal Chemistry*, *3*(8), 1123–1143. doi:10.1016/0968-0896(95)00101-L PMID:7582985

Hara, H., Takemura, A., & Yoshida, R. (2010). On Connectivity of Fibers with Positive Marginals in Multiple Logistic Regression. *Journal of Multivariate Analysis*, *101*(4), 909–925. doi:10.1016/j.jmva.2009.12.014

Hart, H., Chantiluke, K., Cubillo, A. I., Smith, A. B., Simmons, A., Brammer, M. J., ... Rubia, K. (2014). Pattern classification of response inhibition in adhd: Toward the development of neurobiological markers for adhd. *Human Brain Mapping*, *35*(7), 3083–3094. doi:10.1002/hbm.22386 PMID:24123508

Heimer, N. E., Del Sesto, R. E., Meng, Z., Wilkes, J. S., & Carper, W. R. (2006). Vibrational spectra of imidazolium tetrafluoroborate ionic liquids. *Journal of Molecular Liquids*, *124*(1-3), 84–95. doi:10.1016/j.molliq.2005.08.004

He, K., Zhang, X., Ren, S., & Sun, J. (2016). Deep residual learning for image recognition. In *Proceedings of the IEEE conference on computer vision and pattern recognition* (pp. 770-778). IEEE.

Hernandez-Fernandez, F. J., De los Rios, A. P., Tomás-Alonso, F., Gomez, D., & Víllora, G. (2009). Stability of hydrolase enzymes in ionic liquids. *Canadian Journal of Chemical Engineering*, *87*(6), 910–914. doi:10.1002/cjce.20227

Hilfiker, R. (2006). *Polymorphism: in the Pharmaceutical Industry.* Weinheim, Germany: WILEY-VCH Verlag GmbH&Co. doi:10.1002/3527607889

Hill, E. L., & Frith, U. (2003). Understanding autism: insights from mind and brain. *Philosophical Transactions of the Royal Society B: Biological Sciences, 358*(1430), 281.

Hill, E., Berthoz, S., & Frith, U. (2004). Brief report: Cognitive processing of own emotions in individuals with autistic spectrum disorder and in their relatives. *Journal of Autism and Developmental Disabilities, 34*(2), 229–235. doi:10.1023/B:JADD.0000022613.41399.14 PMID:15162941

Homan, R. W., Herman, J., & Purdy, P. (1987). Cerebral location of international 10–20 system electrode placement. *Electroencephalography and Clinical Neurophysiology, 66*(4), 376–382. doi:10.1016/0013-4694(87)90206-9 PMID:2435517

Hoskins, M. (2014). Common Big Data Challenges and How to Overcome Them. *Big Data, 2*(3), 142–143. doi:10.1089/big.2014.0030 PMID:27442494

Hotier, S., Leroy, F., Boisgontier, J., Laidi, C., Mangin, J.-F., Delorme, R., ... Houenou, J. (2017). Social cognition in autism is associated with the neurodevelopment of the posterior superior temporal sulcus. *Acta Psychiatrica Scandinavica, 136*(5), 517–525. doi:10.1111/acps.12814 PMID:28940401

Hough-Troutman, W. L., Smiglak, M., Griffin, S., Reichert, W. M., Mirska, I., Jodynis-Liebert, J., ... Pernak, J. (2009). Ionic liquids with dual biological function: Sweet and anti-microbial, hydrophobic quaternary ammonium-based salts. *New Journal of Chemistry, 33*(1), 26–33. doi:10.1039/B813213P

Hsu, S. C., & Chung, J. G. (2012). Anticancer potential of emodin. *BioMedicine, 2*(3), 108–116. doi:10.1016/j.biomed.2012.03.003

Huang, P. H., & Lin, H. (2010). *Abstract B46: Proliferative suppression of anthraquinone derives emodin and aloe-emodin through selective targeting in prostate and breast cancer cells.* Academic Press.

Huang, H. S., Chiou, J. F., Chiu, H. F., Hwang, J. M., Lin, P. Y., Tao, C. W., ... Jeng, W. R. (2002). Synthesis of symmetrical 1, 5-bis-thio-substituted anthraquinones for cytotoxicity in cultured tumor cells and lipid peroxidation. *Chemical & Pharmaceutical Bulletin, 50*(11), 1491–1494. doi:10.1248/cpb.50.1491 PMID:12419916

Huang, L., Zhang, T., Li, S., Duan, J., Ye, F., Li, H., ... Yang, X. (2014). Anthraquinone G503 induces apoptosis in gastric cancer cells through the mitochondrial pathway. *PLoS One*, *9*(9), e108286. doi:10.1371/journal.pone.0108286 PMID:25268882

Huang, Q., Lu, G., Shen, H. M., Chung, M., & Ong, C. N. (2007). Anti-cancer properties of anthraquinones from rhubarb. *Medicinal Research Reviews*, *27*(5), 609–630. doi:10.1002/med.20094 PMID:17022020

Ibañez, L. V., Grantz, C. J., & Messinger, D. S. (2013). The development of referential communication and autism symptomatology in high-risk infants. *Infancy*, *18*(5), 687–707. doi:10.1111/j.1532-7078.2012.00142.x PMID:24403864

Idowu, P. A., Aladekomo, T. A., & Agbelusi, O. (2016). Prediction of Pediatrics HIV/AIDS Patient's Survival in Nigeria: A Data Mining Approach. *Journal of Research in Science, Technology, Engineering and Management*, *2*(2), 40–45.

Idowu, P. A., Aladekomo, T. A., Agbelusi, O., Alaba, O. B., & Balogun, J. A. (2017a). Prediction of Pediatric HIV/AIDS Survival in Nigeria using Naïve Bayes' Approach. *International Journal of Child Health and Human Development*, *10*(2), 1–12.

Idowu, P. A., Aladekomo, T. A., Agbelusi, O., Alaba, O. B., & Balogun, J. A. (2017b). Prediction of Pediatric HIV/AIDS Survival in Nigeria using C4.5 Decision Trees Algorithm. *International Journal of Child Health and Human Development*, *10*(2), 1–12.

Inamuddin. (2012). Green Solvents II-Properties and Applications of Ionic Liquids. Springer Science+Business Media.

Iwai, N., Nakayama, K., & Kitazume, T. (2011). Antibacterial activities of imidazolium, pyrrolidinium and piperidinium salts. *Bioorganic & Medicinal Chemistry Letters*, *21*(6), 1728–1730. doi:10.1016/j.bmcl.2011.01.081 PMID:21324694

Jacob, R. J. K., & Karn, K. S. (2003). Eye Tracking in Human-Computer Interaction and Usability Research: Ready to Deliver the Promises. In The Mind's Eye: Cognitive and Applied Aspects of Eye Movement Research. Elsevier Science.

Jacobson, J. W., Mulick, J. A., & Green, G. (1998). Cost-benefit estimates for early intensive behavioral intervention for young children with autism – General model and single state case. *Behavioral Interventions, 13*(4), 201–226. doi:10.1002/(SICI)1099-078X(199811)13:4<201::AID-BIN17>3.0.CO;2-R

Jaime, M., Mcmahon, C. M., Davidson, B. C., Newell, L. C., Mundy, P. C., & And Henderson, H. A. (2016). Brief report: Reduced temporal-central EEG alpha coherence during joint attention perception in adolescents with autism spectrum disorder. *Journal of Autism and Developmental Disorders, 46*(4), 1477–1489. doi:10.100710803-015-2667-3 PMID:26659813

Jarrahpour, A., Ebrahimi, E., De Clercq, E., Sinou, V., Latour, C., Bouktab, L. D., & Brunel, J. M. (2011). Synthesis of mono-, bis-spiro-and dispiro-β-lactams and evaluation of their antimalarial activities. *Tetrahedron, 67*(45), 8699–8704. doi:10.1016/j.tet.2011.09.041

Jarrahpour, A., Ebrahimi, E., Khalifeh, R., Sharghi, H., Sahraei, M., Sinou, V., ... Brunel, J. M. (2012). Synthesis of novel β-lactams bearing an anthraquinone moiety, and evaluation of their antimalarial activities. *Tetrahedron, 68*(24), 4740–4744. doi:10.1016/j.tet.2012.04.011

Ji, H., O'saben, E., Boudion, A., & Li, Y. (2015). March madness prediction: A matrix completion approach. *Proceedings of Modeling, Simulation, and Visualization Student Capstone Conference.*

Ji, H., O'Saben, E., Lambi, R., & Li, Y. (2016). Matrix completion based model V2. 0: Predicting the winning probabilities of march madness matches. *Proceedings of Modeling, Simulation, and Visualization Student Capstone Conference.*

Jiang, M., & Zhao, Q. (2017). Learning visual attention to identify people with autism spectrum disorder. *Proceedings of the IEEE International Conference on Computer Vision*, 3267–3276. 10.1109/ICCV.2017.354

Johnson, M. G., Kiyokawa, H., Tani, S., Koyama, J., Morris-Natschke, S. L., Mauger, A., ... Lee, K. H. (1997). Antitumor agents—CLXVII. Synthesis and structure-activity correlations of the cytotoxic anthraquinone 1, 4-bis-(2, 3-epoxypropylamino)-9, 10-anthracenedione, and of related compounds. *Bioorganic & Medicinal Chemistry, 5*(8), 1469–1479. doi:10.1016/S0968-0896(97)00097-7 PMID:9313853

Jones, T. B., Bandettini, P. A., Kenworthy, L., Case, L. K., Milleville, S. C., Martin, A., & And Birn, R. M. (2010). Sources of group differences in functional connectivity: An investigation applied to autism spectrum disorder. *NeuroImage*, *49*(1), 401–414. doi:10.1016/j.neuroimage.2009.07.051 PMID:19646533

Jordheim, L. P., Marton, Z., Rhimi, M., Cros-Perrial, E., Lionne, C., Peyrottes, S., ... Chaloin, L. (2013). Identification and characterization of inhibitors of cytoplasmic 5'-nucleotidase cN-II issued from virtual screening. *Biochemical Pharmacology*, *85*(4), 497–506. doi:10.1016/j.bcp.2012.11.024 PMID:23220537

Juneja, P., & Kashyap, R. (2016). Optimal approach for CT image segmentation using improved energy based method. *International Journal of Control Theory and Applications*, *9*(41), 599–608.

Just, M. A., & Carpenter, P. A. (1976). Eye Fixations and Cognitive Processes. *Cognitive Psychology*, *8*(4), 441–480.

Just, M. A., Cherkassky, V. L., Keller, T. A., Kana, R. K., & Minshew, N. J. (2006). Functional and anatomical cortical underconnectivity in autism: Evidence from an FMRI study of an executive function task and corpus callosum morphometry. *Cerebral Cortex*, *17*(4), 951–961. doi:10.1093/cercor/bhl006 PMID:16772313

Just, M. A., Cherkassky, V. L., Keller, T. A., & Minshew, N. J. (2004). Cortical activation and synchronization during sentence comprehension in high-functioning autism: Evidence of underconnectivity. *Brain*, *127*(8), 1811–1821. doi:10.1093/brain/awh199 PMID:15215213

Kaar, J. L., Jesionowski, A. M., Berberich, J. A., Moulton, R., & Russell, A. J. (2003). Impact of ionic liquid physical properties on lipase activity and stability. *Journal of the American Chemical Society*, *125*(14), 4125–4131. doi:10.1021/ja028557x PMID:12670234

Kahle, D., Yoshida, R., & Garcia-Puente, L. (2017, September). Hybrid Schemes for Exact Conditional Inference in Discrete Exponential Families. *Annals of the Institute of Statistical Mathematics*, 1–29.

Kama, K., & Prem, S. (2013). Utilization of Data Mining Techniques for Prediction and Diagnosis of Major Life Threatening Diseases Survivability-Review. *International Journal of Scientific & Engineering Research*, 4(6), 923–932.

Kana, R. K., Keller, T. A., Cherkassky, V. L., Minshew, N. J., & Just, M. A. (2009). Atypical frontal-posterior synchronization of theory of mind regions in autism during mental state attribution. *Social Neuroscience*, 4(2), 135–152. doi:10.1080/17470910802198510 PMID:18633829

Kana, R. K., Uddin, L. Q., Kenet, T., Chugani, D., & Müller, R.-A. (2014). Brain connectivity in autism. *Frontiers in Human Neuroscience*, 8, 349. doi:10.3389/fnhum.2014.00349 PMID:24917800

Kane, M. J., Bleckley, M. K., Conway, A. R., & Engle, R. W. (2001). A controlled-attention view of working-memory capacity. *Journal of Experimental Psychology: General, 130*(2), 169.

Kapoor, A., Mota, S., & Picard, R. W. (2001). *Towards a learning companion that recognizes affect*. Paper presented at Emotional and Intelligent II: The Tangled Knot of Social Cognition AAAI Fall Symposium.

Kashyap, R., & Piersson, A. (2018b). Big Data Challenges and Solutions in the Medical Industries. In Handbook of Research on Pattern Engineering System Development for Big Data Analytics. IGI Global. doi:10.4018/978-1-5225-3870-7.ch001

Kashyap, R., Gautam, P., & Tiwari, V. (2018). Management and Monitoring Patterns and Future Scope. In Handbook of Research on Pattern Engineering System Development for Big Data Analytics. IGI Global. doi:10.4018/978-1-5225-3870-7.ch014

Kashyap, R., & Gautam, P. (2015). Modified region based segmentation of medical images. In *International Conference on Communication Networks (ICCN)*. IEEE. 10.1109/ICCN.2015.41

Kashyap, R., & Gautam, P. (2016). Fast level set method for segmentation of medical images. In *Proceedings of the International Conference on Informatics and Analytics (ICIA-16)*. ACM. 10.1145/2980258.2980302

Kashyap, R., & Gautam, P. (2017). Fast Medical Image Segmentation Using Energy-Based Method. *Biometrics. Concepts, Methodologies, Tools, and Applications*, *3*(1), 1017–1042. doi:10.4018/978-1-5225-0983-7.ch040

Kashyap, R., & Piersson, A. (2018a). *Impact of Big Data on Security. In Handbook of Research on Network Forensics and Analysis Techniques* (pp. 283–299). IGI Global. doi:10.4018/978-1-5225-4100-4.ch015

Kashyap, R., & Tiwari, V. (2018). Active contours using global models for medical image segmentation. *International Journal of Computational Systems Engineering*, *4*(2/3), 195. doi:10.1504/IJCSYSE.2018.091404

Katsyuba, S. A., Dyson, P. J., Vandyukova, E. E., Chernova, A. V., & Vidiš, A. (2004). Molecular Structure, Vibrational Spectra, and Hydrogen Bonding of the Ionic Liquid 1-Ethyl-3-methyl-1H-imidazolium Tetrafluoroborate. *Helvetica Chimica Acta*, *87*(10), 2556–2565. doi:10.1002/hlca.200490228

Katsyuba, S. A., Griaznova, T. P., Vidis, A., & Dyson, P. J. (2009). Structural studies of the ionic liquid 1-ethyl-3-methylimidazolium tetrafluoroborate in dichloromethane using a combined DFT-NMR spectroscopic approach. *The Journal of Physical Chemistry B*, *113*(15), 5046–5051. doi:10.1021/jp8083327 PMID:19309104

Kaushik, N., Attri, P., Kaushik, N., & Choi, E. (2012). Synthesis and antiproliferative activity of ammonium and imidazolium ionic liquids against T98G brain cancer cells. *Molecules (Basel, Switzerland)*, *17*(12), 13727–13739. doi:10.3390/molecules171213727 PMID:23174892

Keehn, B., Müller, R.-A., & Townsend, J. (2013). Atypical attentional networks and the emergence of autism. *Neuroscience and Biobehavioral Reviews*, *37*(2), 164–183. doi:10.1016/j.neubiorev.2012.11.014 PMID:23206665

Kennedy, D. P., & Adolphs, R. (2012). The social brain in psychiatric and neurological disorders. *Trends in Cognitive Sciences*, *16*(11), 559–572. doi:10.1016/j.tics.2012.09.006 PMID:23047070

Kerr, S., & Durkin, K. (2004). Understanding of thought bubbles as mental representations in children with autism: Implications for theory of mind. *Journal of Autism and Developmental Disorders*, *34*(6), 637–648. doi:10.100710803-004-5285-z PMID:15679184

Kirchner, B. (2009). Ionic Liquids. *Topics in Current Chemistry, 290*. PMID:21107799

Kleinhans, N. M., Richards, T., Sterling, L., Stegbauer, K. C., Mahurin, R., Johnson, L. C., ... Aylward, E. (2008). Abnormal functional connectivity in autism spectrum disorders during face processing. *Brain, 131*(4), 1000–1012. doi:10.1093/brain/awm334 PMID:18234695

Kleinsmith, A., Ravindra De Silva, P., & Bianchi-Berthouze, N. (2005). *Recognizing emotion from postures: cross-cultural differences in user modeling*. Paper presented at User Modeling. 10.1007/11527886_8

Klem, G. H., Lüders, H. O., Jasper, H., & Elger, C. (1999). The ten-twenty electrode system of the international federation. *Electroencephalography and Clinical Neurophysiology, 52*(3), 3–6. PMID:10590970

Klin, A., Lin, D. J., Gorrindo, P., Ramsay, G., & Jones, W. (2009). Two-year-olds with autism orient to non-social contingencies rather than biological motion. *Nature, 459*(7244), 257.

Kokorin, A. (2011). *Ionic Liquids: Applications and Perspectives*. Rijeka: InTech Publishing. doi:10.5772/1782

Komogortsev, O., Holland, C., Jayarathna, S., & Karpov, A. (2013). 2d linear oculomotor plant mathematical model: Verification and biometric applications. *ACM Transactions on Applied Perception (TAP), 10*(4), 27.

Komogortsev, O. V., Jayarathna, S., Aragon, C. R., & Mahmoud, M. 2010. Biometric identification via an oculomotor plant mathematical model. In *Proceedings of the 2010 Symposium on Eye-Tracking Research & Applications*. ACM. 10.1145/1743666.1743679

Koshino, H., Carpenter, P. A., Minshew, N. J., Cherkassky, V. L., Keller, T. A., & Just, M. A. (2005). Functional connectivity in an FMRI working memory task in high-functioning autism. *NeuroImage, 24*(3), 810–821. doi:10.1016/j.neuroimage.2004.09.028 PMID:15652316

Koshino, H., Kana, R. K., Keller, T. A., Cherkassky, V. L., Minshew, N. J., & Just, M. A. (2007). FMRI investigation of working memory for faces in autism: Visual coding and underconnectivity with frontal areas. *Cerebral Cortex, 18*(2), 289–300. doi:10.1093/cercor/bhm054 PMID:17517680

Kozima, H., Michalowski, M. P., & Nakagawa, C. (2009). Keepon: A playful robot for research, therapy, and entertainment. *International Journal of Social Robotics, 1*(1), 3–18. doi:10.100712369-008-0009-8

Kramer, A., Sirevaag, E., & Braune, R. (1987). A Psychophysiological Assessment of Operator Workload during Simulated Flight Missions. *Human Factors, 29*(2), 145–160. doi:10.1177/001872088702900203 PMID:3610180

Krejtz, K., Duchowski, A. T., Niedzielska, A., Biele, C., & Krejtz, I. (2018). Eye tracking cognitive load using pupil diameter and microsaccades with fixed gaze. *PloS One, 13*(9).

Krejtz, K., Duchowski, A. T., Niedzielska, A., Biele, C., & Krejtz, I. (2018a). Eye tracking cognitive load using pupil diameter and micro saccades with fixed gaze. *PloS One, 13*(9).

Krejtz, K., Duchowski, A. T., Niedzielska, A., Biele, C., & Krejtz, I. (2018b). Eye tracking cognitive load using pupil diameter and micro saccades with fixed gaze. *PloS One, 13*(9), 1–23.

Krejtz, K., Duchowski, A., Szmidt, T., Krejtz, I., González Perilli, F., Pires, A., Vilaro, A., & Villalobos, N. (2015). Gaze transition entropy. *ACM Transactions on Applied Perception (TAP), 13*(1), 4.

Krejtz, K., Duchowski, A., Szmidt, T., Krejtz, I., Perilli, F. G., Pires, A., Vilaro, A., & Villalobos, N. (2015). Gaze transition entropy. *Transactions on Applied Perception, 13*(1), 4:1–4:20.

Krejtz, K., Duchowski, A. T., Krejtz, I., Szarkowska, A., & Kopacz, A. (2016). Discerning Ambient/Focal Attention with Coefficient K. *Transactions on Applied Perception, 13*, 3.

Krizhevsky, A., Sutskever, I., & Hinton, G. E. (2012). Imagenet classification with deep convolutional neural networks. In Advances in neural information processing systems (pp. 1097-1105). Academic Press.

Kulic, D., & Croft, E. (2007). Physiological and subjective responses to articulated robot motion. *Robotica, 25*(01), 13–27. doi:10.1017/S0263574706002955

Kumar, V., & Malhotra, S. V. (2009). Study on the potential anti-cancer activity of phosphonium and ammonium-based ionic liquids. *Bioorganic & Medicinal Chemistry Letters*, *19*(16), 4643–4646. doi:10.1016/j.bmcl.2009.06.086 PMID:19615902

Lakshmi, G. S., & Isakki, P. (2017). A Comparative Study of Data Mining Classification Technique Using HIV/AIDS and STD Data. *International Journal of Innovative Research in Computer and Communication Engineering*, *5*(1), 134–139.

Lange, C., Patil, G., & Rudolph, R. (2005). Ionic liquids as refolding additives: N′-alkyl and N′-(ω-hydroxyalkyl) N-methylimidazolium chlorides. *Protein Science*, *14*(10), 2693–2701. doi:10.1110/ps.051596605 PMID:16195554

Lassegues, J. C., Grondin, J., Holomb, R., & Johansson, P. (2007). Raman and ab initio study of the conformational isomerism in the 1-ethyl-3-methyl-imidazolium bis (trifluoromethanesulfonyl) imide ionic liquid. *Journal of Raman Spectroscopy: JRS*, *38*(5), 551–558. doi:10.1002/jrs.1680

Laszlo, J. A., & Compton, D. L. (2001). α-Chymotrypsin catalysis in imidazolium-based ionic liquids. *Biotechnology and Bioengineering*, *75*(2), 181–186. doi:10.1002/bit.1177 PMID:11536140

Lazarev, V. V., Pontes, A., Mitrofanov, A. A., & deAzevedo, L. C. (2015). Reduced interhemispheric connectivity in childhood autism detected by electroencephalographic photic driving coherence. *Journal of Autism and Developmental Disorders*, *45*(2), 537–547. doi:10.100710803-013-1959-8 PMID:24097142

LeCun, Y., Bengio, Y., & Hinton, G. (2015). Deep learning. *Nature*, *521*(7553), 436.

Lee, J. C., & Tan, D. S. (2006). Using a low-cost electroencephalograph for task classification in HCI research. In *Proceedings of the 19th annual ACM symposium on User interface software and technology*. ACM. 10.1145/1166253.1166268

Lee, C. M., & Narayanan, S. S. (2005). Toward detecting emotions in spoken dialogs. *IEEE Transactions on Speech and Audio Processing*, *13*(2), 293–303. doi:10.1109/TSA.2004.838534

Lee, S. H., Ha, S. H., Lee, S. B., & Koo, Y. M. (2006). Adverse effect of chloride impurities on lipase-catalyzed transesterifications in ionic liquids. *Biotechnology Letters*, 28(17), 1335–1339. doi:10.100710529-006-9095-6 PMID:16820978

Lee, S. U., Shin, H. K., Min, Y. K., & Kim, S. H. (2008). Emodin accelerates osteoblast differentiation through phosphatidylinositol 3-kinase activation and bone morphogenetic protein-2 gene expression. *International Immunopharmacology*, 8(5), 741–747. doi:10.1016/j.intimp.2008.01.027 PMID:18387517

Lee, Y.-J., Lee, S., Chang, M., & Kwak, H.-W. (2015). Saccadic movement deficiencies in adults with adhd tendencies. *ADHD Attention Deficit and Hyperactivity Disorders*, 7(4), 271–280. doi:10.100712402-015-0174-1 PMID:25993912

Leigh, R. J., & Zee, D. S. (2015). The neurology of eye movements. Oxford University Press.

Leigh, J. P., & Du, J. (2015). Brief report: Forecasting the economic burden of autism in 2015 and 2025 in the united states. *Journal of Autism and Developmental Disorders*, 45(12), 4135–4139. doi:10.100710803-015-2521-7 PMID:26183723

Leigh, R. J., & Kennard, C. (2004). Using saccades as a research tool in the clinical neurosciences. *Brain*, 127(3), 460–477. doi:10.1093/brain/awh035 PMID:14607787

Lenartowicz, A., & Loo, S. K. (2014). Use of EEG to diagnose ADHD. *Current Psychiatry Reports, 16*(11), 498.

Levinthal, C., Wodak, S. J., Kahn, P., & Dadivanian, A. K. (1975). Hemoglobin interaction in sickle cell fibers. I: Theoretical approaches to the molecular contacts. *Proceedings of the National Academy of Sciences of the United States of America*, 72(4), 1330–1334. doi:10.1073/pnas.72.4.1330 PMID:1055409

Li, B., Zhang, D. M., Luo, Y. M., & Chen, X. G. (2006). Three new and antitumor anthraquinone glycosides from Lasianthus acuminatissimus MERR. *Chemical & Pharmaceutical Bulletin*, 54(3), 297–300. doi:10.1248/cpb.54.297 PMID:16508180

Li, F., Li, X., Shao, J., Chi, P., Chen, J., & Wang, Z. (2010). Estrogenic activity of anthraquinone derivatives: In vitro and in silico studies. *Chemical Research in Toxicology*, *23*(8), 1349–1355. doi:10.1021/tx100118g PMID:20707409

Lin, J. (1991). Divergence measures based on the Shannon entropy. *IEEE Transactions on Information Theory*, *37*(1), 145–151. doi:10.1109/18.61115

Li, R., Zhang, W., Suk, H. I., Wang, L., Li, J., Shen, D., & Ji, S. (2014, September). Deep learning based imaging data completion for improved brain disease diagnosis. In *International Conference on Medical Image Computing and Computer-Assisted Intervention* (pp. 305-312). Springer. 10.1007/978-3-319-10443-0_39

Liu, W., Yu, X., Raj, B., Yi, L., Zou, X., & And Li, M. (2015). Efficient autism spectrum disorder prediction with eye movement: A machine learning framework. In *Affective Computing and Intelligent Interaction (ACII), 2015 International Conference on*. IEEE. 10.1109/ACII.2015.7344638

Liu, C., Conn, K., Sarkar, N., & Stone, W. (2008a). Physiology-based affect recognition for computer-assisted intervention of children with autism spectrum disorder. *International Journal of Human-Computer Studies*, *66*(9), 662–677. doi:10.1016/j.ijhsc.2008.04.003

Liu, C., Conn, K., Sarkar, N., & Stone, W. (2008b). Online Affect Detection and Robot Behavior Adaptation for Intervention of Children with Autism. *IEEE Transactions on Robotics*, *24*(4), 883–896. doi:10.1109/TRO.2008.2001362

Liu, W., Liang, W., & Xu, S. (2011). More information in imaging examination. *European Journal of Radiology*, *80*(2), 325. doi:10.1016/j.ejrad.2010.12.026 PMID:21255954

Li, Y. L., Zhang, J., Min, D., Hongyan, Z., Lin, N., & Li, Q. S. (2016). Anticancer effects of 1, 3-dihydroxy-2-methylanthraquinone and the ethyl acetate fraction of hedyotis diffusa willd against HepG2 carcinoma cells mediated via apoptosis. *PLoS One*, *11*(4), e0151502. doi:10.1371/journal.pone.0151502 PMID:27064569

Lombardo, M. V., Chakrabarti, B., Bullmore, E. T., Baron-Cohen, S., & Consortium, M. A. (2011). Specialization of right temporo-parietal junction for mentalizing and its relation to social impairments in autism. *NeuroImage*, *56*(3), 1832–1838. doi:10.1016/j.neuroimage.2011.02.067 PMID:21356316

Lombardo, M. V., Chakrabarti, B., Bullmore, E. T., Wheelwright, S. J., Sadek, S. A., Suckling, J., ... Baron-Cohen, S. (2010). Shared neural circuits for mentalizing about the self and others. *Journal of Cognitive Neuroscience*, *22*(7), 1623–1635. doi:10.1162/jocn.2009.21287 PMID:19580380

Lown, J. W. (1993). Anthracycline and anthraquinone anticancer agents: Current status and recent developments. *Pharmacology & Therapeutics*, *60*(2), 185–214. doi:10.1016/0163-7258(93)90006-Y PMID:8022857

Lozano, P., de Diego, T., Guegan, J. P., Vaultier, M., & Iborra, J. L. (2001). Stabilization of α-chymotrypsin by ionic liquids in transesterification reactions. *Biotechnology and Bioengineering*, *75*(5), 563–569. doi:10.1002/bit.10089 PMID:11745132

Lue, B. M., Guo, Z., & Xu, X. (2010). Effect of room temperature ionic liquid structure on the enzymatic acylation of flavonoids. *Process Biochemistry*, *45*(8), 1375–1382. doi:10.1016/j.procbio.2010.05.024

Lynch, C. J., Uddin, L. Q., Supekar, K., Khouzam, A., Phillips, J., & Menon, V. (2013). Default mode network in childhood autism: Posteromedial cortex heterogeneity and relationship with social deficits. *Biological Psychiatry*, *74*(3), 212–219. doi:10.1016/j.biopsych.2012.12.013 PMID:23375976

Magassouba, F. B., Diallo, A., Kouyaté, M., Mara, F., Mara, O., Bangoura, O., ... Lamah, K. (2007). Ethnobotanical survey and antibacterial activity of some plants used in Guinean traditional medicine. *Journal of Ethnopharmacology*, *114*(1), 44–53. doi:10.1016/j.jep.2007.07.009 PMID:17825510

Malhotra, S. V. (2010). *Ionic Liquid Applications: Pharmaceuticals, Therapeutics, and Biotechnology*. Washington, DC: ACS. doi:10.1021/bk-2010-1038

Mandryk, R. L., Inkpen, K. M., & Calvert, T. W. (2006). Using physiological techniques to measure user experience with entertainment technologies. *International Journal of Human-Computer Studies*, *25*(2), 141–158.

Manevitz, L., & Yousef, M. (2007). One-class document classification via neural networks. *Neurocomputing*, *70*(7-9), 7–9, 1466–1481. doi:10.1016/j.neucom.2006.05.013

Manlhiot, C. (2018). Machine learning for predictive analytics in medicine: Real opportunity or overblown hype? *European Heart Journal Cardiovascular Imaging, 19*(7), 727–728. doi:10.1093/ehjci/jey041 PMID:29538756

Manojlovic, N. T., Solujic, S., Sukdolak, S., & Milosev, M. (2005). Antifungal activity of Rubia tinctorum, Rhamnus frangula and Caloplaca cerina. *Fitoterapia, 76*(2), 244–246. doi:10.1016/j.fitote.2004.12.002 PMID:15752641

Mao, J. X., Lee, A. S., Kitchin, J. R., Nulwala, H. B., Luebke, D. R., & Damodaran, K. (2013). Interactions in 1-ethyl-3-methyl imidazolium tetracyanoborate ion pair: Spectroscopic and density functional study. *Journal of Molecular Structure, 1038*, 12–18. doi:10.1016/j.molstruc.2013.01.046

Marcano, J. L. L., Bell, M. A., & Beex, A. L. (2016). Classification of adhd and non-adhd using ar models. In *Engineering in Medicine and Biology Society (EMBC), 2016 IEEE 38th Annual International Conference of the.* IEEE. 10.1109/EMBC.2016.7590715

Marrucho, I. M., Branco, L. C., & Rebelo, L. P. N. (2014). Ionic liquids in pharmaceutical applications. *Annual Review of Chemical and Biomolecular Engineering, 5*(1), 527–546. doi:10.1146/annurev-chembioeng-060713-040024 PMID:24910920

Mason, R. A., Williams, D. L., Kana, R. K., Minshew, N., & Just, M. A. (2008). Theory of mind disruption and recruitment of the right hemisphere during narrative comprehension in autism. *Neuropsychologia, 46*(1), 269–280. doi:10.1016/j.neuropsychologia.2007.07.018 PMID:17869314

Matsui, M., Taniguchi, S., Suzuki, M., Wang, M., Funabiki, K., & Shiozaki, H. (2005). Dyes produced by the reaction of 1, 2, 3, 4-tetrafluoro-9, 10-anthraquinones with bifunctional nucleophiles. *Dyes and Pigments, 65*(3), 211–220. doi:10.1016/j.dyepig.2004.07.006

McKenzie, N., McNulty, J., McLeod, D., McFadden, M., & Balachandran, N. (2012). Synthesizing novel anthraquinone natural product-like compounds to investigate protein–ligand interactions in both an in vitro and in vivo assay: An integrated research-based third-year chemical biology laboratory course. *Journal of Chemical Education, 89*(6), 743–749. doi:10.1021/ed200417d

McPhail, G. (2017). Constructivism: Clearing up the confusion between a theory of learning and "constructing" knowledge. *Set: Research Information for Teachers*, (2), 30-22. doi:10.18296et.0081

Meehan, M., Razzaque, S., Insko, B., Whitton, M., & Brooks, F. P. Jr. (2005). Review of four studies on the use of physiological reaction as a measure of presence in stressful virtual environments. *Applied Psychophysiology and Biofeedback*, *30*(3), 239–258. doi:10.100710484-005-6381-3 PMID:16167189

Melin, P., & Sánchez, D. (2017). Multi-objective optimization for modular granular neural networks applied to pattern recognition. *Information Sciences*. doi:10.1016/j.ins.2017.09.031

Micaelo, N. M., & Soares, C. M. (2008). Protein structure and dynamics in ionic liquids. Insights from molecular dynamics simulation studies. *The Journal of Physical Chemistry B*, *112*(9), 2566–2572. doi:10.1021/jp0766050 PMID:18266354

Michalek, A. M., Watson, S. M., Ash, I., Ringleb, S., & Raymer, A. (2014). Effects of noise and audiovisual cues on speech processing in adults with and without adhd. *International Journal of Audiology*, *53*(3), 145–152. doi:10.3109/14992027.2013.866282 PMID:24456181

Michalek, A. P., & And Roche, J. (2017). Pupil dilation as a measure of attention in adhd: A pilot study. *America*, *116*, 2395–2405.

Michaud, F., & Theberge-Turmel, C. (2002). Mobile robotic toys and autism. In K. Dautenhahn, A. H. Bond, L. Canamero, & B. Edmonds (Eds.), *Socially Intelligent Agents: Creating Relationships With Computers and Robots* (pp. 125–132). Norwell, MA: Kluwer. doi:10.1007/0-306-47373-9_15

Mi, H., Petitjean, C., Vera, P., & Ruan, S. (2015). Joint tumor growth prediction and tumor segmentation on therapeutic follow-up PET images. *Medical Image Analysis*, *23*(1), 84–91. doi:10.1016/j.media.2015.04.016 PMID:25988489

Miles-Tribble, V. (2017). Restorative justice as a public theology imperative. *Review & Expositor*, *114*(3), 366–379. doi:10.1177/0034637317721704

Mingle, R. (2017). Machine Learning Techniques on Microbiome -Based Diagnostics. *Advances In Biotechnology & Microbiology*, *6*(4). doi:10.19080/AIBM.2017.06.555695

Mitchell, P., Parsons, S., & Leonard, A. (2007). Using virtual environments for teaching social understanding to adolescents with autistic spectrum disorders. *Journal of Autism and Developmental Disorders, 37*(3), 589–600. doi:10.100710803-006-0189-8 PMID:16900403

Miyagi, T. (2009). Estimation of Inter-regional Trade Coefficients Using Nueral Network Models. *Studies In Regional Science, 39*(3), 519–538. doi:10.2457rs.39.519

Modugu, N. R., & Pittala, P. K. (2017). Ionic liquid mediated and promoted one-pot green synthesis of new isoxazolyl dihydro-1 H-indol-4 (5 H)-one derivatives at ambient temperature. *Cogent Chemistry, 3*(1), 1318693. doi: 10.1080/23312009.2017.1318693

Mohammad-Rezazadeh, I., Frohlich, J., Loo, S. K., & Jeste, S. S. (2016). Brain connectivity in autism spectrum disorder. *Current Opinion in Neurology, 29*(2), 137.

Moniruzzaman, M., & Goto, M. (2011). Ionic Liquids: Future Solvents and Reagents for Pharmaceuticals. *Journal of Chemical Engineering of Japan, 44*(6), 370–381. doi:10.1252/jcej.11we015

Moore, D. J., McGrath, P., & Thorpe, J. (2000). Computer aided learning for people with autism - A framework for research and development. *Innovations in Education & Training International, 37*(3), 218–228. doi:10.1080/13558000050138452

Morgan, D., Mahe, C., Mayanja, B., Whitworth, J. A. G., & Kilmarx, P. H. (2002). Progression to symptomatic disease in people infected with HIV-1 in rural Uganda: Prospective cohort study. *Biomedical Journal, 324*, 193–197. PMID:11809639

Mortimer, J. A. (2012). The Nun Study: Risk Factors for Pathology and Clinical-Pathologic Correlations. *Current Alzheimer Research, 9*(6), 621–627. doi:10.2174/156720512801322546 PMID:22471869

Mostofsky, S. H., Lasker, A., Cutting, L., Denckla, M., & Zee, D. (2001). Oculomotor abnormalities in attention deficit hyperactivity disorder a preliminary study. *Neurology, 57*(3), 423–430. doi:10.1212/WNL.57.3.423 PMID:11502907

Mueller, A., Candrian, G., Kropotov, J. D., Ponomarev, V. A., & Baschera, G.-M. (2010). Classification of adhd patients on the basis of independent erp components using a machine learning system. In Nonlinear biomedical physics (Vol. 4). BioMed Central, S1. doi:10.1186/1753-4631-4-S1-S1

Mueller, S. G., Weiner, M. W., Thal, L. J., Petersen, R. C., Jack, C., Jagust, W., ... Beckett, L. (2005). The Alzheimer's disease neuroimaging initiative. *Neuroimaging Clinics*, *15*(4), 869–877. doi:10.1016/j.nic.2005.09.008 PMID:16443497

Mullen, T. R., Kothe, C. A., Chi, Y. M., Ojeda, A., Kerth, T., Makeig, S., ... Cauwenberghs, G. (2015). Real-time neuroimaging and cognitive monitoring using wearable dry EEG. *IEEE Transactions on Biomedical Engineering*, *62*(11), 2553–2567. doi:10.1109/TBME.2015.2481482 PMID:26415149

Mundy, P. C. (2016). *Autism and joint attention: Development, neuroscience, and clinical fundamentals*. Guilford Publications.

Mundy, P., Block, J., Delgado, C., Pomares, Y., Van Hecke, A. V., & Parlade, M. V. (2007). Individual differences and the development of joint attention in infancy. *Child Development*, *78*(3), 938–954. doi:10.1111/j.1467-8624.2007.01042.x PMID:17517014

Mundy, P., & Newell, L. (2007). Attention, joint attention, and social cognition. *Current Directions in Psychological Science*, *16*(5), 269–274. doi:10.1111/j.1467-8721.2007.00518.x PMID:19343102

Mundy, P., Sigman, M., & Kasari, C. (1990). A longitudinal study of joint attention and language development in autistic children. *Journal of Autism and Developmental Disorders*, *20*(1), 115–128. doi:10.1007/BF02206861 PMID:2324051

Mundy, P., Sigman, M., Ungerer, J., & Sherman, T. (1986). Defining the social deficits of autism: The contribution of non-verbal communication measures. *Journal of Child Psychology and Psychiatry, and Allied Disciplines*, *27*(5), 657–669. doi:10.1111/j.1469-7610.1986.tb00190.x PMID:3771682

Mundy, P., Sullivan, L., & Mastergeorge, A. M. (2009). A parallel and distributed-processing model of joint attention, social cognition and autism. *Autism Research*, *2*(1), 1, 2–21. doi:10.1002/aur.61 PMID:19358304

Munoz, D. P., Armstrong, I. T., Hampton, K. A., & Moore, K. D. (2003). Altered control of visual fixation and saccadic eye movements in attention-deficit hyperactivity disorder. *Journal of Neurophysiology*, *90*(1), 503–514. doi:10.1152/jn.00192.2003 PMID:12672781

Mutula, S. (2009). Ethical, Legal, and Social Issues in Medical Informatics. Online Information Review, 33(5), 1009-1010. doi:10.1108/14684520911001981

Mwamburi, D. M., Ghosh, M., Fauntleroy, J., Gorbach, S. L., & Wanke, C. A. (2005). Predicting CD4 count using total lymphocyte count: A sustainable tool for clinical decisions during HAART use. *The American Journal of Tropical Medicine and Hygiene*, *73*(1), 58–62. doi:10.4269/ajtmh.2005.73.58 PMID:16014833

Myers, S. M., & Johnson, C. P. (2007). Management of children with autism spectrum disorders. *Pediatrics*, *120*(5), 1162–1182. doi:10.1542/peds.2007-2362 PMID:17967921

Naimur Rahman, M., Esmailpour, A., & Zhao, J. (2016). Machine Learning with Big Data An Efficient Electricity Generation Forecasting System. *Big Data Research*, *5*, 9–15. doi:10.1016/j.bdr.2016.02.002

Nara, S. J., Harjani, J. R., & Salunkhe, M. M. (2002). Lipase-catalysed transesterification in ionic liquids and organic solvents: A comparative study. *Tetrahedron Letters*, *43*(16), 2979–2982. doi:10.1016/S0040-4039(02)00420-3

Nasoz, F., Alvarez, K., Lisetti, C., & Finkelstein, N. (2004). Emotion recognition from physiological signals using wireless sensors for presence technologies. *International Journal of Cognition, Technology, and Work*, *6*(1), 4-14.

National Academies Of Sciences. E., Medicine. (2016). Improving diagnosis in health care. National Academies Press.

Noonan, S. K., Haist, F., & Müller, R.-A. (2009). Aberrant functional connectivity in autism: Evidence from low frequency bold signal fluctuations. *Brain Research*, *1262*, 48–63. doi:10.1016/j.brainres.2008.12.076 PMID:19401185

Norbury, C. F., Brock, J., Cragg, L., Einav, S., Griffiths, H., & Nation, K. (2009). Eye-movement patterns are associated with communicative competence in autistic spectrum disorders. *Journal of Child Psychology and Psychiatry, and Allied Disciplines*, *50*(7), 834–842. doi:10.1111/j.1469-7610.2009.02073.x PMID:19298477

Noritomi, H., Minamisawa, K., Kamiya, R., & Kato, S. (2011). Thermal stability of proteins in the presence of aprotic ionic liquids. *Journal of Biomedical Science and Engineering*, *4*(2), 94–99. doi:10.4236/jbise.2011.42013

NRC (National Research Council). (2001). *Educating Children with Autism*. Washington, DC: National Academy Press.

Nunez, P. L., & Srinivasan, R. (2006). A theoretical basis for standing and traveling brain waves measured with human EEG with implications for an integrated consciousness. *Clinical Neurophysiology*, *117*(11), 2424–2435. doi:10.1016/j.clinph.2006.06.754 PMID:16996303

Ojunga, N., Peter, M., Otulo, W., Omollo, O., & Edgar, O. (2014). The Application of Logistic Regression in Modeling of Survival Chances of HIV-Positive Patients under Highly Active Antiretroviral Therapy (HAART): A Case of Nyakach District, Kenya. *Journal of Medicine and Clinical Sciences*, *3*(3), 14–20.

Olayemi, O. C., Olasehinde, O. O., & Agbelusi, O. (2016). Predictive Model of Pediatric HIV/AIDS Survival in Nigeria using Support Vector Machines. *Communications on Applied Electronics*, *5*(8), 29–36. doi:10.5120/cae2016652349

Ozkok, F., & Sahin, Y. M. (2016). *Development of Original Method for Synthesis of Bioactive Anthraquine Anologues*. Patent No: 2016/19610 (Turkish Patent Institute).

Ozokwelu, D., Zhang, S., Okafor, O. C., Cheng, W., & Litombe, N. (2017). *Novel Catalytic and Separation Processes Based On Ionic Liquids*. Elsevier Inc.

Palojoki, S., Pajunen, T., Saranto, K., & Lehtonen, L. (2016). Electronic Health Record-Related Safety Concerns: A Cross-Sectional Survey of Electronic Health Record Users. *JMIR Medical Informatics*, *4*(2), e13. doi:10.2196/medinform.5238 PMID:27154599

Panigrahi, G. K., Verma, N., Singh, N., Asthana, S., Gupta, S. K., Tripathi, A., & Das, M. (2018). Interaction of anthraquinones of Cassia occidentalis seeds with DNA and Glutathione. *Toxicology Reports*, *5*, 164–172. doi:10.1016/j. toxrep.2017.12.024 PMID:29326881

Pankiewicz, F., Zöllmer, A., Gräser, Y., & Hilker, M. (2007). Article. *Archives of Insect Biochemistry and Physiology*, (66), 98–108.

Pantic, M., & Rothkrantz, L. J. M. (2003). Toward an affect-sensitive multimodal human–computer interaction. *Proceedings of the IEEE*, *91*(9), 1370–1390. doi:10.1109/JPROC.2003.817122

Papaiconomou, N., Estager, J., Traore, Y., Bauduin, P., Bas, C., Legeai, S., ... Draye, M. (2010). Synthesis, physicochemical properties, and toxicity data of new hydrophobic ionic liquids containing dimethylpyridinium and trimethylpyridinium cations. *Journal of Chemical & Engineering Data*, *55*(5), 1971–1979. doi:10.1021/je9009283

Papert, S. (1993). *Mindstorms: Children, Computers, and Powerful Ideas* (2nd ed.). New York: Basic Books.

Paramaguru, G., Kathiravan, A., Selvaraj, S., Venuvanalingam, P., & Renganathan, R. (2010). Interaction of anthraquinone dyes with lysozyme: Evidences from spectroscopic and docking studies. *Journal of Hazardous Materials*, *175*(1-3), 985–991. doi:10.1016/j.jhazmat.2009.10.107 PMID:19939563

Park, S., & Kazlauskas, R. J. (2003). Biocatalysis in ionic liquids–advantages beyond green technology. *Current Opinion in Biotechnology*, *14*(4), 432–437. doi:10.1016/S0958-1669(03)00100-9 PMID:12943854

Parsons, S., & Mitchell, P. (2002). The potential of virtual reality in social skills training for people with autistic spectrum disorders. *Journal of Intellectual Disability Research*, *46*(5), 430–443. doi:10.1046/j.1365-2788.2002.00425.x PMID:12031025

Parsons, S., Mitchell, P., & Leonard, A. (2004). The use and understanding of virtual environments by adolescents with autistic spectrum disorders. *Journal of Autism and Developmental Disorders*, *34*(4), 449–466. doi:10.1023/ B:JADD.0000037421.98517.8d PMID:15449520

Parsons, S., Mitchell, P., & Leonard, A. (2005). Do adolescents with autistic spectrum disorders adhere to social conventions in virtual environments? *Autism, 9*(1), 95–117. doi:10.1177/1362361305049032 PMID:15618265

Patai, S. (1988). *The Chemistry of Quinones Compounds*. New York: Wiley.

Patel, R., Kumari, M., & Khan, A. B. (2014). Recent advances in the applications of ionic liquids in protein stability and activity: A review. *Applied Biochemistry and Biotechnology, 172*(8), 3701–3720. doi:10.100712010-014-0813-6 PMID:24599667

Pecchinenda, A., & Smith, C. A. (1996). The affective significance of skin conductance activity during a difficult problem-solving task. *Cognition and Emotion, 10*(5), 481–504. doi:10.1080/026999396380123

Peng, X., Lin, P., Zhang, T., & Wang, J. (2013). Extreme learning machine-based classification of adhd using brain structural mri data. *PloS One, 8*(11).

Perchellet, E. M., Magill, M. J., Huang, X., Dalke, D. M., Hua, D. H., & Perchellet, J. P. (2000). 1, 4-Anthraquinone: An anticancer drug that blocks nucleoside transport, inhibits macromolecule synthesis, induces DNA fragmentation, and decreases the growth and viability of L1210 leukemic cells in the same nanomolar range as daunorubicin in vitro. *Anti-Cancer Drugs, 11*(5), 339–352. doi:10.1097/00001813-200006000-00004 PMID:10912950

Pernak, J., Syguda, A., Mirska, I., Pernak, A., Nawrot, J., Prądzyńska, A., ... Rogers, R. D. (2007). Choline-derivative-based ionic liquids. *Chemistry (Weinheim an der Bergstrasse, Germany), 13*(24), 6817–6827. doi:10.1002/chem.200700285 PMID:17534999

Pesewu, G. A., Cutler, R. R., & Humber, D. P. (2008). Antibacterial activity of plants used in traditional medicines of Ghana with particular reference to MRSA. *Journal of Ethnopharmacology, 116*(1), 102–111. doi:10.1016/j.jep.2007.11.005 PMID:18096337

Phone, D. (2018). Proactive medicines management supports more patient centric services. *International Journal of Integrated Care, 18*(s1), 31. doi:10.5334/ijic.s1031

Picard, R. W. (1997). *Affective Computing*. Cambridge, MA: MIT Press.

Pieme, C. A., Penlap, V. N., Ngogang, J., Kuete, V., Catros, V., & Moulinoux, J. P. (2009). In vitro effects of extract of Senna alata (Ceasalpiniaceae) on the polyamines produced by Leukaemia cells (L1210). *Pharmacognosy Magazine*, 5(17), 8.

Pioggia, G., Igliozzi, R., Ferro, M., Ahluwalia, A., Muratori, F., & De Rossi, D. (2005). An android for enhancing social skills and emotion recognition in people with autism. *IEEE Transactions on Neural Systems and Rehabilitation Engineering*, *13*(4), 507–515. doi:10.1109/TNSRE.2005.856076 PMID:16425833

Plechkova, N. V., & Seddon, K. R. (2014). *Ionic Liquids Further UnCOILed: Critical Expert Overviews.* John Wiley & Sons, Inc. doi:10.1002/9781118839706

Post, F. A., Wood, R., & Maartens, G. (1996). CD4 and total lymphocyte counts as predictors of HIV disease progression. *The Quarterly Journal of Medicine*, 89(7), 505–508. doi:10.1093/qjmed/89.7.505 PMID:8759490

Prendinger, H., Mori, J., & Ishizuka, M. (2005). Using human physiology to evaluate subtle expressivity of a virtual quizmaster in a mathematical game. *International Journal of Human-Computer Studies*, 62(2), 231–245. doi:10.1016/j.ijhcs.2004.11.009

Pretti, C., Renzi, M., Focardi, S. E., Giovani, A., Monni, G., Melai, B., ... Chiappe, C. (2011). Acute toxicity and biodegradability of N-alkyl-N-methylmorpholinium and N-alkyl-DABCO based ionic liquids. *Ecotoxicology and Environmental Safety*, 74(4), 748–753. doi:10.1016/j.ecoenv.2010.10.032 PMID:21093055

Rajathi, K., & Rajendran, A. (2013). Synthesis, Characterization and Biological Evaluation of Imidazolium Based Ionic Liquids. *RRJC*, *2*(1), 36–41.

Ramalingam, A., Hizaddin, H. F., Jayakumar, N. S., & Hashim, M. A. B. (2013). A quantum chemical study on interaction energy between halogen free ionic liquid and aromatic nitrogen compounds. *Journal of Innovative Engineering*, *1*(1), 3.

Rani, P., Sarkar, N., Smith, C. A., & Kirby, L. D. (2004). Anxiety detecting robotic system – towards implicit human-robot collaboration. *Robotica*, 22(1), 85–95. doi:10.1017/S0263574703005319

Rarey, M. (2001). Protein–ligand docking in drug design. *Bioinformatics-from genomes to drugs*, 315-360.

Rath, G., Ndonzao, M., & Hostettmann, K. (1995). Antifungal anthraquinones from Morinda lucida. *International Journal of Pharmacognosy, 33*(2), 107-114.

Recio, M. (2017). Practitioner's Corner • Data Protection Officer: The Key Figure to Ensure Data Protection and Accountability. *European Data Protection Law Review, 3*(1), 114–118. doi:10.21552/edpl/2017/1/18

Redcay, E., Kleiner, M., & Saxe, R. (2012). Look at this: The neural correlates of initiating and responding to bids for joint attention. *Frontiers in Human Neuroscience, 6*, 169. doi:10.3389/fnhum.2012.00169 PMID:22737112

Rey-del-Castillo, P., & Cardeñosa, J. (2016). An Exercise in Exploring Big Data for Producing Reliable Statistical Information. *Big Data, 4*(2), 120–128. doi:10.1089/big.2015.0045 PMID:27441716

Richmond, J., & Nelson, C. A. (2009). Relational memory during infancy: Evidence from eye tracking. *Developmental Science, 12*(4), 549–556. doi:10.1111/j.1467-7687.2009.00795.x PMID:19635082

Roberts, W., Fillmore, M. T., & Milich, R. (2011). Separating automatic and intentional inhibitory mechanisms of attention in adults with attention-deficit/hyperactivity disorder. *Journal of Abnormal Psychology, 120*(1), 223.

Robins, B., Dickerson, P., & Dautenhahn, K. (2005). *Robots as embodied beings – Interactionally sensitive body movements in interactions among autistic children and a robot.* Paper presented at the IEEE International Workshop on Robot and Human Interactive Communication, Nashville, TN. 10.1109/ROMAN.2005.1513756

Rogers, S. J. (2000). Interventions that facilitate socialization in children with autism. *Journal of Autism and Developmental Disorders, 30*(5), 399–409. doi:10.1023/A:1005543321840 PMID:11098875

Rommelse, N., Van Der Stigchel, S., Witlox, J., Geldof, C., Deijen, J.-B., Theeuwes, J., ... Sergeant, J. (2008). Deficits in visuo-spatial working memory, inhibition and oculomotor control in boys with adhd and their non-affected brothers. *Journal of Neural Transmission (Vienna, Austria), 115*(2), 249–260. doi:10.100700702-007-0865-7 PMID:18253811

Rönnberg, J., Lunner, T., Zekveld, A., Sörqvist, P., Danielsson, H., Lyxell, B., ... Rudner, M. (2013). The ease of language understanding (elu) model: Theoretical, empirical, and clinical advances. *Frontiers in Systems Neuroscience*, *7*, 31. doi:10.3389/fnsys.2013.00031 PMID:23874273

Rosma, M. D., Sameem, A. K., Basir, A., Adeeba, K., & Annapurni, K. (2012). The Prediction of AIDS Survival: A Data Mining Approach. *Proceedings of the 2nd WSEAS International Conference on Multivariate Analysis and Its Application in Science and Engineering*, 48 – 53.

Roth, C., Chatzipapadopoulos, S., Kerle, D., Friedriszik, F., Lütgens, M., Lochbrunner, S., ... Ludwig, R. (2012). Hydrogen bonding in ionic liquids probed by linear and nonlinear vibrational spectroscopy. *New Journal of Physics*, *14*(10), 105026. doi:10.1088/1367-2630/14/10/105026

Ruan, G., & Zhang, H. (2017). Closed-loop Big Data Analysis with Visualization and Scalable Computing. *Big Data Research*, *8*, 12–26. doi:10.1016/j.bdr.2017.01.002

Rubia, K. (2018). Cognitive neuroscience of attention deficit hyperactivity disorder (adhd) and its clinical translation. *Frontiers in Human Neuroscience*, *12*, 100. doi:10.3389/fnhum.2018.00100 PMID:29651240

Ruble, L. A., & Robson, D. M. (2006). Individual and environmental determinants of engagement in autism. *Journal of Autism and Developmental Disorders*, *37*(8), 1457–1468. doi:10.100710803-006-0222-y PMID:17151800

Rudie, J. D., Shehzad, Z., Hernandez, L. M., Colich, N. L., Bookheimer, S. Y., Iacoboni, M., & Dapretto, M. (2011). Reduced functional integration and segregation of distributed neural systems underlying social and emotional information processing in autism spectrum disorders. *Cerebral Cortex*, *22*(5), 1025–1037. doi:10.1093/cercor/bhr171 PMID:21784971

Rutter, M. (2006). Autism: Its recognition, early diagnosis, and service implications. *Journal of Developmental and Behavioral Pediatrics*, *27*(Supplement 2), S54–S58. doi:10.1097/00004703-200604002-00002 PMID:16685186

Ryan, A., Kaplan, E., Nebel, J. C., Polycarpou, E., Crescente, V., Lowe, E., ... Sim, E. (2014). Identification of NAD (P) H quinone oxidoreductase activity in azoreductases from P. aeruginosa: Azoreductases and NAD (P) H quinone oxidoreductases belong to the same FMN-dependent superfamily of enzymes. *PLoS One, 9*(6), e98551. doi:10.1371/journal.pone.0098551 PMID:24915188

Salazar, J. C., Schmitt, F. A., Yu, L., Mendiondo, M., & Kryscio, R. J. (2007). Shared Random Effects Analysis of Multi-State Markov Models: Application to a Longitudinal Study of Transitions to Dementia. *Statistics in Medicine, 26*(3), 568–580. doi:10.1002im.2437 PMID:16345024

Samorì, C., Malferrari, D., Valbonesi, P., Montecavalli, A., Moretti, F., Galletti, P., ... Pasteris, A. (2010). Introduction of oxygenated side chain into imidazolium ionic liquids: Evaluation of the effects at different biological organization levels. *Ecotoxicology and Environmental Safety, 73*(6), 1456–1464. doi:10.1016/j.ecoenv.2010.07.020 PMID:20674022

Sasson, N. J., Pinkham, A. E., Weittenhiller, L. P., Faso, D. J., & Simpson, C. (2016). Context Effects on Facial Affect Recognition in Schizophrenia and Autism: Behavioral and Eye-Tracking Evidence. *Schizophrenia Bulletin, 42*(3), 675–683. doi:10.1093chbulbv176 PMID:26645375

Saturnino, C., Fusco, B., Saturnino, P., De Martino, G., Rocco, F., & Lancelot, J. C. (2000). Evaluation of analgesic and anti-inflammatory activity of novel β-lactam monocyclic compounds. *Biological & Pharmaceutical Bulletin, 23*(5), 654–656. doi:10.1248/bpb.23.654 PMID:10823683

Sawyer, A. C. P., Williamson, P., & Young, R. L. (2012). Can Gaze Avoidance Explain Why Individuals with Asperger's Syndrome Can't Recognize Emotions from Facial Expressions? *Journal of Autism and Developmental Disorders, 42*(4), 606–618.

Saxe, R. (2006). Uniquely human social cognition. *Current Opinion in Neurobiology, 16*(2), 235–239. doi:10.1016/j.conb.2006.03.001 PMID:16546372

Scassellati, B. (2005). *Quantitative metrics of social response for autism diagnosis*. Paper presented at the IEEE International Workshop on Robot and Human Interactive Communication, Nashville, TN. 10.1109/ROMAN.2005.1513843

Schechter, M., Zajdenverg, R., Machado, L. L., Pinto, M. E., Lima, L. A., & Perez, M. A. (1994). Predicting CD4 Counts in HIV-infected Brazilian Individuals: A Model Based on the World Health Organization Staging System. *Journal of Acquired Immune Deficiency Syndromes*, *7*(2), 163–168. PMID:7905525

Schilbach, L., Wilms, M., Eickhoff, S. B., Romanzetti, S., Tepest, R., Bente, G., ... Vogeley, K. (2010). Minds made for sharing: Initiating joint attention recruits reward-related neurocircuitry. *Journal of Cognitive Neuroscience*, *22*(12), 2702–2715. doi:10.1162/jocn.2009.21401 PMID:19929761

Schinazi, R. F., Chu, C. K., Babu, J. R., Oswald, B. J., Saalmann, V., Cannon, D. L., ... Nasr, M. (1990). Anthraquinones as a new class of antiviral agents against human immunodeficiency virus. *Antiviral Research*, *13*(5), 265–272. doi:10.1016/0166-3542(90)90071-E PMID:1697740

Schneiderman, M. H., & Ewens, W. L. (1971). The Cognitive Effects of Spatial Invasion. *Pacific Sociological Review*, *14*(4), 469–486. doi:10.2307/1388543

Schottenfeld, D., & Fraumeni, J. F. (2018). *Cancer Epidemiology and Prevention* (4th ed.). Oxford University Press.

Schultz, R. T. (2005). Developmental deficits in social perception in autism: The role of the amygdala and fusiform face area. *International Journal of Developmental Neuroscience*, *23*(2-3), 125–141. doi:10.1016/j.ijdevneu.2004.12.012 PMID:15749240

Schurz, M., Radua, J., Aichhorn, M., Richlan, F., & Perner, J. (2014). Fractionating theory of mind: A meta-analysis of functional brain imaging studies. *Neuroscience and Biobehavioral Reviews*, *42*, 9–34. doi:10.1016/j.neubiorev.2014.01.009 PMID:24486722

Seip, J. (1996). *Teaching the Autistic and Developmentally Delayed: A Guide for Staff Training and Development*. Delta, BC: Author.

Senapati, S., Mahanta, A. K., Kumar, S., & Maiti, P. (2018). Controlled drug delivery vehicles for cancer treatment and their performance. *Signal Transduction and Targeted Therapy, 3*(1), 7.

Shao, J. (1998). *Mathematical Statistics*. New York: Springer Verlag.

Sharpe, D. L., & Baker, D. L. (2007). Financial issues associated with having a child with autism. *Journal of Family and Economic Issues, 28*(2), 247–264. doi:10.100710834-007-9059-6

Sheldon, R. A., Lau, R. M., Sorgedrager, M. J., van Rantwijk, F., & Seddon, K. R. (2002). Biocatalysis in ionic liquids. *Green Chemistry, 4*(2), 147–151. doi:10.1039/b110008b

Shen, Z. L., Zhou, W. J., Liu, Y. T., Ji, S. J., & Loh, T. P. (2008). One-pot chemoenzymatic syntheses of enantiomerically-enriched O-acetyl cyanohydrins from aldehydes in ionic liquid. *Green Chemistry, 10*(3), 283–286. doi:10.1039/b717235d

Sherer, M. R., & Schreibman, L. (2005). Individual behavioral profiles and predictors of treatment effectiveness for children with autism. *Journal of Consulting and Clinical Psychology, 73*(3), 525–538. doi:10.1037/0022-006X.73.3.525 PMID:15982150

Sherman, W. R., & Craig, A. B. (2003). *Understanding virtual reality: interface, application, and design.* Boston: Morgan Kaufmann Publishers.

Shih, P., Shen, M., Öttl, B., Keehn, B., Gaffrey, M. S., & Müller, R.-A. (2010). Atypical network connectivity for imitation in autism spectrum disorder. *Neuropsychologia, 48*(10), 2931–2939. doi:10.1016/j.neuropsychologia.2010.05.035 PMID:20558187

Silva, P. R. D., Osano, M., Marasinghe, A., & Madurapperuma, A. P. (2006). A computational model for recognizing emotion with intensity for machine vision applications. *IEICE Transactions on Information and Systems, E89-D*(7), 2171–2179. doi:10.1093/ietisy/e89-d.7.2171

Simonyan, K., & Zisserman, A. (2014). *Very deep convolutional networks for large-scale image recognition.* arXiv preprint arXiv:1409.1556.

Singh, D. N., Verma, N., Raghuwanshi, S., Shukla, P. K., & Kulshreshtha, D. K. (2006). Antifungal anthraquinones from Saprosma fragrans. *Bioorganic & Medicinal Chemistry Letters, 16*(17), 4512–4514. doi:10.1016/j.bmcl.2006.06.027 PMID:16824761

Singh, Y., Narsai, N., & Mars, M. (2013). Applying Machine Learning to predict Patient-Specific Current CD4 Cell Count in order to determine the Progression of Human Immunodeficiency Virus (HIV) Infection. *African Journal of Biotechnology*, *12*(23), 3724–3750.

Skiera, B., & Ringel, D. (2017). Using Big Search Data to Map Your Market: Marketing in a Digital Age. *IESE Insight*, (32), 31-37. doi:10.15581/002. art-2982

Smith, C. A. (1989). Dimensions of appraisal and physiological response in emotion. *Journal of Personality and Social Psychology*, *56*(3), 339–353. doi:10.1037/0022-3514.56.3.339 PMID:2926633

Snyder, S. M., Rugino, T. A., Hornig, M., & Stein, M. A. (2015). Integration of an EEG biomarker with a clinician's ADHD evaluation. *Brain and Behavior*, *5*(4), 3–30. doi:10.1002/brb3.330 PMID:25798338

Sparks, B., Friedman, S., Shaw, D., Aylward, E., Echelard, D., Artru, A., ... Dager, S. R. (2002). Brain structural abnormalities in young children with autism spectrum disorder. *Neurology*, *59*(2), 184–192. doi:10.1212/WNL.59.2.184 PMID:12136055

Spence, S. J., Sharifi, P., & Wiznitzer, M. (2004). Autism spectrum disorder: screening, diagnosis, and medical evaluation. In *Seminars in Pediatric Neurology* (Vol. 11, pp. 186–195). Elsevier. doi:10.1016/j.spen.2004.07.002

Sperka, T., Pitlik, J., Bagossi, P., & Tözsér, J. (2005). Beta-lactam compounds as apparently uncompetitive inhibitors of HIV-1 protease. *Bioorganic & Medicinal Chemistry Letters*, *15*(12), 3086–3090. doi:10.1016/j. bmcl.2005.04.020 PMID:15893929

Standen, P. J., & Brown, D. J. (2005). Virtual reality in the rehabilitation of people with intellectual disabilities [review]. *Cyberpsychology & Behavior*, *8*(3), 272–282, discussion 283–288. doi:10.1089/cpb.2005.8.272 PMID:15971976

Stapleton, M., Liao, G., Brokstein, P., Hong, L., Carninci, P., Shiraki, T., ... Yu, C. (2002). The Drosophila gene collection: Identification of putative full-length cDNAs for 70% of D. melanogaster genes. *Genome Research*, *12*(8), 1294–1300. doi:10.1101/gr.269102 PMID:12176937

Sternberg, M. J., & Moont, G. (2002). Modelling protein–protein and protein–DNA docking. *Bioinformatics-From Genomes to Drugs*, 361-404.

Stokes, S. (2000). *Assistive technology for children with autism*. Published under a CESA 7 contract funded by the Wisconsin Department of Public Instruction.

Stolte, S., Arning, J., Bottin-Weber, U., Müller, A., Pitner, W. R., Welz-Biermann, U., ... Ranke, J. (2007). Effects of different head groups and functionalised side chains on the cytotoxicity of ionic liquids. *Green Chemistry*, 9(7), 760–767. doi:10.1039/B615326G

Strickland, D. (1997). Virtual reality for the treatment of autism. In G. Riva (Ed.), *Virtual reality in neuropsycho-physiology* (pp. 81–86). Amsterdam: IOS Press.

Strickland, D., Marcus, L. M., Mesibov, G. B., & Hogan, K. (1996). Brief report: Two case studies using virtual reality as a learning tool for autistic children. *Journal of Autism and Developmental Disorders*, 26(6), 651–659. doi:10.1007/BF02172354 PMID:8986851

Sun, Q., Muckatira, S., Yuan, L., Ji, S., Newfeld, S., Kumar, S., & Ye, J. (2013). Image-level and group-level models for Drosophila gene expression pattern annotation. *BMC Bioinformatics*, 14(1), 350. doi:10.1186/1471-2105-14-350 PMID:24299119

Swanson, M. R., Serlin, G. C., & Siller, M. (2013). Broad Autism Phenotype in Typically Developing Children Predicts Performance on an Eye-Tracking Measure of Joint Attention. *Journal of Autism and Developmental Disorders*, 43(3), 707–718.

Swettenham, J. (1996). Can children with autism be taught to understand false belief using computers? *Journal of Child Psychology and Psychiatry, and Allied Disciplines*, 37(2), 157–165. doi:10.1111/j.1469-7610.1996.tb01387.x PMID:8682895

Symeonidou, I., Dumontheil, I., Chow, W.-Y., & Breheny, R. (2016). Development of online use of theory of mind during adolescence: An eye-tracking study. *Journal of Experimental Child Psychology*, 149, 81–97. doi:10.1016/j.jecp.2015.11.007 PMID:26723471

Szegedy, C., Liu, W., Jia, Y., Sermanet, P., Reed, S., Anguelov, D., ... Rabinovich, A. (2015, June). *Going deeper with convolutions*. CVPR.

Takemura, A., & Yoshida, R. (2008). A Generalization of the Integer Linear Infeasibility Problem. *Discrete Optimization*, *5*(1), 36–52. doi:10.1016/j.disopt.2007.10.004

Talaty, E. R., Raja, S., Storhaug, V. J., Dölle, A., & Carper, W. R. (2004). Raman and infrared spectra and ab initio calculations of C2-4MIM imidazolium hexafluorophosphate ionic liquids. *The Journal of Physical Chemistry B*, *108*(35), 13177–13184. doi:10.1021/jp040199s

Tarekegn, G. B., & Sreenivasarao, V. (2016). Application of Data Mining Techniques on Pre ART Data: The Case of Felege Hiwot Referral Hospital. *International Journal of Research Studies in Computer Science and Engineering*, *3*(2), 1–9.

Tarkan, L. (2002). Autism therapy is called effective, but rare. *New York Times*.

Tartaro, A., & Cassell, J. (2007). Using virtual peer technology as an intervention for children with autism. In J. Lazar (Ed.), *Towards Universal Usability: Designing Computer Interfaces for Diverse User Populations*. Chichester, UK: John Wiley and Sons.

Thapaliya, S., Jayarathna, S., & Jaime, M. (2018). *Evaluating the EEG and eye movements for autism spectrum disorder*. Academic Press.

The World Health Report. (1996). *Fighting disase, Fostering development*. WHO.

Thorup, E., Nyström, P., Gredebäck, G., Bölte, S., & Falck-Ytter, T. (2016). Altered gaze following during live interaction in infants at risk for autism: an eye tracking study. *Molecular Autism*, *7*(1), 12.

Thorup, E., Nyström, P., Gredebäck, G., Bölte, S., & Falck-Ytter, T. (2018). Reduced Alternating Gaze During Social Interaction in Infancy is Associated with Elevated Symptoms of Autism in Toddlerhood. *Journal of Abnormal Child Psychology*, *46*(7), 1547–1561.

Tian, Y., & Peng, Y. (2011). Study on Communication of Massive 3D Spatial Data Based on ACE. *Geo-Information Science*, *12*(6), 819–827. doi:10.3724/SP.J.1047.2010.00819

Toichi, M., & Kamio, Y. (2003). Paradoxical autonomic response to mental tasks in autism. *Journal of Autism and Developmental Disorders*, *33*(4), 417–426. doi:10.1023/A:1025062812374 PMID:12959420

Tomancak, P., Beaton, A., Weiszmann, R., Kwan, E., Shu, S., Lewis, S. E., ... Rubin, G. M. (2002). Systematic determination of patterns of gene expression during Drosophila embryogenesis. *Genome Biology, 3*(12).

Tomancak, P., Berman, B. P., Beaton, A., Weiszmann, R., Kwan, E., Hartenstein, V., ... Rubin, G. M. (2007). Global analysis of patterns of gene expression during Drosophila embryogenesis. *Genome Biology*, *8*(7), R145. doi:10.1186/gb-2007-8-7-r145 PMID:17645804

Trepagnier, C. Y., Sebrechts, M. M., Finkelmeyer, A., Stewart, W., Woodford, J., & Coleman, M. (2006). Simulating social interaction to address deficits of autistic spectrum disorder in children. *Cyberpsychology & Behavior*, *9*(2), 213–217. doi:10.1089/cpb.2006.9.213 PMID:16640482

Tsang, S. W., Zhang, H., Lin, C., Xiao, H., Wong, M., Shang, H., ... Bian, Z. (2013). Rhein, a natural anthraquinone derivative, attenuates the activation of pancreatic stellate cells and ameliorates pancreatic fibrosis in mice with experimental chronic pancreatitis. *PLoS One*, *8*(12), e82201. doi:10.1371/journal.pone.0082201 PMID:24312641

Tsang, V. (2018). Eye-tracking study on facial emotion recognition tasks in individuals with high-functioning autism spectrum disorders. *Autism*, *22*(2), 161–170. doi:10.1177/1362361316667830 PMID:29490486

Tseng, P.-H., Cameron, I. G., Pari, G., Reynolds, J. N., Munoz, D. P., & Itti, L. (2013). High-throughput classification of clinical populations from natural viewing eye movements. *Journal of Neurology*, *260*(1), 275–284. doi:10.100700415-012-6631-2 PMID:22926163

Tyas, S. L., Salazar, J., Snowdon, D., Desrosiers, M., Riley, K., Mendiondo, M., & Kryscio, R. (2007). Transitions to Mild Cognitive Impairments, Dementia, and Death: Findings from the Nun Study. *American Journal of Epidemiology*, *165*(11), 1231–1238. doi:10.1093/aje/kwm085 PMID:17431012

Uddin, L. Q., Supekar, K., Lynch, C. J., Khouzam, A., Phillips, J., Feinstein, C., ... Menon, V. (2013). Salience network–based classification and prediction of symptom severity in children with autism. *JAMA Psychiatry, 70*(8), 869–879. doi:10.1001/jamapsychiatry.2013.104 PMID:23803651

Van Der Stigchel, S., Rommelse, N., Deijen, J., Geldof, C., Witlox, J., Oosterlaan, J., ... Theeuwes, J. (2007). Oculomotor capture in adhd. *Cognitive Neuropsychology, 24*(5), 535–549. doi:10.1080/02643290701523546 PMID:18416506

Ventura, S. P., de Barros, R. L., Sintra, T., Soares, C. M., Lima, Á. S., & Coutinho, J. A. (2012). Simple screening method to identify toxic/non-toxic ionic liquids: Agar diffusion test adaptation. *Ecotoxicology and Environmental Safety, 83*, 55–62. doi:10.1016/j.ecoenv.2012.06.002 PMID:22742861

Ventura, S. P., Marques, C. S., Rosatella, A. A., Afonso, C. A., Gonçalves, F., & Coutinho, J. A. (2012). Toxicity assessment of various ionic liquid families towards Vibrio fischeri marine bacteria. *Ecotoxicology and Environmental Safety, 76*, 162–168. doi:10.1016/j.ecoenv.2011.10.006 PMID:22019310

Ventura, S. P., Silva, F. A., Gonçalves, A. M., Pereira, J. L., Gonçalves, F., & Coutinho, J. A. (2014). Ecotoxicity analysis of cholinium-based ionic liquids to Vibrio fischeri marine bacteria. *Ecotoxicology and Environmental Safety, 102*, 48–54. doi:10.1016/j.ecoenv.2014.01.003 PMID:24580821

Vicente, K., Thornton, D., & Moray, N. (1987). Spectral-Analysis of Sinus Arrhythmia - a Measure of Mental Effort. *Human Factors, 29*(2), 171–182. doi:10.1177/001872088702900205 PMID:3610182

Vivanti, G., Fanning, P. A. J., Hocking, D. R., Sievers, S., & Dissanayake, C. (2017). Social Attention, Joint Attention and Sustained Attention in Autism Spectrum Disorder and Williams Syndrome: Convergences and Divergences. *Journal of Autism and Developmental Disorders, 47*(6), 1866–1877.

Wagner, J. B., Luyster, R. J., Tager-Flusberg, H., & Nelson, C. A. (2016). Greater Pupil Size in Response to Emotional Faces as an Early Marker of Social-Communicative Difficulties in Infants at High Risk for Autism. *Infancy, 21*(5), 560–581. doi:10.1111/infa.12128 PMID:27616938

Wang, J., Barstein, J., Ethridge, L. E., Mosconi, M. W., Takarae, Y., & Sweeney, J. A. (2013). Resting state EEG abnormalities in autism spectrum disorders. *Journal of Neurodevelopmental Disorders, 5*(1), 24.

Wang, H., Malhotra, S. V., & Francis, A. J. (2011). Toxicity of various anions associated with methoxyethyl methyl imidazolium-based ionic liquids on Clostridium sp. *Chemosphere, 82*(11), 1597–1603. doi:10.1016/j. chemosphere.2010.11.049 PMID:21159360

Wang, W., Chen, R., Luo, Z., Wang, W., & Chen, J. (2018). Antimicrobial activity and molecular docking studies of a novel anthraquinone from a marine-derived fungus Aspergillus versicolor. *Natural Product Research, 32*(5), 558–563. doi:10.1080/14786419.2017.1329732 PMID:28511613

Waoo, N., Kashyap, R., & Jaiswal, A. (2010). DNA nano array analysis using hierarchical quality threshold clustering. In *2010 2nd IEEE International Conference on Information Management and Engineering.* IEEE. 10.1109/ICIME.2010.5477579

Wasserscheid, P., & Welton, T. (2002). *Ionic Liquids in Synthesis.* Weinheim, Germany: Wiley-VCH Verlag GmbH&Co. KgaA. doi:10.1002/3527600701

Wei, S., & Kryscio, R. J. (2016). Semi-Markov Models for Interval Censored Transient Cognitive States with Back Transitions and a Competing Risk. *Statistical Methods in Medical Research, 25*(6), 2909–2924. doi:10.1177/0962280214534412 PMID:24821001

Welchew, D. E., Ashwin, C., Berkouk, K., Salvador, R., Suckling, J., Baron-Cohen, S., & Bullmore, E. (2005). Functional Disconnectivity of the medial temporal lobe in Asperger's syndrome. *Biological Psychiatry, 57*(9), 991–998. doi:10.1016/j.biopsych.2005.01.028 PMID:15860339

Wieckowski, A. T., & White, S. W. (2017). Eye-Gaze Analysis of Facial Emotion Recognition and Expression in Adolescents with ASD. *Journal of Clinical Child and Adolescent Psychology, 46*(1), 110–124. doi:10.1080/15 374416.2016.1204924 PMID:27654330

Wieder, S., & Greenspan, S. (2005). Can children with autism master the core deficits and become empathetic, creative, and reflective? *The Journal of Developmental and Learning Disorders, 9*, 1–29.

Wijesiriwardana, R., Mitcham, K., & Dias, T. (2004). *Fibre-meshed transducers based real time wearable physiological information monitoring system.* Paper presented at the International Symposium on Wearable Computers, Washington, DC. 10.1109/ISWC.2004.20

Willcutt, E. G. (2012). The prevalence of dsm-iv attention-deficit/hyperactivity disorder: A meta-analytic review. *Neurotherapeutics; the Journal of the American Society for Experimental NeuroTherapeutics*, *9*(3), 490–499. doi:10.100713311-012-0135-8 PMID:22976615

Wuthi-Udomlert, M., Prathanturarug, S., & Soonthornchareonnon, N. (2001, July). Antifungal activities of Senna alata extracts using different methods of extraction. In *International Conference on Medicinal and Aromatic Plants (Part II) 597* (pp. 205-208). Academic Press.

Wuthi-udomlert, M., Kupittayanant, P., & Gritsanapan, W. (2010). In vitro evaluation of antifungal activity of anthraquinone derivatives of Senna alata. *J Health Res*, *24*(3), 117–122.

Xie, Z. (2016). *Topics in Logistic Regression Analysis* (PhD thesis). Lexington, KY: Dept. Statistics, Univ. Kentucky.

Xu, G., Strathearn, L., Liu, B., Yang, B., & Bao, W. (2018). Twenty-year trends in diagnosed attentiondeficit/hyperactivity disorder among us children and adolescents, 1997-2016. *JAMA Network Open*, *1*(4), e181471–e181471. doi:10.1001/jamanetworkopen.2018.1471 PMID:30646132

Yamamoto, E., Yamaguchi, S., & Nagamune, T. (2011). Protein refolding by N-alkylpyridinium and N-alkyl-N-methylpyrrolidinium ionic liquids. *Applied Biochemistry and Biotechnology*, *164*(6), 957–967. doi:10.100712010-011-9187-1 PMID:21302144

Yang, K. L., Wei, M. Y., Shao, C. L., Fu, X. M., Guo, Z. Y., Xu, R. F., ... Wang, C. Y. (2012). Antibacterial anthraquinone derivatives from a sea anemone-derived fungus Nigrospora sp. *Journal of Natural Products*, *75*(5), 935–941. doi:10.1021/np300103w PMID:22545792

Yang, Z., & Pan, W. (2005). Ionic liquids: Green solvents for nonaqueous biocatalysis. *Enzyme and Microbial Technology*, *37*(1), 19–28. doi:10.1016/j.enzmictec.2005.02.014

Yan, H., Wu, J., Dai, G., Zhong, A., Chen, H., Yang, J., & Han, D. (2012). Interaction mechanisms of ionic liquids [Cnmim] Br (n=4, 6, 8, 10) with bovine serum albumin. *Journal of Luminescence*, *132*(3), 622–628. doi:10.1016/j.jlumin.2011.10.026

Yen, G. C., Duh, P. D., & Chuang, D. Y. (2000). Antioxidant activity of anthraquinones and anthrone. *Food Chemistry, 70*(4), 437–441. doi:10.1016/S0308-8146(00)00108-4

Yoder, P., Stone, W. L., Walden, T., & Malesa, E. (2009). Predicting social impairment and ASD diagnosis in younger siblings of children with autism spectrum disorder. *Journal of Autism and Developmental Disorders, 39*(10), 1381–1391. doi:10.100710803-009-0753-0 PMID:19449096

Yuan, L., Wang, Y., Thompson, P. M., Narayan, V. A., & Ye, J. (2012). Multi-source feature learning for joint analysis of incomplete multiple heterogeneous neuroimaging data. *NeuroImage, 61*(3), 622–632. doi:10.1016/j.neuroimage.2012.03.059 PMID:22498655

Yu, J., Zhang, S., Dai, Y., Lu, X., Lei, Q., & Fang, W. (2016). Antimicrobial activity and cytotoxicity of piperazinium-and guanidinium-based ionic liquids. *Journal of Hazardous Materials, 307*, 73–81. doi:10.1016/j.jhazmat.2015.12.028 PMID:26775108

Zarzeczanska, D., Niedzialkowski, P., Wcislo, A., Chomicz, L., Rak, J., & Ossowski, T. (2014). Synthesis, redox properties, and basicity of substituted 1-aminoanthraquinones: Spectroscopic, electrochemical, and computational studies in acetonitrile solutions. *Structural Chemistry, 25*(2), 625–634. doi:10.100711224-013-0332-z

Zhai, J., Barreto, A., Chin, C., & Li, C. (2005). User Stress Detection in Human-Computer Interactions. *Biomedical Sciences Instrumentation, 41*, 277–286. PMID:15850118

Zhang, J., Redman, N., Litke, A. P., Zeng, J., Zhan, J., Chan, K. Y., & Chang, C. W. T. (2011). Synthesis and antibacterial activity study of a novel class of cationic anthraquinone analogs. *Bioorganic & Medicinal Chemistry, 19*(1), 498–503. doi:10.1016/j.bmc.2010.11.001 PMID:21111625

Zhang, L., Saleh, I., Thapaliya, S., Louie, J., Figueroa-Hernandez, J., & Ji, H. (2018). An Empirical Evaluation of Machine Learning Approaches for Species Identification through Bioacoustics. *Proceedings of the 2017 International Conference on Computational Science and Computational Intelligence.*

Zhang, Q. G., Wang, N. N., & Yu, Z. W. (2010). The hydrogen bonding interactions between the ionic liquid 1-ethyl-3-methylimidazolium ethyl sulfate and water. *The Journal of Physical Chemistry B, 114*(14), 4747–4754. doi:10.1021/jp1009498 PMID:20337406

Zhang, W., Li, R., Deng, H., Wang, L., Lin, W., Ji, S., & Shen, D. (2015). Deep convolutional neural networks for multi-modality isointense infant brain image segmentation. *NeuroImage*, *108*, 214–224. doi:10.1016/j. neuroimage.2014.12.061 PMID:25562829

Zhang, W., Li, R., Zeng, T., Sun, Q., Kumar, S., Ye, J., & Ji, S. (2016). *Deep model based transfer and multi-task learning for biological image analysis. IEEE Transactions on Big Data.* doi:10.1109/TBDATA.2016.2573280

Zhang, X., Thuong, P. T., Jin, W., Su, N. D., Bae, K., & Kang, S. S. (2005). Antioxidant Activity of Anthraquinones and Flavonoids from Flower ofReynoutria sachalinensis. *Archives of Pharmacal Research*, *28*(1), 22–27. doi:10.1007/BF02975130 PMID:15742803

Zhao, H. (2010). Methods for stabilizing and activating enzymes in ionic liquids—A review. *Journal of Chemical Technology and Biotechnology (Oxford, Oxfordshire)*, *85*(7), 891–907. doi:10.1002/jctb.2375

Zhao, H., Olubajo, O., Song, Z., Sims, A. L., Person, T. E., Lawal, R. A., & Holley, L. A. (2006). Effect of kosmotropicity of ionic liquids on the enzyme stability in aqueous solutions. *Bioorganic Chemistry*, *34*(1), 15–25. doi:10.1016/j.bioorg.2005.10.004 PMID:16325223

Zheng, Y., Zhu, L., Fan, L., Zhao, W., Wang, J., Hao, X., ... Wang, W. (2017). Synthesis, SAR and pharmacological characterization of novel anthraquinone cation compounds as potential anticancer agents. *European Journal of Medicinal Chemistry*, *125*, 902–913. doi:10.1016/j.ejmech.2016.10.012 PMID:27769031

Zhu, H., Lee, Y., & Rosenthal, A. (2016). Data Standards Challenges for Interoperable and Quality Data. *Journal Of Data And Information Quality*, *7*(1-2), 1–3. doi:10.1145/2903723

Zorn, D. D., Boatz, J. A., & Gordon, M. S. (2006). Electronic structure studies of tetrazolium-based ionic liquids. *The Journal of Physical Chemistry B*, *110*(23), 11110–11119. doi:10.1021/jp060854r PMID:16771373

Related References

To continue our tradition of advancing information science and technology research, we have compiled a list of recommended IGI Global readings. These references will provide additional information and guidance to further enrich your knowledge and assist you with your own research and future publications.

Abu Seman, S. A., & Ramayah, T. (2017). Are We Ready to App?: A Study on mHealth Apps, Its Future, and Trends in Malaysia Context. In J. Pelet (Ed.), *Mobile Platforms, Design, and Apps for Social Commerce* (pp. 69–83). Hershey, PA: IGI Global. doi:10.4018/978-1-5225-2469-4.ch005

Aggarwal, S., & Azad, V. (2017). A Hybrid System Based on FMM and MLP to Diagnose Heart Disease. In S. Bhattacharyya, S. De, I. Pan, & P. Dutta (Eds.), *Intelligent Multidimensional Data Clustering and Analysis* (pp. 293–325). Hershey, PA: IGI Global. doi:10.4018/978-1-5225-1776-4.ch011

Akaichi, J., & Mhadhbi, L. (2016). A Clinical Decision Support System: Ontology-Driven Approach for Effective Emergency Management. In J. Moon & M. Galea (Eds.), *Improving Health Management through Clinical Decision Support Systems* (pp. 270–294). Hershey, PA: IGI Global. doi:10.4018/978-1-4666-9432-3.ch013

Akerkar, R. (2016). Towards an Intelligent Integrated Approach for Clinical Decision Support. In A. Aggarwal (Ed.), *Managing Big Data Integration in the Public Sector* (pp. 187–205). Hershey, PA: IGI Global. doi:10.4018/978-1-4666-9649-5.ch011

Al-Busaidi, S. S. (2018). Interdisciplinary Relationships Between Medicine and Social Sciences. In M. Al-Suqri, A. Al-Kindi, S. AlKindi, & N. Saleem (Eds.), *Promoting Interdisciplinarity in Knowledge Generation and Problem Solving* (pp. 124–137). Hershey, PA: IGI Global. doi:10.4018/978-1-5225-3878-3.ch009

Al Kareh, T., & Thoumy, M. (2018). The Impact of Health Information Digitization on the Physiotherapist-Patient Relationship: A Pilot Study of the Lebanese Community. *International Journal of Healthcare Information Systems and Informatics*, *13*(2), 29–53. doi:10.4018/IJHISI.2018040103

Alenzuela, R. (2017). Research, Leadership, and Resource-Sharing Initiatives: The Role of Local Library Consortia in Access to Medical Information. In S. Ram (Ed.), *Library and Information Services for Bioinformatics Education and Research* (pp. 199–211). Hershey, PA: IGI Global. doi:10.4018/978-1-5225-1871-6.ch012

Ameri, H., Alizadeh, S., & Noughabi, E. A. (2017). Application of Data Mining Techniques in Clinical Decision Making: A Literature Review and Classification. In E. Noughabi, B. Raahemi, A. Albadvi, & B. Far (Eds.), *Handbook of Research on Data Science for Effective Healthcare Practice and Administration* (pp. 257–295). Hershey, PA: IGI Global. doi:10.4018/978-1-5225-2515-8.ch012

Anand, S. (2017). Medical Image Enhancement Using Edge Information-Based Methods. In B. Singh (Ed.), *Computational Tools and Techniques for Biomedical Signal Processing* (pp. 123–148). Hershey, PA: IGI Global. doi:10.4018/978-1-5225-0660-7.ch006

Angjellari-Dajci, F., Sapienza, C., Lawless, W. F., & Kavanagh, K. (2016). Human Capital Accumulation in Medical Simulated Learning Environments: A Framework for Economic Evaluation. In M. Russ (Ed.), *Quantitative Multidisciplinary Approaches in Human Capital and Asset Management* (pp. 65–88). Hershey, PA: IGI Global. doi:10.4018/978-1-4666-9652-5.ch004

Anil, M., Ayyildiz-Tamis, D., Tasdemir, S., Sendemir-Urkmez, A., & Gulce-Iz, S. (2016). Bioinspired Materials and Biocompatibility. In M. Bououdina (Ed.), *Emerging Research on Bioinspired Materials Engineering* (pp. 294–322). Hershey, PA: IGI Global. doi:10.4018/978-1-4666-9811-6.ch011

Anton, J. L., Soriano, J. V., Martinez, M. I., & Garcia, F. B. (2018). Comprehensive E-Learning Appraisal System. In M. Khosrow-Pour, D.B.A. (Ed.), Encyclopedia of Information Science and Technology, Fourth Edition (pp. 5787-5799). Hershey, PA: IGI Global. doi:10.4018/978-1-5225-2255-3.ch503

Arabi, M. (2016). Redesigning the Organizational Structure to Reach Efficiency: The Case of Ministry of Health and Medical Education of Iran. In R. Gholipour & K. Rouzbehani (Eds.), *Social, Economic, and Political Perspectives on Public Health Policy-Making* (pp. 257–294). Hershey, PA: IGI Global. doi:10.4018/978-1-4666-9944-1.ch012

Assis-Hassid, S., Heart, T., Reychav, I., & Pliskin, J. S. (2016). Modelling Factors Affecting Patient-Doctor-Computer Communication in Primary Care. *International Journal of Reliable and Quality E-Healthcare*, 5(1), 1–17. doi:10.4018/IJRQEH.2016010101

Atzori, B., Hoffman, H. G., Vagnoli, L., Messeri, A., & Grotto, R. L. (2018). Virtual Reality as Distraction Technique for Pain Management in Children and Adolescents. In M. Khosrow-Pour, D.B.A. (Ed.), Encyclopedia of Information Science and Technology, Fourth Edition (pp. 5955-5965). Hershey, PA: IGI Global. doi:10.4018/978-1-5225-2255-3.ch518

Audibert, M., Mathonnat, J., Pélissier, A., & Huang, X. X. (2018). The Impact of the New Rural Cooperative Medical Scheme on Township Hospitals' Utilization and Income Structure in Weifang Prefecture, China. In I. Management Association (Ed.), Health Economics and Healthcare Reform: Breakthroughs in Research and Practice (pp. 109-121). Hershey, PA: IGI Global. doi:10.4018/978-1-5225-3168-5.ch007

Ayyachamy, S. (2016). Analysis and Comparison of Developed 2D Medical Image Database Design using Registration Scheme, Retrieval Scheme, and Bag-of-Visual-Words. In N. Dey & A. Ashour (Eds.), *Classification and Clustering in Biomedical Signal Processing* (pp. 149–168). Hershey, PA: IGI Global. doi:10.4018/978-1-5225-0140-4.ch007

Babalola, A. C. (2016). Literacy and Decision Making on Health Issues among Married Women in Southwest Nigeria. In V. Wang (Ed.), *Handbook of Research on Advancing Health Education through Technology* (pp. 191–212). Hershey, PA: IGI Global. doi:10.4018/978-1-4666-9494-1.ch009

Babu, A., & Ayyappan, S. (2017). A Methodological Evaluation of Crypto-Watermarking System for Medical Images. In C. Bhatt & S. Peddoju (Eds.), *Cloud Computing Systems and Applications in Healthcare* (pp. 189–217). Hershey, PA: IGI Global. doi:10.4018/978-1-5225-1002-4.ch010

Bakke, A. (2017). Ethos in E-Health: From Informational to Interactive Websites. In M. Folk & S. Apostel (Eds.), *Establishing and Evaluating Digital Ethos and Online Credibility* (pp. 85–103). Hershey, PA: IGI Global. doi:10.4018/978-1-5225-1072-7.ch005

Bali, S. (2018). Enhancing the Reach of Health Care Through Telemedicine: Status and New Possibilities in Developing Countries. In U. Pandey & V. Indrakanti (Eds.), *Open and Distance Learning Initiatives for Sustainable Development* (pp. 339–354). Hershey, PA: IGI Global. doi:10.4018/978-1-5225-2621-6.ch019

Barrett, T. E. (2018). Essentials for Education and Training for Tomorrow's Physicians. In C. Smith (Ed.), *Exploring the Pressures of Medical Education From a Mental Health and Wellness Perspective* (pp. 230–252). Hershey, PA: IGI Global. doi:10.4018/978-1-5225-2811-1.ch010

Barrett, T. J. (2016). Knowledge in Action: Fostering Health Education through Technology. In V. Wang (Ed.), *Handbook of Research on Advancing Health Education through Technology* (pp. 39–62). Hershey, PA: IGI Global. doi:10.4018/978-1-4666-9494-1.ch003

Berrahal, S., & Boudriga, N. (2017). The Risks of Wearable Technologies to Individuals and Organizations. In A. Marrington, D. Kerr, & J. Gammack (Eds.), *Managing Security Issues and the Hidden Dangers of Wearable Technologies* (pp. 18–46). Hershey, PA: IGI Global. doi:10.4018/978-1-5225-1016-1.ch002

Bhagat, A. P., & Atique, M. (2016). Medical Image Mining Using Fuzzy Connectedness Image Segmentation: Efficient Retrieval of Patients' Stored Images. In W. Karâa & N. Dey (Eds.), *Biomedical Image Analysis and Mining Techniques for Improved Health Outcomes* (pp. 184–209). Hershey, PA: IGI Global. doi:10.4018/978-1-4666-8811-7.ch009

Bhargava, P. (2018). Blended Learning: An Effective Application to Clinical Teaching. In S. Tang & C. Lim (Eds.), *Preparing the Next Generation of Teachers for 21st Century Education* (pp. 302–320). Hershey, PA: IGI Global. doi:10.4018/978-1-5225-4080-9.ch018

Binh, N. T., & Tuyet, V. T. (2016). The Combination of Adaptive Filters to Improve the Quality of Medical Images in New Wavelet Domain. In N. Dey & A. Ashour (Eds.), *Classification and Clustering in Biomedical Signal Processing* (pp. 46–76). Hershey, PA: IGI Global. doi:10.4018/978-1-5225-0140-4.ch003

Bird, J. L. (2017). Writing Healing Narratives. In V. Bryan & J. Bird (Eds.), *Healthcare Community Synergism between Patients, Practitioners, and Researchers* (pp. 1–28). Hershey, PA: IGI Global. doi:10.4018/978-1-5225-0640-9.ch001

Bottrighi, A., Leonardi, G., Piovesan, L., & Terenziani, P. (2016). Knowledge-Based Support to the Treatment of Exceptions in Computer Interpretable Clinical Guidelines. *International Journal of Knowledge-Based Organizations*, 6(3), 1–27. doi:10.4018/IJKBO.2016070101

Bougoulias, K., Kouris, I., Prasinos, M., Giokas, K., & Koutsouris, D. (2017). Ob/Gyn EMR Software: A Solution for Obstetricians and Gynecologists. In A. Moumtzoglou (Ed.), *Design, Development, and Integration of Reliable Electronic Healthcare Platforms* (pp. 101–111). Hershey, PA: IGI Global. doi:10.4018/978-1-5225-1724-5.ch006

Bouslimi, R., Ayadi, M. G., & Akaichi, J. (2018). Medical Image Retrieval in Healthcare Social Networks. *International Journal of Healthcare Information Systems and Informatics*, 13(2), 13–28. doi:10.4018/IJHISI.2018040102

Bouzaabia, O., Bouzaabia, R., & Mejri, K. (2017). Role of Internet in the Development of Medical Tourism Service in Tunisia. In A. Capatina & E. Rancati (Eds.), *Key Challenges and Opportunities in Web Entrepreneurship* (pp. 211–241). Hershey, PA: IGI Global. doi:10.4018/978-1-5225-2466-3.ch009

Briz-Ponce, L., Juanes-Méndez, J. A., & García-Peñalvo, F. J. (2016). The Role of Gender in Technology Acceptance for Medical Education. In M. Cruz-Cunha, I. Miranda, R. Martinho, & R. Rijo (Eds.), *Encyclopedia of E-Health and Telemedicine* (pp. 1013–1027). Hershey, PA: IGI Global. doi:10.4018/978-1-4666-9978-6.ch079

Briz-Ponce, L., Juanes-Méndez, J. A., & García-Peñalvo, F. J. (2016). A Research Contribution to the Analysis of Mobile Devices in Higher Education from Medical Students' Point of View. In L. Briz-Ponce, J. Juanes-Méndez, & F. García-Peñalvo (Eds.), *Handbook of Research on Mobile Devices and Applications in Higher Education Settings* (pp. 196–221). Hershey, PA: IGI Global. doi:10.4018/978-1-5225-0256-2.ch009

Brown-Jackson, K. L. (2018). Telemedicine and Telehealth: Academics Engaging the Community in a Call to Action. In S. Burton (Ed.), *Engaged Scholarship and Civic Responsibility in Higher Education* (pp. 166–193). Hershey, PA: IGI Global. doi:10.4018/978-1-5225-3649-9.ch008

Bwalya, K. J. (2017). Next Wave of Tele-Medicine: Virtual Presence of Medical Personnel. In K. Moahi, K. Bwalya, & P. Sebina (Eds.), *Health Information Systems and the Advancement of Medical Practice in Developing Countries* (pp. 168–180). Hershey, PA: IGI Global. doi:10.4018/978-1-5225-2262-1.ch010

Carlton, E. L., Holsinger, J. W. Jr, & Anunobi, N. (2016). Physician Engagement with Health Information Technology: Implications for Practice and Professionalism. *International Journal of Computers in Clinical Practice*, *1*(2), 51–73. doi:10.4018/IJCCP.2016070103

Castillo-Page, L., Eliason, J., Conrad, S. S., & Nivet, M. A. (2016). Diversity in Undergraduate Medical Education: An Examination of Organizational Culture and Climate in Medical Schools. In C. Scott & J. Sims (Eds.), *Developing Workforce Diversity Programs, Curriculum, and Degrees in Higher Education* (pp. 304–326). Hershey, PA: IGI Global. doi:10.4018/978-1-5225-0209-8.ch016

Cebeci, H. I., & Hiziroglu, A. (2016). Review of Business Intelligence and Intelligent Systems in Healthcare Domain. In N. Celebi (Ed.), *Intelligent Techniques for Data Analysis in Diverse Settings* (pp. 192–206). Hershey, PA: IGI Global. doi:10.4018/978-1-5225-0075-9.ch009

Celik, G. (2018). Determining Headache Diseases With Genetic Algorithm. In U. Kose, G. Guraksin, & O. Deperlioglu (Eds.), *Nature-Inspired Intelligent Techniques for Solving Biomedical Engineering Problems* (pp. 249–262). Hershey, PA: IGI Global. doi:10.4018/978-1-5225-4769-3.ch012

Chakraborty, C., Gupta, B., & Ghosh, S. K. (2016). Mobile Telemedicine Systems for Remote Patient's Chronic Wound Monitoring. In A. Moumtzoglou (Ed.), *M-Health Innovations for Patient-Centered Care* (pp. 213–239). Hershey, PA: IGI Global. doi:10.4018/978-1-4666-9861-1.ch011

Chakraborty, S., Chatterjee, S., Ashour, A. S., Mali, K., & Dey, N. (2018). Intelligent Computing in Medical Imaging: A Study. In N. Dey (Ed.), *Advancements in Applied Metaheuristic Computing* (pp. 143–163). Hershey, PA: IGI Global. doi:10.4018/978-1-5225-4151-6.ch006

Chavez, A., & Kovarik, C. (2017). Open Source Technology for Medical Practice in Developing Countries. In K. Moahi, K. Bwalya, & P. Sebina (Eds.), *Health Information Systems and the Advancement of Medical Practice in Developing Countries* (pp. 33–59). Hershey, PA: IGI Global. doi:10.4018/978-1-5225-2262-1.ch003

Chen, E. T. (2016). Examining the Influence of Information Technology on Modern Health Care. In P. Manolitzas, E. Grigoroudis, N. Matsatsinis, & D. Yannacopoulos (Eds.), *Effective Methods for Modern Healthcare Service Quality and Evaluation* (pp. 110–136). Hershey, PA: IGI Global. doi:10.4018/978-1-4666-9961-8.ch006

Chin, S. (2016). Surviving Sandy: Recovering Collections after a Natural Disaster. In E. Decker & J. Townes (Eds.), *Handbook of Research on Disaster Management and Contingency Planning in Modern Libraries* (pp. 366–388). Hershey, PA: IGI Global. doi:10.4018/978-1-4666-8624-3.ch016

Chojnacki, M., & Wójcik, A. (2016). Security and the Role of New Technologies and Innovation in Medical Ethics. In A. Rosiek & K. Leksowski (Eds.), *Organizational Culture and Ethics in Modern Medicine* (pp. 52–77). Hershey, PA: IGI Global. doi:10.4018/978-1-4666-9658-7.ch003

Cılız, N., Yıldırım, H., & Temizel, Ş. (2016). Structure Development for Effective Medical Waste and Hazardous Waste Management System. In U. Akkucuk (Ed.), *Handbook of Research on Waste Management Techniques for Sustainability* (pp. 303–327). Hershey, PA: IGI Global. doi:10.4018/978-1-4666-9723-2.ch016

Ciufudean, C. (2018). Innovative Formalism for Biological Data Analysis. In M. Khosrow-Pour, D.B.A. (Ed.), Encyclopedia of Information Science and Technology, Fourth Edition (pp. 1814-1824). Hershey, PA: IGI Global. doi:10.4018/978-1-5225-2255-3.ch158

Ciufudean, C., & Ciufudean, O. (2016). Tele-Monitoring for Medical Diagnosis Availability. In M. Cruz-Cunha, I. Miranda, R. Martinho, & R. Rijo (Eds.), *Encyclopedia of E-Health and Telemedicine* (pp. 401–411). Hershey, PA: IGI Global. doi:10.4018/978-1-4666-9978-6.ch032

Colaguori, R., & Danesi, M. (2017). Medical Semiotics: A Revisitation and an Exhortation. *International Journal of Semiotics and Visual Rhetoric, 1*(1), 11–18. doi:10.4018/IJSVR.2017010102

Cole, A. W., & Salek, T. A. (2017). Adopting a Parasocial Connection to Overcome Professional Kakoethos in Online Health Information. In M. Folk & S. Apostel (Eds.), *Establishing and Evaluating Digital Ethos and Online Credibility* (pp. 104–120). Hershey, PA: IGI Global. doi:10.4018/978-1-5225-1072-7.ch006

Contreras, E. C., & Puente, G. J. (2016). How to Identify Rheumatic Diseases by General Physicians. In T. Gasmelseid (Ed.), *Advancing Pharmaceutical Processes and Tools for Improved Health Outcomes* (pp. 136–166). Hershey, PA: IGI Global. doi:10.4018/978-1-5225-0248-7.ch006

D'Andrea, A., Ferri, F., & Grifoni, P. (2016). RFID Technologies in Healthcare Setting: Applications and Future Perspectives. *International Journal of Computers in Clinical Practice, 1*(1), 15–27. doi:10.4018/IJCCP.2016010102

Damianakis, A., Kallonis, P., Loudos, G., Tsatsos, D., & Tsoukalis, A. (2016). Exploiting 3D Medical Equipment Simulations to Support Biomedical Engineering Academic Courses: Design Methodology and Implementation in a Small Scale National Project. In B. Khan (Ed.), *Revolutionizing Modern Education through Meaningful E-Learning Implementation* (pp. 277–295). Hershey, PA: IGI Global. doi:10.4018/978-1-5225-0466-5.ch015

Demiroz, E. (2016). Principles of Instructional Design for E-Learning and Online Learning Practices: Implications for Medical Education. In V. Wang (Ed.), *Handbook of Research on Advancing Health Education through Technology* (pp. 419–451). Hershey, PA: IGI Global. doi:10.4018/978-1-4666-9494-1.ch018

Deperlioglu, O. (2018). Intelligent Techniques Inspired by Nature and Used in Biomedical Engineering. In U. Kose, G. Guraksin, & O. Deperlioglu (Eds.), *Nature-Inspired Intelligent Techniques for Solving Biomedical Engineering Problems* (pp. 51–77). Hershey, PA: IGI Global. doi:10.4018/978-1-5225-4769-3.ch003

Dey, N., & Ashour, A. S. (2018). Meta-Heuristic Algorithms in Medical Image Segmentation: A Review. In N. Dey (Ed.), *Advancements in Applied Metaheuristic Computing* (pp. 185–203). Hershey, PA: IGI Global. doi:10.4018/978-1-5225-4151-6.ch008

Dey, N., Ashour, A. S., & Althoupety, A. S. (2017). Thermal Imaging in Medical Science. In V. Santhi (Ed.), *Recent Advances in Applied Thermal Imaging for Industrial Applications* (pp. 87–117). Hershey, PA: IGI Global. doi:10.4018/978-1-5225-2423-6.ch004

Di Virgilio, F., Camillo, A. A., & Camillo, I. C. (2017). The Impact of Social Network on Italian Users' Behavioural Intention for the Choice of a Medical Tourist Destination. *International Journal of Tourism and Hospitality Management in the Digital Age, 1*(1), 36–49. doi:10.4018/IJTHMDA.2017010103

Dias, C. M., Ribeiro, A. G., & Furtado, S. F. (2016). An Overview about the Use of Healthcare Applications on Mobile Devices. In M. Cruz-Cunha, I. Miranda, R. Martinho, & R. Rijo (Eds.), *Encyclopedia of E-Health and Telemedicine* (pp. 285–298). Hershey, PA: IGI Global. doi:10.4018/978-1-4666-9978-6.ch024

Dogra, A. K., & Dogra, P. (2017). The Medical Tourism Industry in the BRIC Nations: An Indian Analysis. In M. Dhiman (Ed.), *Opportunities and Challenges for Tourism and Hospitality in the BRIC Nations* (pp. 320–336). Hershey, PA: IGI Global. doi:10.4018/978-1-5225-0708-6.ch020

Drowos, J. L., & Wood, S. K. (2017). Preparing Future Physicians to Adapt to the Changing Health Care System: Promoting Humanism through Curricular Design. In V. Bryan & J. Bird (Eds.), *Healthcare Community Synergism between Patients, Practitioners, and Researchers* (pp. 106–125). Hershey, PA: IGI Global. doi:10.4018/978-1-5225-0640-9.ch006

Dulam, K. (2017). Medical Patents and Impact on Availability and Affordability of Essential Medicines in India. In R. Aggarwal & R. Kaur (Eds.), *Patent Law and Intellectual Property in the Medical Field* (pp. 41–57). Hershey, PA: IGI Global. doi:10.4018/978-1-5225-2414-4.ch003

Dutta, P. (2017). Decision Making in Medical Diagnosis via Distance Measures on Interval Valued Fuzzy Sets. *International Journal of System Dynamics Applications, 6*(4), 63–83. doi:10.4018/IJSDA.2017100104

318

Edoh, T. O., Pawar, P. A., Brügge, B., & Teege, G. (2016). A Multidisciplinary Remote Healthcare Delivery System to Increase Health Care Access, Pathology Screening, and Treatment in Developing Countries: The Case of Benin. *International Journal of Healthcare Information Systems and Informatics*, *11*(4), 1–31. doi:10.4018/IJHISI.2016100101

El Guemhioui, K., & Demurjian, S. A. (2017). Semantic Reconciliation of Electronic Health Records Using Semantic Web Technologies. *International Journal of Information Technology and Web Engineering*, *12*(2), 26–48. doi:10.4018/IJITWE.2017040102

Ellouze, N., Rekhis, S., & Boudriga, N. (2016). Forensic Investigation of Digital Crimes in Healthcare Applications. In O. Isafiade & A. Bagula (Eds.), *Data Mining Trends and Applications in Criminal Science and Investigations* (pp. 169–210). Hershey, PA: IGI Global. doi:10.4018/978-1-5225-0463-4.ch007

Eneanya, A. N. (2016). Health Policy Implementation and Its Barriers: The Case Study of US Health System. In R. Gholipour & K. Rouzbehani (Eds.), *Social, Economic, and Political Perspectives on Public Health Policy-Making* (pp. 42–63). Hershey, PA: IGI Global. doi:10.4018/978-1-4666-9944-1.ch003

Entico, G. J. (2016). Knowledge Management and the Medical Health Librarians: A Perception Study. In J. Yap, M. Perez, M. Ayson, & G. Entico (Eds.), *Special Library Administration, Standardization and Technological Integration* (pp. 52–77). Hershey, PA: IGI Global. doi:10.4018/978-1-4666-9542-9.ch003

Ferradji, M. A., & Zidani, A. (2016). Collaborative Environment for Remote Clinical Reasoning Learning. *International Journal of E-Health and Medical Communications*, *7*(4), 62–81. doi:10.4018/IJEHMC.2016100104

Fisher, J. (2018). Sociological Perspectives on Improving Medical Diagnosis Emphasizing CAD. In M. Khosrow-Pour, D.B.A. (Ed.), Encyclopedia of Information Science and Technology, Fourth Edition (pp. 1017-1024). Hershey, PA: IGI Global. doi:10.4018/978-1-5225-2255-3.ch088

Flores, C. D., Respício, A., Coelho, H., Bez, M. R., & Fonseca, J. M. (2016). Simulation for Medical Training. In M. Cruz-Cunha, I. Miranda, R. Martinho, & R. Rijo (Eds.), *Encyclopedia of E-Health and Telemedicine* (pp. 827–842). Hershey, PA: IGI Global. doi:10.4018/978-1-4666-9978-6.ch064

Frank, E. M. (2018). Healthcare Education: Integrating Simulation Technologies. In V. Bryan, A. Musgrove, & J. Powers (Eds.), *Handbook of Research on Human Development in the Digital Age* (pp. 163–182). Hershey, PA: IGI Global. doi:10.4018/978-1-5225-2838-8.ch008

Garner, G. (2018). Foundations for Yoga Practice in Rehabilitation. In S. Telles & N. Singh (Eds.), *Research-Based Perspectives on the Psychophysiology of Yoga* (pp. 263–307). Hershey, PA: IGI Global. doi:10.4018/978-1-5225-2788-6.ch015

Gasmelseid, T. M. (2016). Improving Pharmaceutical Care through the Use of Intelligent Pharmacoinformatics. In T. Gasmelseid (Ed.), *Advancing Pharmaceutical Processes and Tools for Improved Health Outcomes* (pp. 167–188). Hershey, PA: IGI Global. doi:10.4018/978-1-5225-0248-7.ch007

Gavurová, B., Kováč, V., & Šoltés, M. (2018). Medical Equipment and Economic Determinants of Its Structure and Regulation in the Slovak Republic. In M. Khosrow-Pour, D.B.A. (Ed.), Encyclopedia of Information Science and Technology, Fourth Edition (pp. 5841-5852). Hershey, PA: IGI Global. doi:10.4018/978-1-5225-2255-3.ch508

Ge, X., Wang, Q., Huang, K., Law, V., & Thomas, D. C. (2017). Designing Simulated Learning Environments and Facilitating Authentic Learning Experiences in Medical Education. In J. Stefaniak (Ed.), *Advancing Medical Education Through Strategic Instructional Design* (pp. 77–100). Hershey, PA: IGI Global. doi:10.4018/978-1-5225-2098-6.ch004

Gewald, H., & Gewald, C. (2018). Inhibitors of Physicians' Use of Mandatory Hospital Information Systems (HIS). *International Journal of Healthcare Information Systems and Informatics, 13*(1), 29–44. doi:10.4018/IJHISI.2018010103

Ghosh, D., & Dinda, S. (2017). Health Infrastructure and Economic Development in India. In R. Das (Ed.), *Social, Health, and Environmental Infrastructures for Economic Growth* (pp. 99–119). Hershey, PA: IGI Global. doi:10.4018/978-1-5225-2364-2.ch006

Ghosh, K., & Sen, K. C. (2017). The Potential of Crowdsourcing in the Health Care Industry. In N. Wickramasinghe (Ed.), *Handbook of Research on Healthcare Administration and Management* (pp. 418–427). Hershey, PA: IGI Global. doi:10.4018/978-1-5225-0920-2.ch024

Ghrab, S., & Saad, I. (2016). Identifying Crucial Know-How and Knowing-That for Medical Decision Support. *International Journal of Decision Support System Technology*, 8(4), 14–33. doi:10.4018/IJDSST.2016100102

Giokas, K., Tsirmpas, C., Anastasiou, A., Iliopoulou, D., Costarides, V., & Koutsouris, D. (2016). Contemporary Heart Failure Treatment Based on Improved Knowledge and Personalized Care of Comorbidities. In D. Fotiadis (Ed.), *Handbook of Research on Trends in the Diagnosis and Treatment of Chronic Conditions* (pp. 301–314). Hershey, PA: IGI Global. doi:10.4018/978-1-4666-8828-5.ch014

Gopalan, V., Chan, E., & Ho, D. T. (2018). Deliberate Self-Harm and Suicide Ideology in Medical Students. In C. Smith (Ed.), *Exploring the Pressures of Medical Education From a Mental Health and Wellness Perspective* (pp. 122–143). Hershey, PA: IGI Global. doi:10.4018/978-1-5225-2811-1.ch005

Goswami, S., Dey, U., Roy, P., Ashour, A., & Dey, N. (2017). Medical Video Processing: Concept and Applications. In N. Dey, A. Ashour, & P. Patra (Eds.), *Feature Detectors and Motion Detection in Video Processing* (pp. 1–17). Hershey, PA: IGI Global. doi:10.4018/978-1-5225-1025-3.ch001

Goswami, S., Mahanta, K., Goswami, S., Jigdung, T., & Devi, T. P. (2018). Ageing and Cancer: The Epigenetic Basis, Alternative Treatment, and Care. In B. Prasad & S. Akbar (Eds.), *Handbook of Research on Geriatric Health, Treatment, and Care* (pp. 206–235). Hershey, PA: IGI Global. doi:10.4018/978-1-5225-3480-8.ch012

Gouva, M. I. (2017). The Psychological Impact of Medical Error on Patients, Family Members, and Health Professionals. In M. Riga (Ed.), *Impact of Medical Errors and Malpractice on Health Economics, Quality, and Patient Safety* (pp. 171–196). Hershey, PA: IGI Global. doi:10.4018/978-1-5225-2337-6.ch007

Gürcü, M., & Tengilimoğlu, D. (2017). Health Tourism-Based Destination Marketing. In A. Bayraktar & C. Uslay (Eds.), *Strategic Place Branding Methodologies and Theory for Tourist Attraction* (pp. 308–331). Hershey, PA: IGI Global. doi:10.4018/978-1-5225-0579-2.ch015

Gürsel, G. (2016). Mobility in Healthcare: M-Health. In A. Panagopoulos (Ed.), *Handbook of Research on Next Generation Mobile Communication Systems* (pp. 485–511). Hershey, PA: IGI Global. doi:10.4018/978-1-4666-8732-5.ch019

Gürsel, G. (2017). For Better Healthcare Mining Health Data. In S. Bhattacharyya, S. De, I. Pan, & P. Dutta (Eds.), *Intelligent Multidimensional Data Clustering and Analysis* (pp. 135–158). Hershey, PA: IGI Global. doi:10.4018/978-1-5225-1776-4.ch006

Guzman-Lugo, G., Lopez-Martinez, M., Lopez-Ramirez, B., & Avila-Vazquez, D. (2016). City-Driven Approach to Determine Health Services Based on Current User Location and Collaborative Information. *International Journal of Knowledge Society Research, 7*(1), 53–62. doi:10.4018/IJKSR.2016010104

Gyaase, P. O., Darko-Lartey, R., William, H., & Borkloe, F. (2017). Towards an Integrated Electronic Medical Records System for Quality Healthcare in Ghana: An Exploratory Factor Analysis. *International Journal of Computers in Clinical Practice, 2*(2), 38–55. doi:10.4018/IJCCP.2017070103

Handayani, P. W., Sandhyaduhita, P. I., Hidayanto, A. N., Pinem, A. A., Fajrina, H. R., Junus, K. M., ... Ayuningtyas, D. (2016). Integrated Hospital Information System Architecture Design in Indonesia. In T. Iyamu & A. Tatnall (Eds.), *Maximizing Healthcare Delivery and Management through Technology Integration* (pp. 207–236). Hershey, PA: IGI Global. doi:10.4018/978-1-4666-9446-0.ch013

Hanel, P. (2017). Is China Catching Up?: Health-Related Applications of Biotechnology. In T. Bas & J. Zhao (Eds.), *Comparative Approaches to Biotechnology Development and Use in Developed and Emerging Nations* (pp. 465–520). Hershey, PA: IGI Global. doi:10.4018/978-1-5225-1040-6.ch016

Harmsen, C. A., & Royle, R. N. (2016). St. Stephen's Hospital Hervey Bay: Study of Developing a Digital Hospital. In J. Moon & M. Galea (Eds.), *Improving Health Management through Clinical Decision Support Systems* (pp. 127–153). Hershey, PA: IGI Global. doi:10.4018/978-1-4666-9432-3.ch006

Harp, D., Shim, R. S., Johnson, J., Harp, J. A., Wilcox, W. C., & Wilcox, J. K. (2016). Race and Gender Inequalities in Medicine and Biomedical Research. In U. Thomas & J. Drake (Eds.), *Critical Research on Sexism and Racism in STEM Fields* (pp. 115–134). Hershey, PA: IGI Global. doi:10.4018/978-1-5225-0174-9.ch006

Hartman, A., & Brown, S. (2017). Synergism through Therapeutic Visual Arts. In V. Bryan & J. Bird (Eds.), *Healthcare Community Synergism between Patients, Practitioners, and Researchers* (pp. 29–48). Hershey, PA: IGI Global. doi:10.4018/978-1-5225-0640-9.ch002

Hazra, J., Chowdhury, A. R., & Dutta, P. (2016). Cluster Based Medical Image Registration Using Optimized Neural Network. In S. Bhattacharyya, P. Banerjee, D. Majumdar, & P. Dutta (Eds.), *Handbook of Research on Advanced Hybrid Intelligent Techniques and Applications* (pp. 551–581). Hershey, PA: IGI Global. doi:10.4018/978-1-4666-9474-3.ch018

Hung, S., Huang, W., Yen, D. C., Chang, S., & Lu, C. (2016). Effect of Information Service Competence and Contextual Factors on the Effectiveness of Strategic Information Systems Planning in Hospitals. *Journal of Global Information Management, 24*(1), 14–36. doi:10.4018/JGIM.2016010102

Iltchev, P., Śliwczyński, A., Szynkiewicz, P., & Marczak, M. (2016). Mobile Health Applications Assisting Patients with Chronic Diseases: Examples from Asthma Care. In A. Moumtzoglou (Ed.), *M-Health Innovations for Patient-Centered Care* (pp. 170–196). Hershey, PA: IGI Global. doi:10.4018/978-1-4666-9861-1.ch009

Iqbal, S., Ahmad, S., & Willis, I. (2017). Influencing Factors for Adopting Technology Enhanced Learning in the Medical Schools of Punjab, Pakistan. *International Journal of Information and Communication Technology Education, 13*(3), 27–39. doi:10.4018/IJICTE.2017070103

Jagan, J., Dalkiliç, Y., & Samui, P. (2016). Utilization of SVM, LSSVM and GP for Predicting the Medical Waste Generation. In G. Hua (Ed.), *Smart Cities as a Solution for Reducing Urban Waste and Pollution* (pp. 224–251). Hershey, PA: IGI Global. doi:10.4018/978-1-5225-0302-6.ch008

Jagiello, K., Sosnowska, A., Mikolajczyk, A., & Puzyn, T. (2017). Nanomaterials in Medical Devices: Regulations' Review and Future Perspectives. *Journal of Nanotoxicology and Nanomedicine, 2*(2), 1–11. doi:10.4018/JNN.2017070101

Jena, T. K. (2018). Skill Training Process in Medicine Through Distance Mode. In U. Pandey & V. Indrakanti (Eds.), *Optimizing Open and Distance Learning in Higher Education Institutions* (pp. 228–243). Hershey, PA: IGI Global. doi:10.4018/978-1-5225-2624-7.ch010

Jesus, Â., & Gomes, M. J. (2016). Web 2.0 Tools in Biomedical and Pharmaceutical Education: Updated Review and Commentary. In T. Gasmelseid (Ed.), *Advancing Pharmaceutical Processes and Tools for Improved Health Outcomes* (pp. 52–78). Hershey, PA: IGI Global. doi:10.4018/978-1-5225-0248-7.ch003

Joseph, V., & Miller, J. M. (2018). Medical Students' Perceived Stigma in Seeking Care: A Cultural Perspective. In C. Smith (Ed.), *Exploring the Pressures of Medical Education From a Mental Health and Wellness Perspective* (pp. 44–67). Hershey, PA: IGI Global. doi:10.4018/978-1-5225-2811-1.ch002

Joyce, B. L., & Swanberg, S. M. (2017). Using Backward Design for Competency-Based Undergraduate Medical Education. In J. Stefaniak (Ed.), *Advancing Medical Education Through Strategic Instructional Design* (pp. 53–76). Hershey, PA: IGI Global. doi:10.4018/978-1-5225-2098-6.ch003

Kaljo, K., & Jacques, L. (2018). Flipping the Medical School Classroom. In M. Khosrow-Pour, D.B.A. (Ed.), Encyclopedia of Information Science and Technology, Fourth Edition (pp. 5800-5809). Hershey, PA: IGI Global. doi:10.4018/978-1-5225-2255-3.ch504

Karon, R. (2016). Utilisation of Health Information Systems for Service Delivery in the Namibian Environment. In T. Iyamu & A. Tatnall (Eds.), *Maximizing Healthcare Delivery and Management through Technology Integration* (pp. 169–183). Hershey, PA: IGI Global. doi:10.4018/978-1-4666-9446-0.ch011

Kasina, H., Bahubalendruni, M. V., & Botcha, R. (2017). Robots in Medicine: Past, Present and Future. *International Journal of Manufacturing, Materials, and Mechanical Engineering*, 7(4), 44–64. doi:10.4018/IJMMME.2017100104

Katehakis, D. G. (2018). Electronic Medical Record Implementation Challenges for the National Health System in Greece. *International Journal of Reliable and Quality E-Healthcare*, 7(1), 16–30. doi:10.4018/IJRQEH.2018010102

Katz, A., & Shtub, A. (2016). Design and Build a Wizard of Oz (WOZ) Telemedicine Simulator Platform. In M. Cruz-Cunha, I. Miranda, R. Martinho, & R. Rijo (Eds.), *Encyclopedia of E-Health and Telemedicine* (pp. 128–141). Hershey, PA: IGI Global. doi:10.4018/978-1-4666-9978-6.ch011

Kaur, P. D., & Sharma, P. (2017). Success Dimensions of ICTs in Healthcare. In B. Singh (Ed.), *Computational Tools and Techniques for Biomedical Signal Processing* (pp. 149–173). Hershey, PA: IGI Global. doi:10.4018/978-1-5225-0660-7.ch007

Kaushik, P. (2018). Comorbidity of Medical and Psychiatric Disorders in Geriatric Population: Treatment and Care. In B. Prasad & S. Akbar (Eds.), *Handbook of Research on Geriatric Health, Treatment, and Care* (pp. 448–474). Hershey, PA: IGI Global. doi:10.4018/978-1-5225-3480-8.ch025

Khachane, M. Y. (2017). Organ-Based Medical Image Classification Using Support Vector Machine. *International Journal of Synthetic Emotions*, 8(1), 18–30. doi:10.4018/IJSE.2017010102

Kirci, P. (2018). Intelligent Techniques for Analysis of Big Data About Healthcare and Medical Records. In N. Shah & M. Mittal (Eds.), *Handbook of Research on Promoting Business Process Improvement Through Inventory Control Techniques* (pp. 559–582). Hershey, PA: IGI Global. doi:10.4018/978-1-5225-3232-3.ch029

Kldiashvili, E. (2016). Cloud Computing as the Useful Resource for Application of the Medical Information System for Quality Assurance Purposes. *International Journal of Computers in Clinical Practice*, 1(2), 1–23. doi:10.4018/IJCCP.2016070101

Kldiashvili, E. (2018). Cloud Approach for the Medical Information System: MIS on Cloud. In M. Khosrow-Pour (Ed.), *Incorporating Nature-Inspired Paradigms in Computational Applications* (pp. 238–261). Hershey, PA: IGI Global. doi:10.4018/978-1-5225-5020-4.ch008

Kldiashvili, E., Burduli, A., Ghortlishvili, G., & Sheklashvili, I. (2016). Georgian Experience in Telecytology. In M. Cruz-Cunha, I. Miranda, R. Martinho, & R. Rijo (Eds.), *Encyclopedia of E-Health and Telemedicine* (pp. 62–71). Hershey, PA: IGI Global. doi:10.4018/978-1-4666-9978-6.ch006

Ko, H., Mesicek, L., Choi, J., Choi, J., & Hwang, S. (2018). A Study on Secure Contents Strategies for Applications With DRM on Cloud Computing. *International Journal of Cloud Applications and Computing*, 8(1), 143–153. doi:10.4018/IJCAC.2018010107

Komendziński, T., Dreszer-Drogorób, J., Mikołajewska, E., Mikołajewski, D., & Bałaj, B. (2016). Interdisciplinary Education for Research and Everyday Clinical Practice: Lessons Learned from InteRDoCTor Project. In A. Rosiek & K. Leksowski (Eds.), *Organizational Culture and Ethics in Modern Medicine* (pp. 78–110). Hershey, PA: IGI Global. doi:10.4018/978-1-4666-9658-7.ch004

Komendziński, T., Mikołajewska, E., & Mikołajewski, D. (2018). Cross-Cultural Decision-Making in Healthcare: Theory and Practical Application in Real Clinical Conditions. In A. Rosiek-Kryszewska & K. Leksowski (Eds.), *Healthcare Administration for Patient Safety and Engagement* (pp. 276–298). Hershey, PA: IGI Global. doi:10.4018/978-1-5225-3946-9.ch015

Konecny, L. T. (2018). Medical School Wellness Initiatives. In C. Smith (Ed.), *Exploring the Pressures of Medical Education From a Mental Health and Wellness Perspective* (pp. 209–228). Hershey, PA: IGI Global. doi:10.4018/978-1-5225-2811-1.ch009

Konieczna, A., & Słomkowski, P. (2016). Confrontation of Human Rights in Daily Clinical Situations. In A. Rosiek & K. Leksowski (Eds.), *Organizational Culture and Ethics in Modern Medicine* (pp. 255–281). Hershey, PA: IGI Global. doi:10.4018/978-1-4666-9658-7.ch011

Kromrei, H., Solomonson, W. L., & Juzych, M. S. (2017). Teaching Residents How to Teach. In J. Stefaniak (Ed.), *Advancing Medical Education Through Strategic Instructional Design* (pp. 164–185). Hershey, PA: IGI Global. doi:10.4018/978-1-5225-2098-6.ch008

Kulkarni, S., Savyanavar, A., Kulkarni, P., Stranieri, A., & Ghorpade, V. (2018). Framework for Integration of Medical Image and Text-Based Report Retrieval to Support Radiological Diagnosis. In M. Kolekar & V. Kumar (Eds.), *Biomedical Signal and Image Processing in Patient Care* (pp. 86–122). Hershey, PA: IGI Global. doi:10.4018/978-1-5225-2829-6.ch006

Kumar, A., & Sarkar, B. K. (2018). Performance Analysis of Nature-Inspired Algorithms-Based Bayesian Prediction Models for Medical Data Sets. In U. Singh, A. Tiwari, & R. Singh (Eds.), *Soft-Computing-Based Nonlinear Control Systems Design* (pp. 134–155). Hershey, PA: IGI Global. doi:10.4018/978-1-5225-3531-7.ch007

Kurtz, R. S. (2016). Fortitude: A Study of African Americans in Surgery in New York City. In U. Thomas & J. Drake (Eds.), *Critical Research on Sexism and Racism in STEM Fields* (pp. 153–169). Hershey, PA: IGI Global. doi:10.4018/978-1-5225-0174-9.ch009

Labbadi, W., & Akaichi, J. (2017). Efficient Algorithm for Answering Fuzzy Medical Requests in Pervasive Healthcare Information Systems. *International Journal of Healthcare Information Systems and Informatics*, *12*(2), 46–64. doi:10.4018/IJHISI.2017040103

Lagumdzija, A., & Swing, V. K. (2017). Health, Digitalization, and Individual Empowerment. In F. Topor (Ed.), *Handbook of Research on Individualism and Identity in the Globalized Digital Age* (pp. 380–402). Hershey, PA: IGI Global. doi:10.4018/978-1-5225-0522-8.ch017

Lamey, T. W., & Davidson-Shivers, G. V. (2017). Instructional Strategies and Sequencing. In J. Stefaniak (Ed.), *Advancing Medical Education Through Strategic Instructional Design* (pp. 30–52). Hershey, PA: IGI Global. doi:10.4018/978-1-5225-2098-6.ch002

Leon, G. (2017). The Role of Forensic Medicine in Medical Errors. In M. Riga (Ed.), *Impact of Medical Errors and Malpractice on Health Economics, Quality, and Patient Safety* (pp. 144–170). Hershey, PA: IGI Global. doi:10.4018/978-1-5225-2337-6.ch006

Lidia, B., Federica, G., & Maria, V. E. (2016). The Patient-Centered Medicine as the Theoretical Framework for Patient Engagement. In G. Graffigna (Ed.), *Promoting Patient Engagement and Participation for Effective Healthcare Reform* (pp. 25–39). Hershey, PA: IGI Global. doi:10.4018/978-1-4666-9992-2.ch002

Love, L., & McDowelle, D. (2018). Developing a Comprehensive Wellness Program for Medical Students. In C. Smith (Ed.), *Exploring the Pressures of Medical Education From a Mental Health and Wellness Perspective* (pp. 190–208). Hershey, PA: IGI Global. doi:10.4018/978-1-5225-2811-1.ch008

Lovell, K. L. (2017). Development and Evaluation of Neuroscience Computer-Based Modules for Medical Students: Instructional Design Principles and Effectiveness. In J. Stefaniak (Ed.), *Advancing Medical Education Through Strategic Instructional Design* (pp. 262–276). Hershey, PA: IGI Global. doi:10.4018/978-1-5225-2098-6.ch013

Lubin, R., & Hamlin, M. D. (2018). Medical Student Burnout: A Social Cognitive Learning Perspective on Medical Student Mental Health and Wellness. In C. Smith (Ed.), *Exploring the Pressures of Medical Education From a Mental Health and Wellness Perspective* (pp. 92–121). Hershey, PA: IGI Global. doi:10.4018/978-1-5225-2811-1.ch004

Luk, C. Y. (2018). Moving Towards Universal Health Coverage: Challenges for the Present and Future in China. In B. Fong, A. Ng, & P. Yuen (Eds.), *Sustainable Health and Long-Term Care Solutions for an Aging Population* (pp. 19–45). Hershey, PA: IGI Global. doi:10.4018/978-1-5225-2633-9.ch002

Mahat, M., & Pettigrew, A. (2017). The Regulatory Environment of Non-Profit Higher Education and Research Institutions and Its Implications for Managerial Strategy: The Case of Medical Education and Research. In L. West & A. Worthington (Eds.), *Handbook of Research on Emerging Business Models and Managerial Strategies in the Nonprofit Sector* (pp. 336–351). Hershey, PA: IGI Global. doi:10.4018/978-1-5225-2537-0.ch017

Maitra, I. K., & Bandhyopadhyaay, S. K. (2017). Adaptive Edge Detection Method towards Features Extraction from Diverse Medical Imaging Technologies. In S. Bhattacharyya, S. De, I. Pan, & P. Dutta (Eds.), *Intelligent Multidimensional Data Clustering and Analysis* (pp. 159–192). Hershey, PA: IGI Global. doi:10.4018/978-1-5225-1776-4.ch007

Mangu, V. P. (2017). Mobile Health Care: A Technology View. In C. Bhatt & S. Peddoju (Eds.), *Cloud Computing Systems and Applications in Healthcare* (pp. 1–18). Hershey, PA: IGI Global. doi:10.4018/978-1-5225-1002-4.ch001

Manirabona, A., Fourati, L. C., & Boudjit, S. (2017). Investigation on Healthcare Monitoring Systems: Innovative Services and Applications. *International Journal of E-Health and Medical Communications, 8*(1), 1–18. doi:10.4018/IJEHMC.2017010101

Mannai, M. M., & Karâa, W. B. (2016). Biomedical Image Processing Overview. In W. Karâa & N. Dey (Eds.), *Biomedical Image Analysis and Mining Techniques for Improved Health Outcomes* (pp. 1–12). Hershey, PA: IGI Global. doi:10.4018/978-1-4666-8811-7.ch001

Manzoor, A. (2016). RFID in Health Care-Building Smart Hospitals for Quality Healthcare. *International Journal of User-Driven Healthcare, 6*(2), 21–45. doi:10.4018/IJUDH.2016070102

Marwan, M., Kartit, A., & Ouahmane, H. (2018). A Framework to Secure Medical Image Storage in Cloud Computing Environment. *Journal of Electronic Commerce in Organizations*, *16*(1), 1–16. doi:10.4018/JECO.2018010101

Masoud, M. P., Nejad, M. K., Darebaghi, H., Chavoshi, M., & Farahani, M. (2018). The Decision Support System and Conventional Method of Telephone Triage by Nurses in Emergency Medical Services: A Comparative Investigation. *International Journal of E-Business Research*, *14*(1), 77–88. doi:10.4018/IJEBR.2018010105

McDonald, W. G., Martin, M., & Salzberg, L. D. (2018). From Medical Student to Medical Resident: Graduate Medical Education and Mental Health in the United States. In C. Smith (Ed.), *Exploring the Pressures of Medical Education From a Mental Health and Wellness Perspective* (pp. 145–169). Hershey, PA: IGI Global. doi:10.4018/978-1-5225-2811-1.ch006

Medhekar, A. (2017). The Role of Social Media for Knowledge Dissemination in Medical Tourism: A Case of India. In R. Chugh (Ed.), *Harnessing Social Media as a Knowledge Management Tool* (pp. 25–54). Hershey, PA: IGI Global. doi:10.4018/978-1-5225-0495-5.ch002

Medhekar, A., & Haq, F. (2018). Urbanization and New Jobs Creation in Healthcare Services in India: Challenges and Opportunities. In U. Benna & I. Benna (Eds.), *Urbanization and Its Impact on Socio-Economic Growth in Developing Regions* (pp. 198–218). Hershey, PA: IGI Global. doi:10.4018/978-1-5225-2659-9.ch010

Mehta, G., Dutta, M. K., & Kim, P. S. (2016). An Efficient and Lossless Cryptosystem for Security in Tele-Ophthalmology Applications Using Chaotic Theory. *International Journal of E-Health and Medical Communications*, *7*(4), 28–47. doi:10.4018/IJEHMC.2016100102

Mehta, P. (2017). Framework of Indian Healthcare System and its Challenges: An Insight. In V. Bryan & J. Bird (Eds.), *Healthcare Community Synergism between Patients, Practitioners, and Researchers* (pp. 247–271). Hershey, PA: IGI Global. doi:10.4018/978-1-5225-0640-9.ch011

Metelmann, B., & Metelmann, C. (2016). M-Health in Prehospital Emergency Medicine: Experiences from the EU funded Project LiveCity. In A. Moumtzoglou (Ed.), *M-Health Innovations for Patient-Centered Care* (pp. 197–212). Hershey, PA: IGI Global. doi:10.4018/978-1-4666-9861-1.ch010

Mi, M. (2017). Informal Learning in Medical Education. In J. Stefaniak (Ed.), *Advancing Medical Education Through Strategic Instructional Design* (pp. 225–244). Hershey, PA: IGI Global. doi:10.4018/978-1-5225-2098-6.ch011

Miglioretti, M., Mariani, F., & Vecchio, L. (2016). Could Patient Engagement Promote a Health System Free From Malpractice Litigation Risk? In G. Graffigna (Ed.), *Promoting Patient Engagement and Participation for Effective Healthcare Reform* (pp. 240–264). Hershey, PA: IGI Global. doi:10.4018/978-1-4666-9992-2.ch012

Misra, S. C., & Bisui, S. (2016). Feasibility of Large Scale Implementation of Personalized Medicine in the Current Scenario. *International Journal of E-Health and Medical Communications*, 7(2), 30–49. doi:10.4018/IJEHMC.2016040103

Misra, S. C., Bisui, S., & Fantazy, K. (2016). Identifying Critical Changes in Adoption of Personalized Medicine (PM) in Healthcare Management. *International Journal of E-Health and Medical Communications*, 7(3), 1–15. doi:10.4018/IJEHMC.2016070101

Mohammadian, M., Hatzinakos, D., Spachos, P., & Jentzsh, R. (2016). An Intelligent and Secure Framework for Wireless Information Technology in Healthcare for User and Data Classification in Hospitals. In V. Wang (Ed.), *Handbook of Research on Advancing Health Education through Technology* (pp. 452–479). Hershey, PA: IGI Global. doi:10.4018/978-1-4666-9494-1.ch019

Mokeddem, S., & Atmani, B. (2016). Assessment of Clinical Decision Support Systems for Predicting Coronary Heart Disease. *International Journal of Operations Research and Information Systems*, 7(3), 57–73. doi:10.4018/IJORIS.2016070104

Mokrzycka, A., & Kowalska-Bobko, I. (2016). Public Health Legislation and Patient's Rights: Health2020 Strategy, European Perspective. In A. Rosiek & K. Leksowski (Eds.), *Organizational Culture and Ethics in Modern Medicine* (pp. 298–322). Hershey, PA: IGI Global. doi:10.4018/978-1-4666-9658-7.ch013

Moon, J. D., & Galea, M. P. (2016). Overview of Clinical Decision Support Systems in Healthcare. In J. Moon & M. Galea (Eds.), *Improving Health Management through Clinical Decision Support Systems* (pp. 1–27). Hershey, PA: IGI Global. doi:10.4018/978-1-4666-9432-3.ch001

Mosadeghrad, A. M., & Woldemichael, A. (2017). Application of Quality Management in Promoting Patient Safety and Preventing Medical Errors. In M. Riga (Ed.), *Impact of Medical Errors and Malpractice on Health Economics, Quality, and Patient Safety* (pp. 91–112). Hershey, PA: IGI Global. doi:10.4018/978-1-5225-2337-6.ch004

Moumtzoglou, A. (2017). Digital Medicine: The Quality Standpoint. In A. Moumtzoglou (Ed.), *Design, Development, and Integration of Reliable Electronic Healthcare Platforms* (pp. 179–195). Hershey, PA: IGI Global. doi:10.4018/978-1-5225-1724-5.ch011

Moumtzoglou, A., & Pouliakis, A. (2018). Population Health Management and the Science of Individuality. *International Journal of Reliable and Quality E-Healthcare*, 7(2), 1–26. doi:10.4018/IJRQEH.2018040101

Mpofu, C. (2016). International Medical Experiences Outbound New Zealand: An Economic and Medical Workforce Strategy. In D. Velliaris & D. Coleman-George (Eds.), *Handbook of Research on Study Abroad Programs and Outbound Mobility* (pp. 446–469). Hershey, PA: IGI Global. doi:10.4018/978-1-5225-0169-5.ch018

Mukhtar, W. F., & Abuelyaman, E. S. (2017). Opportunities and Challenges of Big Data in Healthcare. In N. Wickramasinghe (Ed.), *Handbook of Research on Healthcare Administration and Management* (pp. 47–58). Hershey, PA: IGI Global. doi:10.4018/978-1-5225-0920-2.ch004

Munugala, S., Brar, G. K., Syed, A., Mohammad, A., & Halgamuge, M. N. (2018). The Much Needed Security and Data Reforms of Cloud Computing in Medical Data Storage. In M. Lytras & P. Papadopoulou (Eds.), *Applying Big Data Analytics in Bioinformatics and Medicine* (pp. 99–113). Hershey, PA: IGI Global. doi:10.4018/978-1-5225-2607-0.ch005

Narasimhamurthy, A. (2016). An Overview of Machine Learning in Medical Image Analysis: Trends in Health Informatics. In N. Dey & A. Ashour (Eds.), *Classification and Clustering in Biomedical Signal Processing* (pp. 23–45). Hershey, PA: IGI Global. doi:10.4018/978-1-5225-0140-4.ch002

Ngara, R. (2017). Multiple Voices, Multiple Paths: Towards Dialogue between Western and Indigenous Medical Knowledge Systems. In P. Ngulube (Ed.), *Handbook of Research on Theoretical Perspectives on Indigenous Knowledge Systems in Developing Countries* (pp. 332–358). Hershey, PA: IGI Global. doi:10.4018/978-1-5225-0833-5.ch015

O'Connor, Y., & Heavin, C. (2018). Defining and Characterising the Landscape of eHealth. In M. Khosrow-Pour, D.B.A. (Ed.), Encyclopedia of Information Science and Technology, Fourth Edition (pp. 5864-5875). Hershey, PA: IGI Global. doi:10.4018/978-1-5225-2255-3.ch510

Ochonogor, W. C., & Okite-Amughoro, F. A. (2018). Building an Effective Digital Library in a University Teaching Hospital (UTH) in Nigeria. In A. Tella & T. Kwanya (Eds.), *Handbook of Research on Managing Intellectual Property in Digital Libraries* (pp. 184–204). Hershey, PA: IGI Global. doi:10.4018/978-1-5225-3093-0.ch010

Olaniran, B. A. (2016). ICTs, E-health, and Multidisciplinary Healthcare Teams: Promises and Challenges. *International Journal of Privacy and Health Information Management, 4*(2), 62–75. doi:10.4018/IJPHIM.2016070105

Olaniran, B. A. (2016). ICT Use and Multidisciplinary Healthcare Teams in the Age of e-Health. *International Journal of Reliable and Quality E-Healthcare, 5*(1), 18–31. doi:10.4018/IJRQEH.2016010102

Olivares, S. L., Cruz, A. G., Cabrera, M. V., Regalado, A. I., & García, J. E. (2017). An Assessment Study of Quality Model for Medical Schools in Mexico. In S. Mukerji & P. Tripathi (Eds.), *Handbook of Research on Administration, Policy, and Leadership in Higher Education* (pp. 404–439). Hershey, PA: IGI Global. doi:10.4018/978-1-5225-0672-0.ch016

Omidoyin, E. O., Opeke, R. O., & Osagbemi, G. K. (2016). Utilization Pattern and Privacy Issues in the use of Health Records for Research Practice by Doctors: Selected Nigerian Teaching Hospitals as Case Study. *International Journal of Privacy and Health Information Management, 4*(1), 1–11. doi:10.4018/IJPHIM.2016010101

Omoruyi, E. A., & Omidele, F. (2018). Resident Physician and Medical Academic Faculty Burnout: A Review of Current Literature. In C. Smith (Ed.), *Exploring the Pressures of Medical Education From a Mental Health and Wellness Perspective* (pp. 171–189). Hershey, PA: IGI Global. doi:10.4018/978-1-5225-2811-1.ch007

Osop, H., & Sahama, T. (2016). Data-Driven and Practice-Based Evidence: Design and Development of Efficient and Effective Clinical Decision Support System. In J. Moon & M. Galea (Eds.), *Improving Health Management through Clinical Decision Support Systems* (pp. 295–328). Hershey, PA: IGI Global. doi:10.4018/978-1-4666-9432-3.ch014

Ossowski, R., & Izdebski, P. (2016). Ethical Aspects of Talking to a Patient. In A. Rosiek & K. Leksowski (Eds.), *Organizational Culture and Ethics in Modern Medicine* (pp. 203–235). Hershey, PA: IGI Global. doi:10.4018/978-1-4666-9658-7.ch009

Pandian, P. S. (2016). An Overview of Telemedicine Technologies for Healthcare Applications. *International Journal of Biomedical and Clinical Engineering*, 5(2), 29–52. doi:10.4018/IJBCE.2016070103

Papadopoulou, P., Lytras, M., & Marouli, C. (2018). Bioinformatics as Applied to Medicine: Challenges Faced Moving from Big Data to Smart Data to Wise Data. In M. Lytras & P. Papadopoulou (Eds.), *Applying Big Data Analytics in Bioinformatics and Medicine* (pp. 1–25). Hershey, PA: IGI Global. doi:10.4018/978-1-5225-2607-0.ch001

Paraskou, A., & George, B. P. (2018). An Overview of Reproductive Tourism. In *Legal and Economic Considerations Surrounding Reproductive Tourism: Emerging Research and Opportunities* (pp. 1–17). Hershey, PA: IGI Global. doi:10.4018/978-1-5225-2694-0.ch001

Park, S., & Moon, J. (2016). Strategic Approach towards Clinical Information Security. In J. Moon & M. Galea (Eds.), *Improving Health Management through Clinical Decision Support Systems* (pp. 329–359). Hershey, PA: IGI Global. doi:10.4018/978-1-4666-9432-3.ch015

Pereira, D., Castro, A., Gomes, P., Areias, J. C., Reis, Z. S., Coimbra, M. T., & Cruz-Correia, R. (2016). Digital Auscultation: Challenges and Perspectives. In M. Cruz-Cunha, I. Miranda, R. Martinho, & R. Rijo (Eds.), *Encyclopedia of E-Health and Telemedicine* (pp. 910–927). Hershey, PA: IGI Global. doi:10.4018/978-1-4666-9978-6.ch070

Peters, R. A., & Cruz, M. (2016). The States as Generators of Incremental Change in American Health Care Policy: 1935 to 1965. In R. Gholipour & K. Rouzbehani (Eds.), *Social, Economic, and Political Perspectives on Public Health Policy-Making* (pp. 86–114). Hershey, PA: IGI Global. doi:10.4018/978-1-4666-9944-1.ch005

Phuritsabam, B., & Devi, A. B. (2017). Information Seeking Behavior of Medical Scientists at Jawaharlal Nehru Institute of Medical Science: A Study. In S. Ram (Ed.), *Library and Information Services for Bioinformatics Education and Research* (pp. 177–187). Hershey, PA: IGI Global. doi:10.4018/978-1-5225-1871-6.ch010

Pieczka, B. (2018). Management of Risk and Adverse Events in Medical Entities. In A. Rosiek-Kryszewska & K. Leksowski (Eds.), *Healthcare Administration for Patient Safety and Engagement* (pp. 31–46). Hershey, PA: IGI Global. doi:10.4018/978-1-5225-3946-9.ch003

Poduval, J. (2016). Curriculum Development. In *Optimizing Medicine Residency Training Programs* (pp. 45–102). Hershey, PA: IGI Global. doi:10.4018/978-1-4666-9527-6.ch003

Poduval, J. (2016). Ethics and Professionalism. In *Optimizing Medicine Residency Training Programs* (pp. 103–133). Hershey, PA: IGI Global. doi:10.4018/978-1-4666-9527-6.ch004

Poduval, J. (2016). Management Skills and Leadership. In *Optimizing Medicine Residency Training Programs* (pp. 182–205). Hershey, PA: IGI Global. doi:10.4018/978-1-4666-9527-6.ch008

Poduval, J. (2016). Medicine Residency Training. In *Optimizing Medicine Residency Training Programs* (pp. 1–27). Hershey, PA: IGI Global. doi:10.4018/978-1-4666-9527-6.ch001

Poduval, J. (2016). Personal Issues. In *Optimizing Medicine Residency Training Programs* (pp. 206–221). Hershey, PA: IGI Global. doi:10.4018/978-1-4666-9527-6.ch009

Poduval, J. (2017). Medical Errors: Impact on Health Care Quality. In M. Riga (Ed.), *Impact of Medical Errors and Malpractice on Health Economics, Quality, and Patient Safety* (pp. 33–60). Hershey, PA: IGI Global. doi:10.4018/978-1-5225-2337-6.ch002

Politis, D., Stagiopoulos, P., Aidona, S., Kyriafinis, G., & Constantinidis, I. (2018). Autonomous Learning and Skill Accreditation: A Paradigm for Medical Studies. In A. Kumar (Ed.), *Optimizing Student Engagement in Online Learning Environments* (pp. 266–296). Hershey, PA: IGI Global. doi:10.4018/978-1-5225-3634-5.ch012

Pomares-Quimbaya, A., Gonzalez, R. A., Quintero, S., Muñoz, O. M., Bohórquez, W. R., García, O. M., & Londoño, D. (2016). A Review of Existing Applications and Techniques for Narrative Text Analysis in Electronic Medical Records. In M. Cruz-Cunha, I. Miranda, R. Martinho, & R. Rijo (Eds.), *Encyclopedia of E-Health and Telemedicine* (pp. 796–811). Hershey, PA: IGI Global. doi:10.4018/978-1-4666-9978-6.ch062

Pomares-Quimbaya, A., González, R. A., Sierra, A., Daza, J. C., Muñoz, O., García, A., ... Bohórquez, W. R. (2017). ICT for Enabling the Quality Evaluation of Health Care Services: A Case Study in a General Hospital. In A. Moumtzoglou (Ed.), *Design, Development, and Integration of Reliable Electronic Healthcare Platforms* (pp. 196–210). Hershey, PA: IGI Global. doi:10.4018/978-1-5225-1724-5.ch012

Pouliakis, A., Margari, N., Karakitsou, E., Archondakis, S., & Karakitsos, P. (2018). Emerging Technologies Serving Cytopathology: Big Data, the Cloud, and Mobile Computing. In I. El Naqa (Ed.), *Emerging Developments and Practices in Oncology* (pp. 114–152). Hershey, PA: IGI Global. doi:10.4018/978-1-5225-3085-5.ch005

Queirós, A., Silva, A. G., Ferreira, A., Caravau, H., Cerqueira, M., & Rocha, N. P. (2016). Assessing Mobile Applications Considered Medical Devices. In M. Cruz-Cunha, I. Miranda, R. Martinho, & R. Rijo (Eds.), *Encyclopedia of E-Health and Telemedicine* (pp. 111–127). Hershey, PA: IGI Global. doi:10.4018/978-1-4666-9978-6.ch010

Raffaeli, L., Spinsante, S., & Gambi, E. (2016). Integrated Smart TV-Based Personal e-Health System. *International Journal of E-Health and Medical Communications*, 7(1), 48–64. doi:10.4018/IJEHMC.2016010103

Rai, A., Kothari, R., & Singh, D. P. (2017). Assessment of Available Technologies for Hospital Waste Management: A Need for Society. In R. Singh, A. Singh, & V. Srivastava (Eds.), *Environmental Issues Surrounding Human Overpopulation* (pp. 172–188). Hershey, PA: IGI Global. doi:10.4018/978-1-5225-1683-5.ch010

Ramamoorthy, S., & Sivasubramaniam, R. (2018). Image Processing Including Medical Liver Imaging: Medical Image Processing from Big Data Perspective, Ultrasound Liver Images, Challenges. In M. Lytras & P. Papadopoulou (Eds.), *Applying Big Data Analytics in Bioinformatics and Medicine* (pp. 380–392). Hershey, PA: IGI Global. doi:10.4018/978-1-5225-2607-0.ch016

Rathor, G. P., & Gupta, S. K. (2017). Improving Multimodality Image Fusion through Integrate AFL and Wavelet Transform. In V. Tiwari, B. Tiwari, R. Thakur, & S. Gupta (Eds.), *Pattern and Data Analysis in Healthcare Settings* (pp. 143–157). Hershey, PA: IGI Global. doi:10.4018/978-1-5225-0536-5.ch008

Rawat, D. B., & Bhattacharya, S. (2016). Wireless Body Area Network for Healthcare Applications. In N. Meghanathan (Ed.), *Advanced Methods for Complex Network Analysis* (pp. 343–358). Hershey, PA: IGI Global. doi:10.4018/978-1-4666-9964-9.ch014

Rea, P. M. (2016). Advances in Anatomical and Medical Visualisation. In M. Pinheiro & D. Simões (Eds.), *Handbook of Research on Engaging Digital Natives in Higher Education Settings* (pp. 244–264). Hershey, PA: IGI Global. doi:10.4018/978-1-5225-0039-1.ch011

Rexhepi, H., & Persson, A. (2017). Challenges to Implementing IT Support for Evidence Based Practice Among Nurses and Assistant Nurses: A Qualitative Study. *Journal of Electronic Commerce in Organizations*, *15*(2), 61–76. doi:10.4018/JECO.2017040105

Reychav, I., & Azuri, J. (2016). Including Elderly Patients in Decision Making via Electronic Health Literacy. In M. Cruz-Cunha, I. Miranda, R. Martinho, & R. Rijo (Eds.), *Encyclopedia of E-Health and Telemedicine* (pp. 241–249). Hershey, PA: IGI Global. doi:10.4018/978-1-4666-9978-6.ch020

Richards, D., & Caldwell, P. H. (2016). Gamification to Improve Adherence to Clinical Treatment Advice: Improving Adherence to Clinical Treatment. In D. Novák, B. Tulu, & H. Brendryen (Eds.), *Handbook of Research on Holistic Perspectives in Gamification for Clinical Practice* (pp. 47–77). Hershey, PA: IGI Global. doi:10.4018/978-1-4666-9522-1.ch004

Rissman, B. (2016). Medical Conditions Associated with NLD. In B. Rissman (Ed.), *Medical and Educational Perspectives on Nonverbal Learning Disability in Children and Young Adults* (pp. 27–66). Hershey, PA: IGI Global. doi:10.4018/978-1-4666-9539-9.ch002

Rosiek, A. (2018). The Assessment of Actions of the Environment and the Impact of Preventive Medicine for Public Health in Poland. In A. Rosiek-Kryszewska & K. Leksowski (Eds.), *Healthcare Administration for Patient Safety and Engagement* (pp. 106–119). Hershey, PA: IGI Global. doi:10.4018/978-1-5225-3946-9.ch006

Rosiek, A., Leksowski, K., Goch, A., Rosiek-Kryszewska, A., & Leksowski, Ł. (2016). Medical Treatment and Difficult Ethical Decisions in Interdisciplinary Hospital Teams. In A. Rosiek & K. Leksowski (Eds.), *Organizational Culture and Ethics in Modern Medicine* (pp. 121–153). Hershey, PA: IGI Global. doi:10.4018/978-1-4666-9658-7.ch006

Rosiek, A., & Rosiek-Kryszewska, A. (2018). Managed Healthcare: Doctor Life Satisfaction and Its Impact on the Process of Communicating With the Patient. In A. Rosiek-Kryszewska & K. Leksowski (Eds.), *Healthcare Administration for Patient Safety and Engagement* (pp. 244–261). Hershey, PA: IGI Global. doi:10.4018/978-1-5225-3946-9.ch013

Rosiek-Kryszewska, A., Leksowski, Ł., Rosiek, A., Leksowski, K., & Goch, A. (2016). Clinical Communication in the Aspect of Development of New Technologies and E-Health in the Doctor-Patient Relationship. In A. Rosiek & K. Leksowski (Eds.), *Organizational Culture and Ethics in Modern Medicine* (pp. 18–51). Hershey, PA: IGI Global. doi:10.4018/978-1-4666-9658-7.ch002

Rosiek-Kryszewska, A., & Rosiek, A. (2018). The Involvement of the Patient and his Perspective Evaluation of the Quality of Healthcare. In A. Rosiek-Kryszewska & K. Leksowski (Eds.), *Healthcare Administration for Patient Safety and Engagement* (pp. 121–144). Hershey, PA: IGI Global. doi:10.4018/978-1-5225-3946-9.ch007

Rosiek-Kryszewska, A., & Rosiek, A. (2018). The Impact of Management and Leadership Roles in Building Competitive Healthcare Units. In A. Rosiek-Kryszewska & K. Leksowski (Eds.), *Healthcare Administration for Patient Safety and Engagement* (pp. 13–30). Hershey, PA: IGI Global. doi:10.4018/978-1-5225-3946-9.ch002

Roşu, S. M., Păvăloiu, I. B., Dragoi, G., Apostol, C. G., & Munteanu, D. (2016). Telemedicine Based on LMDS in the Urban/Metropolitan Area: A Romanian Case Study. In M. Cruz-Cunha, I. Miranda, R. Martinho, & R. Rijo (Eds.), *Encyclopedia of E-Health and Telemedicine* (pp. 96–109). Hershey, PA: IGI Global. doi:10.4018/978-1-4666-9978-6.ch009

Rouzbehani, K. (2017). Health Policy Implementation: Moving Beyond Its Barriers in United States. In N. Wickramasinghe (Ed.), *Handbook of Research on Healthcare Administration and Management* (pp. 541–552). Hershey, PA: IGI Global. doi:10.4018/978-1-5225-0920-2.ch032

Ruiz, I. M., Cohen, D. S., & Marco, Á. M. (2016). ISO/IEEE11073 Family of Standards: Trends and Applications on E-Health Monitoring. In M. Cruz-Cunha, I. Miranda, R. Martinho, & R. Rijo (Eds.), *Encyclopedia of E-Health and Telemedicine* (pp. 646–660). Hershey, PA: IGI Global. doi:10.4018/978-1-4666-9978-6.ch050

Sam, S. (2017). Mobile Phones and Expanding Human Capabilities in Plural Health Systems. In K. Moahi, K. Bwalya, & P. Sebina (Eds.), *Health Information Systems and the Advancement of Medical Practice in Developing Countries* (pp. 93–114). Hershey, PA: IGI Global. doi:10.4018/978-1-5225-2262-1.ch006

Sankaranarayanan, S., & Ganesan, S. (2016). Applications of Intelligent Agents in Health Sector-A Review. *International Journal of E-Health and Medical Communications*, 7(1), 1–30. doi:10.4018/IJEHMC.2016010101

Santos-Trigo, M., Suaste, E., & Figuerola, P. (2018). Technology Design and Routes for Tool Appropriation in Medical Practices. In M. Khosrow-Pour, D.B.A. (Ed.), Encyclopedia of Information Science and Technology, Fourth Edition (pp. 3794-3804). Hershey, PA: IGI Global. doi:10.4018/978-1-5225-2255-3.ch329

Sarivougioukas, J., Vagelatos, A., Parsopoulos, K. E., & Lagaris, I. E. (2018). Home UbiHealth. In M. Khosrow-Pour, D.B.A. (Ed.), Encyclopedia of Information Science and Technology, Fourth Edition (pp. 7765-7774). Hershey, PA: IGI Global. doi:10.4018/978-1-5225-2255-3.ch675

Sarkar, B. K. (2017). Big Data and Healthcare Data: A Survey. *International Journal of Knowledge-Based Organizations*, 7(4), 50–77. doi:10.4018/IJKBO.2017100104

Saxena, K., & Banodha, U. (2017). An Essence of the SOA on Healthcare. In R. Bhadoria, N. Chaudhari, G. Tomar, & S. Singh (Eds.), *Exploring Enterprise Service Bus in the Service-Oriented Architecture Paradigm* (pp. 283–304). Hershey, PA: IGI Global. doi:10.4018/978-1-5225-2157-0.ch018

Schmeida, M., & McNeal, R. (2016). Consulting Online Healthcare Information: E-Caregivers as Knowledgeable Decision Makers. *International Journal of Computers in Clinical Practice*, 1(1), 42–52. doi:10.4018/IJCCP.2016010104

Sen, K., & Ghosh, K. (2018). Incorporating Global Medical Knowledge to Solve Healthcare Problems: A Framework for a Crowdsourcing System. *International Journal of Healthcare Information Systems and Informatics*, 13(1), 1–14. doi:10.4018/IJHISI.2018010101

Shakdher, A., & Pandey, K. (2017). REDAlert+: Medical/Fire Emergency and Warning System using Android Devices. *International Journal of E-Health and Medical Communications*, 8(1), 37–51. doi:10.4018/IJEHMC.2017010103

Shekarian, E., Abdul-Rashid, S. H., & Olugu, E. U. (2017). An Integrated Fuzzy VIKOR Method for Performance Management in Healthcare. In M. Tavana, K. Szabat, & K. Puranam (Eds.), *Organizational Productivity and Performance Measurements Using Predictive Modeling and Analytics* (pp. 40–61). Hershey, PA: IGI Global. doi:10.4018/978-1-5225-0654-6.ch003

Shi, J., Erdem, E., & Liu, H. (2016). Expanding Role of Telephone Systems in Healthcare: Developments and Opportunities. In A. Dwivedi (Ed.), *Reshaping Medical Practice and Care with Health Information Systems* (pp. 87–131). Hershey, PA: IGI Global. doi:10.4018/978-1-4666-9870-3.ch004

Shijina, V., & John, S. J. (2017). Multiple Relations and its Application in Medical Diagnosis. *International Journal of Fuzzy System Applications*, 6(4), 47–62. doi:10.4018/IJFSA.2017100104

Shipley, N., & Chakraborty, J. (2018). Big Data and mHealth: Increasing the Usability of Healthcare Through the Customization of Pinterest – Literary Perspective. In J. Machado, A. Abelha, M. Santos, & F. Portela (Eds.), *Next-Generation Mobile and Pervasive Healthcare Solutions* (pp. 46–66). Hershey, PA: IGI Global. doi:10.4018/978-1-5225-2851-7.ch004

Singh, A., & Dutta, M. K. (2017). A Reversible Data Hiding Scheme for Efficient Management of Tele-Ophthalmological Data. *International Journal of E-Health and Medical Communications*, 8(3), 38–54. doi:10.4018/IJEHMC.2017070103

Sivaji, A., Radjo, H. K., Amin, M., & Abu Hashim, M. A. (2016). Design of a Hospital Interactive Wayfinding System: Designing for Malaysian Users. In N. Mohamed, T. Mantoro, M. Ayu, & M. Mahmud (Eds.), *Critical Socio-Technical Issues Surrounding Mobile Computing* (pp. 88–123). Hershey, PA: IGI Global. doi:10.4018/978-1-4666-9438-5.ch005

Skourti, P. K., & Pavlakis, A. (2017). The Second Victim Phenomenon: The Way Out. In M. Riga (Ed.), *Impact of Medical Errors and Malpractice on Health Economics, Quality, and Patient Safety* (pp. 197–222). Hershey, PA: IGI Global. doi:10.4018/978-1-5225-2337-6.ch008

Smith, C. R. (2018). Medical Students' Quest Towards the Long White Coat: Impact on Mental Health and Well-Being. In C. Smith (Ed.), *Exploring the Pressures of Medical Education From a Mental Health and Wellness Perspective* (pp. 1–42). Hershey, PA: IGI Global. doi:10.4018/978-1-5225-2811-1.ch001

Smith, S. I., & Dandignac, M. (2018). Perfectionism: Addressing Lofty Expectations in Medical School. In C. Smith (Ed.), *Exploring the Pressures of Medical Education From a Mental Health and Wellness Perspective* (pp. 68–91). Hershey, PA: IGI Global. doi:10.4018/978-1-5225-2811-1.ch003

Sobrinho, Á. A., Dias da Silva, L., Perkusich, A., Cunha, P., Pinheiro, M. E., & Melo de Medeiros, L. (2016). Towards Medical Systems to Aid the Detection and Treatment of Chronic Diseases. In D. Fotiadis (Ed.), *Handbook of Research on Trends in the Diagnosis and Treatment of Chronic Conditions* (pp. 50–69). Hershey, PA: IGI Global. doi:10.4018/978-1-4666-8828-5.ch003

Soczywko, J., & Rutkowska, D. (2018). The Patient/Provider Relationship in Emergency Medicine: Organization, Communication, and Understanding. In A. Rosiek-Kryszewska & K. Leksowski (Eds.), *Healthcare Administration for Patient Safety and Engagement* (pp. 74–105). Hershey, PA: IGI Global. doi:10.4018/978-1-5225-3946-9.ch005

Sołtysik-Piorunkiewicz, A., Furmankiewicz, M., & Ziuziański, P. (2016). Web Healthcare Applications in Poland: Trends, Standards, Barriers and Possibilities of Implementation and Usage of E-Health Systems. In I. Deliyannis, P. Kostagiolas, & C. Banou (Eds.), *Experimental Multimedia Systems for Interactivity and Strategic Innovation* (pp. 258–283). Hershey, PA: IGI Global. doi:10.4018/978-1-4666-8659-5.ch013

Soni, P. (2018). Implications of HIPAA and Subsequent Regulations on Information Technology. In M. Gupta, R. Sharman, J. Walp, & P. Mulgund (Eds.), *Information Technology Risk Management and Compliance in Modern Organizations* (pp. 71–98). Hershey, PA: IGI Global. doi:10.4018/978-1-5225-2604-9.ch004

Spinelli, R., & Benevolo, C. (2016). From Healthcare Services to E-Health Applications: A Delivery System-Based Taxonomy. In A. Dwivedi (Ed.), *Reshaping Medical Practice and Care with Health Information Systems* (pp. 205–245). Hershey, PA: IGI Global. doi:10.4018/978-1-4666-9870-3.ch007

Srivastava, A., & Aggarwal, A. K. (2018). Medical Image Fusion in Spatial and Transform Domain: A Comparative Analysis. In M. Anwar, A. Khosla, & R. Kapoor (Eds.), *Handbook of Research on Advanced Concepts in Real-Time Image and Video Processing* (pp. 281–300). Hershey, PA: IGI Global. doi:10.4018/978-1-5225-2848-7.ch011

Srivastava, S. K., & Roy, S. N. (2018). Recommendation System: A Potential Tool for Achieving Pervasive Health Care. In J. Machado, A. Abelha, M. Santos, & F. Portela (Eds.), *Next-Generation Mobile and Pervasive Healthcare Solutions* (pp. 111–127). Hershey, PA: IGI Global. doi:10.4018/978-1-5225-2851-7.ch008

Stancu, A. (2016). Correlations and Patterns of Food and Health Consumer Expenditure. In A. Jean-Vasile (Ed.), *Food Science, Production, and Engineering in Contemporary Economies* (pp. 44–101). Hershey, PA: IGI Global. doi:10.4018/978-1-5225-0341-5.ch003

Stanimirovic, D. (2017). Digitalization of Death Certification Model: Transformation Issues and Implementation Concerns. In S. Saeed, Y. Bamarouf, T. Ramayah, & S. Iqbal (Eds.), *Design Solutions for User-Centric Information Systems* (pp. 22–43). Hershey, PA: IGI Global. doi:10.4018/978-1-5225-1944-7.ch002

Stavros, A., Vavoulidis, E., & Nasioutziki, M. (2016). The Use of Mobile Health Applications for Quality Control and Accreditational Purposes in a Cytopathology Laboratory. In A. Moumtzoglou (Ed.), *M-Health Innovations for Patient-Centered Care* (pp. 262–283). Hershey, PA: IGI Global. doi:10.4018/978-1-4666-9861-1.ch013

Sukkird, V., & Shirahada, K. (2018). E-Health Service Model for Asian Developing Countries: A Case of Emergency Medical Service for Elderly People in Thailand. In M. Khosrow-Pour (Ed.), *Optimizing Current Practices in E-Services and Mobile Applications* (pp. 214–232). Hershey, PA: IGI Global. doi:10.4018/978-1-5225-5026-6.ch011

Sygit, B., & Wąsik, D. (2016). Patients' Rights and Medical Personnel Duties in the Field of Hospital Care. In A. Rosiek & K. Leksowski (Eds.), *Organizational Culture and Ethics in Modern Medicine* (pp. 282–297). Hershey, PA: IGI Global. doi:10.4018/978-1-4666-9658-7.ch012

Sygit, B., & Wąsik, D. (2016). The Idea of Human Rights in Conditions of Hospital Treatment. In A. Rosiek & K. Leksowski (Eds.), *Organizational Culture and Ethics in Modern Medicine* (pp. 236–254). Hershey, PA: IGI Global. doi:10.4018/978-1-4666-9658-7.ch010

Talbot, T. B. (2017). Making Lifelike Medical Games in the Age of Virtual Reality: An Update on "Playing Games with Biology" from 2013. In B. Dubbels (Ed.), *Transforming Gaming and Computer Simulation Technologies across Industries* (pp. 103–119). Hershey, PA: IGI Global. doi:10.4018/978-1-5225-1817-4.ch006

Tamposis, I., Pouliakis, A., Fezoulidis, I., & Karakitsos, P. (2016). Mobile Platforms Supporting Health Professionals: Need, Technical Requirements, and Applications. In A. Moumtzoglou (Ed.), *M-Health Innovations for Patient-Centered Care* (pp. 91–114). Hershey, PA: IGI Global. doi:10.4018/978-1-4666-9861-1.ch005

Tiago, M. T., Tiago, F., Amaral, F. E., & Silva, S. (2016). Healthy 3.0: Healthcare Digital Dimensions. In A. Dwivedi (Ed.), *Reshaping Medical Practice and Care with Health Information Systems* (pp. 287–322). Hershey, PA: IGI Global. doi:10.4018/978-1-4666-9870-3.ch010

Tripathy, B. (2016). Application of Rough Set Based Models in Medical Diagnosis. In S. Dash & B. Subudhi (Eds.), *Handbook of Research on Computational Intelligence Applications in Bioinformatics* (pp. 144–168). Hershey, PA: IGI Global. doi:10.4018/978-1-5225-0427-6.ch008

Turcu, C. E., & Turcu, C. O. (2017). Social Internet of Things in Healthcare: From Things to Social Things in Internet of Things. In C. Reis & M. Maximiano (Eds.), *Internet of Things and Advanced Application in Healthcare* (pp. 266–295). Hershey, PA: IGI Global. doi:10.4018/978-1-5225-1820-4.ch010

Unwin, D. W., Sanzogni, L., & Sandhu, K. (2017). Developing and Measuring the Business Case for Health Information Technology. In K. Moahi, K. Bwalya, & P. Sebina (Eds.), *Health Information Systems and the Advancement of Medical Practice in Developing Countries* (pp. 262–290). Hershey, PA: IGI Global. doi:10.4018/978-1-5225-2262-1.ch015

Urooj, S., & Singh, S. P. (2016). Wavelet Transform-Based Soft Computational Techniques and Applications in Medical Imaging. In P. Saxena, D. Singh, & M. Pant (Eds.), *Problem Solving and Uncertainty Modeling through Optimization and Soft Computing Applications* (pp. 339–363). Hershey, PA: IGI Global. doi:10.4018/978-1-4666-9885-7.ch016

Vasant, P. (2018). A General Medical Diagnosis System Formed by Artificial Neural Networks and Swarm Intelligence Techniques. In U. Kose, G. Guraksin, & O. Deperlioglu (Eds.), *Nature-Inspired Intelligent Techniques for Solving Biomedical Engineering Problems* (pp. 130–145). Hershey, PA: IGI Global. doi:10.4018/978-1-5225-4769-3.ch006

Waegemann, C. P. (2016). mHealth: History, Analysis, and Implementation. In A. Moumtzoglou (Ed.), M-Health Innovations for Patient-Centered Care (pp. 1-19). Hershey, PA: IGI Global. doi:10.4018/978-1-4666-9861-1.ch001

Watfa, M. K., Majeed, H., & Salahuddin, T. (2016). Computer Based E-Healthcare Clinical Systems: A Comprehensive Survey. *International Journal of Privacy and Health Information Management*, 4(1), 50–69. doi:10.4018/IJPHIM.2016010104

Wietholter, J. P., Coetzee, R., Nardella, B., Kincaid, S. E., & Slain, D. (2016). International Healthcare Experiences: Caring While Learning and Learning While Caring. In D. Velliaris & D. Coleman-George (Eds.), *Handbook of Research on Study Abroad Programs and Outbound Mobility* (pp. 470–496). Hershey, PA: IGI Global. doi:10.4018/978-1-5225-0169-5.ch019

Witzke, K., & Specht, O. (2017). M-Health Telemedicine and Telepresence in Oral and Maxillofacial Surgery: An Innovative Prehospital Healthcare Concept in Structurally Weak Areas. *International Journal of Reliable and Quality E-Healthcare*, 6(4), 37–48. doi:10.4018/IJRQEH.2017100105

Wójcik, A., & Chojnacki, M. (2016). Behavior and Ethical Problems in the Functioning of the Operating Theater (Case Study). In A. Rosiek & K. Leksowski (Eds.), *Organizational Culture and Ethics in Modern Medicine* (pp. 154–179). Hershey, PA: IGI Global. doi:10.4018/978-1-4666-9658-7.ch007

Wolk, K., & Marasek, K. P. (2016). Translation of Medical Texts using Neural Networks. *International Journal of Reliable and Quality E-Healthcare*, 5(4), 51–66. doi:10.4018/IJRQEH.2016100104

Wong, A. K., & Lo, M. F. (2018). Using Pervasive Computing for Sustainable Healthcare in an Aging Population. In B. Fong, A. Ng, & P. Yuen (Eds.), *Sustainable Health and Long-Term Care Solutions for an Aging Population* (pp. 187–202). Hershey, PA: IGI Global. doi:10.4018/978-1-5225-2633-9.ch010

Wu, W., Martin, B. C., & Ni, C. (2017). A Systematic Review of Competency-Based Education Effort in the Health Professions: Seeking Order Out of Chaos. In K. Rasmussen, P. Northrup, & R. Colson (Eds.), *Handbook of Research on Competency-Based Education in University Settings* (pp. 352–378). Hershey, PA: IGI Global. doi:10.4018/978-1-5225-0932-5.ch018

Yadav, N., Aliasgari, M., & Poellabauer, C. (2016). Mobile Healthcare in an Increasingly Connected Developing World. *International Journal of Privacy and Health Information Management, 4*(2), 76–97. doi:10.4018/IJPHIM.2016070106

Yadav, S., Ekbal, A., Saha, S., Pathak, P. S., & Bhattacharyya, P. (2017). Patient Data De-Identification: A Conditional Random-Field-Based Supervised Approach. In S. Saha, A. Mandal, A. Narasimhamurthy, S. V, & S. Sangam (Eds.), Handbook of Research on Applied Cybernetics and Systems Science (pp. 234-253). Hershey, PA: IGI Global. doi:10.4018/978-1-5225-2498-4.ch011

Yu, B., Wijesekera, D., & Costa, P. C. (2017). Informed Consent in Healthcare: A Study Case of Genetic Services. In A. Moumtzoglou (Ed.), *Design, Development, and Integration of Reliable Electronic Healthcare Platforms* (pp. 211–242). Hershey, PA: IGI Global. doi:10.4018/978-1-5225-1724-5.ch013

Yu, B., Wijesekera, D., & Costa, P. C. (2017). Informed Consent in Electronic Medical Record Systems. In I. Management Association (Ed.), Healthcare Ethics and Training: Concepts, Methodologies, Tools, and Applications (pp. 1029-1049). Hershey, PA: IGI Global. doi:10.4018/978-1-5225-2237-9.ch049

Yu, M., Li, J., & Wang, W. (2017). Creative Life Experience among Students in Medical Education. In C. Zhou (Ed.), *Handbook of Research on Creative Problem-Solving Skill Development in Higher Education* (pp. 158–184). Hershey, PA: IGI Global. doi:10.4018/978-1-5225-0643-0.ch008

Zarour, K. (2017). Towards a Telehomecare in Algeria: Case of Diabetes Measurement and Remote Monitoring. *International Journal of E-Health and Medical Communications, 8*(4), 61–80. doi:10.4018/IJEHMC.2017100104

Zavyalova, Y. V., Korzun, D. G., Meigal, A. Y., & Borodin, A. V. (2017). Towards the Development of Smart Spaces-Based Socio-Cyber-Medicine Systems. *International Journal of Embedded and Real-Time Communication Systems, 8*(1), 45–63. doi:10.4018/IJERTCS.2017010104

Zeinali, A. A. (2018). Word Formation Study in Developing Naming Guidelines in the Translation of English Medical Terms Into Persian. In M. Khosrow-Pour, D.B.A. (Ed.), Encyclopedia of Information Science and Technology, Fourth Edition (pp. 5136-5147). Hershey, PA: IGI Global. doi:10.4018/978-1-5225-2255-3.ch446

Ziminski, T. B., Demurjian, S. A., Sanzi, E., & Agresta, T. (2016). Toward Integrating Healthcare Data and Systems: A Study of Architectural Alternatives. In T. Iyamu & A. Tatnall (Eds.), *Maximizing Healthcare Delivery and Management through Technology Integration* (pp. 270–304). Hershey, PA: IGI Global. doi:10.4018/978-1-4666-9446-0.ch016

Ziminski, T. B., Demurjian, S. A., Sanzi, E., Baihan, M., & Agresta, T. (2016). An Architectural Solution for Health Information Exchange. *International Journal of User-Driven Healthcare*, 6(1), 65–103. doi:10.4018/IJUDH.2016010104

Zineldin, M., & Vasicheva, V. (2018). Reducing Medical Errors and Increasing Patient Safety: TRM and 5 Q's Approaches for Better Quality of Life. In *Technological Tools for Value-Based Sustainable Relationships in Health: Emerging Research and Opportunities* (pp. 87–115). Hershey, PA: IGI Global. doi:10.4018/978-1-5225-4091-5.ch005

About the Contributors

Sevim Akyuz is a professor of physics, currently working at the Physics Department of Istanbul Kultur University (Istanbul-Turkey). Her research interest is on experimental and theoretical molecular spectroscopy and mainly focused on the study of a relationship between the structure and spectral properties of macromolecules using combined theoretical and experimental methods. She has 182 scientific papers as SCI record and total number of citations according to Web of Knowledge is 1335. Her H-index according to Web of Knowledge is 22.

Ali Tugrul Albayrak is Research Assistant Dr. at the Chemical Engineering Department of Istanbul University - Cerrahpasa (Turkey). His research is focused on the elucidation of the structure of ionic liquids using experimental methods. He has 3 scientific papers as SCI record.

Surendar Aravindhan is an Assistant Professor at Vignan's Foundation for Science, Technology and Research, India, and pursuing PhD degree in Anna University, Chennai. His research interests include embedded system and bioinformatics. He has published research outcomes in several IEEE conferences and peer-reviewed international journals and has about 30 research publications to his credit. He is Editor of International Journal of Communication & Computer Technology, International Journal of Pharmaceutical Research and guest editor for many special issues with Inderscience. He is a member of IEEE and ACM.

Jeremiah Ademola Balogun is a Graduate Research Assistant in the Department of Computer Science and Engineering, Obafemi Awolowo University, Nigeria. His focus is in the area of applied computing that is application of computing theories to address and solve health related problems in Sub Saharan Africa. He has published in journals and presented papers in conferences within Nigeria. He is currently researching into Cancer and environmental-related diseases in Nigeria. His research interest includes Health Informatics, Data Mining, Machine Learning, Software Engineering and Geographical Information System. He enjoys reading and brainstorming sessions.

Sefa Celik is an Associate Professor at the Electrical-Electronics Engineering Department of Istanbul University - Cerrahpasa (Turkey). His research is focused on the elucidation of the structure of biomacromolecules using combined experimental (molecular spectroscopy) and theoretical methods (ab initio, molecular dynamics), particularly on the molecular docking studies for shedding light on new drug design. He has 18 scientific papers as SCI record.

Hisayuki Hara is currently a Professor in the Faculty of Culture and Information Science at Doshisha University, Kyoto, Japan. He has been also a Visiting Professor at Institute of Statistical Mathematics. His current research interest focuses on both theoretical and applied statistics, especially on graphical models, Markov bases, statistical computing, statistical decision theory and econometric analysis.

Peter Adebayo Idowu is a senior researcher in the Department of Computer Science and Engineering, Obafemi Awolowo University, Nigeria. His research focus is on applied computing that is application of computing to address and solve health related problems in Sub Saharan Africa. He has over 40 publications to his credit in local journals, international journals and referred conference proceedings. He is currently researching into HIV/ AIDS, disease modelling and cloud computing in health care delivery. He is also a Member of British Computer Society, Nigerian Computer Society, Computer Professional Registration Council of Nigeria, Nigerian Young Academy, International Geospatial Society, International Association of Engineers and International Federation of Information Processing WG 9.4. His research interest includes Health Informatics, Data Modelling, Software Engineering, Geographical Information System, and Informatics. Within the last three years, Dr Idowu has successively trained 13 graduate students. He is blessed with two Research Associates; Praise and Vicky. He enjoys reading and driving. He enjoys reading and driving.

Mark Jaime is Assistant Professor of Psychology at Indiana University-Purdue University, Columbus (IUPUC). Dr. Jaime has been studying the social neurocognitive development of ASD for over 10 years. His research interests focus on how EEG measures of the socially engaged autistic brain may be meaningful for the objective classification of ASD. Dr. Jaime is also the founder and principal investigator of IUPUC's Social Neuroscience lab where he and his team study various aspects of social information processing in ASD and typical development.

Bo Ji is a lecturer in the Department of Computer Science at Nanjing Tech University Pujiang Institute. He received the Bachelor's degree in Automation from Anhui University of Technology in 2010 and the Master's degree in Automation from University of Science and Technology of China in 2013. His research interests include data mining, reinforcement learning, and recommender systems.

Hao Ji is currently an Assistant Professor in the Department of Computer Science at California State Polytechnic University, Pomona. He received the Ph.D. degree in Computer Science from Old Dominion University in 2016. He received the Bachelor's degree in Applied Mathematics and the Master's degree in Computer Science from Hefei University of Technology in 2007 and 2010, respectively.

Ramgopal Kashyap's areas of interest are image processing, pattern recognition, and machine learning. He has published many research papers, and book chapters in international journals and conferences like Springer, Inderscience, Elsevier, ACM, and IGI-Global indexed by Science Citation Index (SCI) and Scopus (Elsevier). He has Reviewed Research Papers in the Science Citation Index Expanded, Springer Journals and Editorial Board Member and conferences programme committee member of the IEEE, Springer international conferences and journals held in countries: Czech Republic, Switzerland, UAE, Australia, Hungary, Poland, Taiwan, Denmark, India, USA, UK, Austria, and Turkey. He has written many book chapters published by IGI Global, USA.

Kavitha Kavitha is working as R&D Head in Synthesishub, Advance scientific Research. She has published more than 12 research papers in various reputed journals and Conferences She is also a Reviewer for many reputed journals.

Uttama Lahiri received her Ph.D. in 2011 from Vanderbilt University, Nashville, Tennessee. She received the M.Tech. degree in Instrumentation engineering in 2004 from Indian Institute of Technology, Kharagpur, India. From 2004 to 2007 she worked for Tata Steel, Jamshedpur in plant automation. She is currently an Associate Professor at Indian Institute of Technology, Gandhinagar, India. Her current research interests include affective computing, adaptive response systems, signal processing, human-computer interaction, and robotics.

Rongjian Li is currently a Quantitative Modeling Associate in KeyBank. Before joining KeyBank, he was a visiting student in the School of Electrical Engineering and Computer Science, Washington State University. He earned his Ph.D. in Computer Science from Old Dominion University in 2016. His research interests include machine learning, data mining, computational biology, and computational neuroscience.

Anne M. P. Michalek is a certified speech-language pathologist and Assistant Professor in the Communication Disorders and Special Education Department at Old Dominion University. Dr. Michalek's research is rooted in a multi-disciplinary approach using biomedical technologies or single subject design to generate empirical evidence that bridges theory and practice and facilitates the design of effective diagnostic and instructional tools for students with ASD, ADHD, and hearing impairments. Primarily, she explores the use of eye gaze metrics as an objective and reliable measure of executive attention, social cognition, or audiovisual speech processing for children or adults with ASD or ADHD. She runs an eye tracking lab and teaches graduate and undergraduate speech-language pathology students.

Isaiah Oke holds a PhD degree in Civil Engineering. His main research Interest is in water Engineering. He has published a number of articles in reputable journals and Conference Proceedings. He is an academic in the Department of Civil Engineering, Obafemi Awolowo University, Ile-Ife, Nigeria.

Ayşen E. Özel is a Professor at the Physics Department of Istanbul University (Turkey). She is a head of Atom and Molecular Physics division. Her research is focused on the molecular spectroscopy and on the molecular modeling. She has 34 scientific papers as SCI record.

Funda Özkök is a Research Assistant at the Chemistry Department of Istanbul University - Cerrahpasa (Turkey). Her research is focused on the synthesis of organic compounds as anticancer agents and determination of structure of these bioactive compounds. She has 6 scientific papers as SCI record.

Nilanjan Sarkar received the Ph.D. degree in mechanical engineering and applied mechanics from the University of Pennsylvania, Philadelphia, in 1993. He was a Postdoctoral Fellow at Queen's University, Canada. Then, he joined the University of Hawaii as an Assistant Professor. In 2000, he joined Vanderbilt University, Nashville, TN, where he is currently Chair of the Department of mechanical engineering and Professor of mechanical engineering and computer engineering. His current research interests include human–robot interaction, rehabilitation robotics, cyber-physical systems, and control.

Zachary Warren received his Ph.D. in clinical psychology from the University of Miami, Miami, Florida in 2005. In 2006 he joined Vanderbilt University as and is an Associate Professor of Pediatrics, Psychiatry & Behavioral Sciences, and Special Education; and Executive Director of TRIAD. His research focuses on early childhood development and intervention for children with autism spectrum disorder.

Karla Conn Welch received her Ph.D. in 2009 from Vanderbilt University, Nashville, Tennessee. In 2005 she was awarded a National Science Foundation Graduate Research Fellowship. She is currently an Associate Professor of electrical and computer engineering at the University of Louisville. Her research interests include human-computer interaction, affective computing, machine learning, adaptive response systems, and robotics.

Ruriko Yoshida is an Associate Professor in the Department of Operations Research at Naval Postgraduate School. Her main interests lie in applications of tools in algebra and combinatorics to problems under graphical models; Graphical Gaussian models, Bayesian networks, and discrete exponential families. She is a mathematical statistician with extensive experience in systematic biology. Her research group has a long track record of developing computational tools and statistical methods for systematic biology.

Wenlu Zhang is currently an assistant professor of Computer Engineering and Computer Science at California State University Long Beach. She leads Machine Learning Lab at CSULB. Before joining CSULB, she was a post-doc in the School of Electrical Engineering and Computer Science, Washington State University. Zhang obtained her Ph.D. degree in Computer Science from Old Dominion University in 2016, advised by Prof. Shuiwang Ji. Her research interests include machine learning, data mining, computational biology, and computational neuroscience.

Index

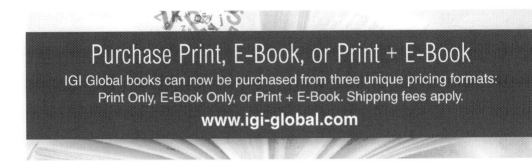
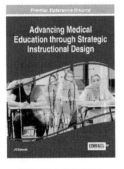
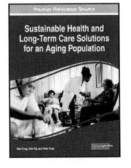
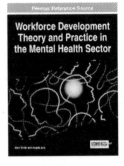
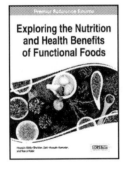
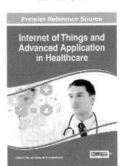
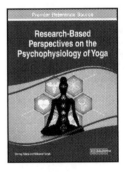
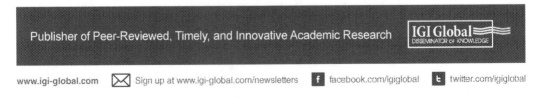

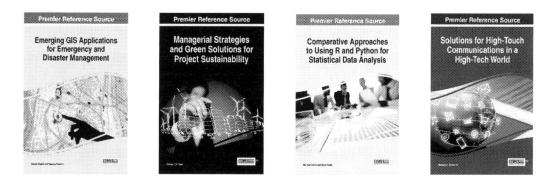

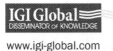

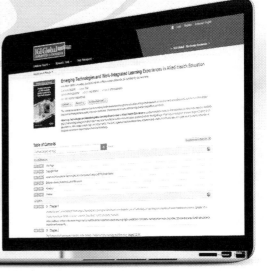

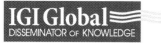
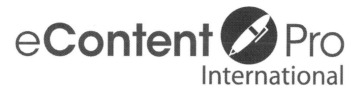

Printed in the United States
By Bookmasters